Overview-Map Key

Other cities in the *60 Hikes Within 60 Miles* series:

Albuquerque

Atlanta

Baltimore

Boston

Chicago

Cincinnati

Cleveland

Dallas and Fort Worth

Denver and Boulder

Harrisburg

Houston

Los Angeles

Madison

Minneapolis and St. Paul

Nashville

New York City

Philadelphia

Phoenix

Pittsburgh

Richmond

Sacramento

Salt Lake City

San Antonio and Austin

San Diego

San Francisco

Seattle

St. Louis

Washington, D.C.

60 HIKES WITHIN 60 MILES

PORTLAND

INCLUDING the Coast,
Mounts Hood and St. Helens,
and the Santiam River

FIFTH EDITION

Paul Gerald

 MENASHA RIDGE PRESS
Birmingham, Alabama

60 Hikes Within 60 Miles: Portland

Copyright © 2014 Paul Gerald
All rights reserved
Printed in the United States of America
Published by Menasha Ridge Press
Distributed by Publishers Group West
Fifth edition, third printing 2016

Project editor: Ritchey Halphen
Cover design and cartography: Scott McGrew
Typesetting and text design: Annie Long
Cover photo of Mount Hood and interior photos: Paul Gerald except where noted
Proofreader: John Michael Arnaud
Indexer: Ann Weik Cassar / Cassar Technical Services

Library of Congress Cataloging-in-Publication Data

Gerald, Paul, 1966–
   60 hikes within 60 miles, Portland : including the coast, Mounts Hood and St. Helens, and the Santiam River / Paul Gerald.
   pages cm
      Summary: "Updated maps, new hikes, even more rankings and categories, fresh photography, and useful backpacking options make the newest edition of this authoritative guide to Portland's best day hikes the most exciting yet. *60 Hikes Within 60 Miles: Portland* by Paul Gerald profiles 60 select trails that give outdoor adventurers a little of everything there is to enjoy around Portland: mountain views, forest solitude, picturesque streams, strenuous workouts, casual strolls, fascinating history, fields of flowers, awesome waterfalls, and ocean beaches. Whether readers want a convenient city bus ride to the flat and fascinating Washington Park, a bumpy drive to Lookout Mountain, or the thigh-burners that are Kings and Elk Mountains, this book lets them know what to bring, how to get to the trailhead, where to go on the trail, and what to look for while hiking."— Provided by publisher.
      ISBN 978-0-89732-512-7 (paperback) — ISBN 0-89732-512-5 — eISBN 978-0-89732-513-4
      1. Hiking—Oregon—Portland Region—Guidebooks. 2. Portland Region (Or.)—Guidebooks.
   I. Title. II. Title: Sixty hikes within sixty miles, Portland.
   GV199.42.O72P6738 2014
   796.5109795'49—dc23
                                        2014011026

 MENASHA RIDGE PRESS
An imprint of AdventureKEEN
2204 First Avenue South, Suite 102
Birmingham, Alabama 35233
menasharidge.com

Disclaimer

Table of Contents

*With immense gratitude and respect, I dedicate this book
to the people who build and maintain the trails.*

*And with love to Maria, who's like
a warm campfire on a cold night.*

Acknowledgments

It blows my mind to think, 14 years after first hearing of this project, that I am now finishing up the fifth edition of this book. So I have to first acknowledge the people who've really made that possible: all of you, who have bought and read this book by the thousands. Your enjoyment of it has turned it from a low-paying ego trip into the basis of a career, as well as a connection to my community. I cherish both, and I thank you for them.

Of course, there are dozens of people behind the scenes who make this happen, starting with all the people at Menasha Ridge Press—none of whom I've even had the chance to meet! First and foremost are Molly Merkle, who for years has patiently answered all my tedious questions and tolerated my somewhat adversarial relationship with deadlines. For the last two editions, it's mainly been project editor Ritchey Halphen putting up with me. Then there are the people who turn my Word files, photos, and GPS tracks into the book you're holding: Annie Long, Scott McGrew, John Michael Arnaud, and Ann Cassar. Thanks to Allison Brown for patiently explaining my royalties reports—many times—and also to Pat LaFleur for letting the world know the book exists. And finally, many thanks to Mike Jones, whom I'm lucky to have right here in Portland so he can act as my publishing guru (though I can see him wincing at that remark right now).

I processed a lot of information for this book, much of which came from the U.S. Forest Service, Oregon State Parks, **portlandhikers.org,** the Columbia Gorge Visitors Center, Washington State Parks, the Mazamas, and the amazing book *Oregon Geographical Names* from the Oregon Historical Society Press. (I am proud to own a signed copy of the seventh edition, revised and updated by Lewis L. McArthur, and I recommend it highly.)

Once I put all the information together, I needed somebody to make sure I wasn't completely out of touch with reality. Enter a small army of patient employees of various federal, state, and private agencies who interrupted their busy schedules to review all the text. My humble thanks to them all: Bob Stillson, Brandon Haraughty, Breanne Jordan, Dean Robertson, Erik Plunkett, Gary McDaniel, Gary Walker, Greg Hawley, Heather Latham, Jacquelyn Oakes, Jane Dooley, J. W. Cleveland, Karen Houston, Kevin Strandberg, Lorie Hutton, Lynn Barlow, Mark Marshall, Pete Marvin, Randy Peterson, Rick Swart, Robin Jensen, Stephen Anderson, Susan Freston, Tom Atiyeh, and Tom Robinson. Special thanks also to [you know who you are!] for all his help

Acknowledgments

th Old Vista Ridge Trail. Jim Thayer's website, **foresthiker.com,** was invaluable in piecing together info on the Salmonberry River, and Gary Riggs contributed some helpful info, too. Ryan Ojerio with the Washington Trails Association was fantastic with Coyote Wall and Cape Horn. And thanks to Becky Schreiber for helping out so much with the trails in Hoyt Arboretum. (I'm serious about Iceland, dang it!)

Of course, a hike is a lonely experience without good friends to share it with. Here—listed alphabetically to avoid controversy—is a list of the folks who made "researching" this fifth edition such an enjoyable experience: Alice Brocum, Amelia Ferrel, Ann Brown, Anna Blumenkron, Annie McCartney, Asani Seawell, Bill Dewsnap, Brian Goldman, Carole Beauclerk, Chris Davis, Daniel Bailey, David Burdick, David Greenlee, David Grennell, David Shaw, Dawn Van Seygen, Diane Caws, Dianne Denotter, Dyanne Foster, Gary Riggs, Gordy Molitor, Ingrid Wehrle, Irhan Ilong, Jane Garbisch, Jim Chase, Judy Mosch, Julie Haykin, Kelly Podshadley, Kyong Bates, Maria Shindler, Mary Lisby, Nancy Chapman, Pam Martin, Regis Krug, Scott Rieders, Sherry Bourdin, Steve Gilbert, and Tracy Groom. I've done a horrendous job of keeping notes on who accompanied me along the way, and I absolutely left people out. I apologize in advance.

And finally, a lifetime of love and thanks to my family back east: Marjorie and Barry Gerald; Lee, Lela, and Jack Gerald and Max Simpson; and Lucy, Becky, David, Jeff, and Charlie Cook. And a big hug to the Monday Meditators, for keeping me (reasonably) sane, one day at a time.

—Paul Gerald

Foreword

Welcome to Menasha Ridge Press's 60 Hikes Within 60 Miles, a series designed to provide hikers with the information they need to find and hike the very best trails surrounding large metropolitan areas.

Our strategy is simple: First, find a hiker who knows the area and loves to hike. Second, ask that person to spend a year researching the most popular and very best trails around. And third, have that person describe each trail in terms of difficulty, scenery, condition, elevation change, and other categories of information that are important to hikers. "Pretend you've just completed a hike and met up with other hikers at the trailhead," we told each author. "Imagine their questions, and be clear in your answers."

An experienced hiker and writer, Paul Gerald has selected 60 of the best hikes in and around the Portland, Oregon, metropolitan area. From greenways and urban hikes that make use of parklands to flora- and fauna-rich treks along the cliffs and hills in the hinterlands, Paul provides hikers (and walkers) with a great variety of hikes—and all within roughly 60 miles of Portland.

You'll get the most from this book if you take a moment to read the Introduction, which explains how to read the trail listings. Though this is a where-to rather than a how-to guide, readers who haven't hiked extensively will find the Introduction of particular value.

As much to free the spirit as to free the body, let these hikes elevate you above the urban fray.

All the best,
The editors at Menasha Ridge Press

About the Author

Paul Gerald's writing career began on the sports desk of the much-missed *Dallas Times Herald* back in 1986. He later worked for the *Commercial Appeal* of Memphis, Tennessee, and the *Memphis Flyer* alternative weekly, as well as the *Santa Barbara News-Press* in California. After leaving newspapers, he wrote some 300 freelance travel articles for the *Flyer;* his work has also appeared in Northwest Airlines' *World Traveler,* Portland's *Willamette Week, The Oregonian,* and more random publications than he can remember.

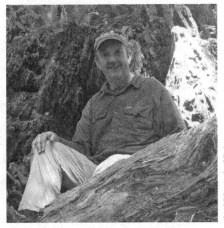

PHOTO: Judy Olivier

He's also worked in and around landscaping, public relations, social work, an amusement park, Alaskan fishing boats, the YMCA, corporate marketing, FedEx, and now Embark Adventures, a Portland-based adventure-travel company.

Paul's hiking life started at age 12, when he went to a summer camp in the Absoraka Mountains of Wyoming, and his hometown of Memphis never looked the same. He's hiked in the Rocky Mountains from New Mexico to Montana, and in Appalachia, Alaska, Argentina, Italy, and Nepal. In 1996 he moved to Portland to be close to the ocean, the mountains, the big trees, and the coffee shops. He leads hikes and outings, both domestic and international, for the Mazamas mountaineering club.

The first edition of *60 Hikes Within 60 Miles: Portland,* published in 2001, was Paul's first book. He also authored *Day and Overnight Hikes: Oregon's Pacific Crest Trail,* and he revised *Best Tent Camping: Oregon* for Menasha Ridge in 2009. In addition, he wrote *Peaceful Places: Portland* for Menasha in 2012, and he wrote and published *Breakfast in Bridgetown: The Definitive Guide to Portland's Favorite Meal,* under his own imprint, Bacon and Eggs Press. The third edition of the latter is due in spring 2014.

Paul greatly enjoys meeting people who use his books out on the trails; he's also grateful that none of them have appeared to be lost or angry. He does hope, however, that any feedback will be directed to him, care of the publisher, or to **paulgerald.com, facebook.com/hikerpaul,** or **twitter.com/60hikesportland.** And he hopes people will continue to enjoy and benefit from the fruits of his labor—if hiking and writing can truly be called labor.

Preface

Here's a funny admission from the author of a hiking book: There comes a time, almost every time I go hiking, when I kind of hate it.

Sometimes it's the weather, of course—I'm pretty much a fair-weather hiker. Sometimes it's the big uphills. Sometimes it's the big downhills. Sometimes it's the tedious drive back home (in particular the stretch of I-84 between Troutdale and I-205). Sometimes it's the early start, or the late return, or all the chatter on the trail.

Maybe I'm just getting old; my 47-year-old legs and back complain a good bit more than their 25-year-old versions did. Maybe it's the pounds I put on while writing a breakfast guidebook. And maybe I fell into the trap of letting my favorite pastime become part of my job; slogging up a viewless hill in the rain because "I have to do it for my book" hardly screams "glamorous life of a writer."

So why do it?

For the little moments in between.

Take Multnomah Falls, for example. You drive there, you see the falls, you fight the crowds, and maybe you drag yourself up the paved trail to the top of the falls for a look around. And yes, I am being a horribly jaded Oregonian, but there's an element of "been there, done that."

Ah, but if you keep going, there's a place just a little farther up, right past the old bridge over the creek, where the pavement ends, the crowds turn around, and it turns into a trail, a path leading into the woods, bound for miles away. And every time I go there, there's a little moment waiting for me, like a present I'm always getting for the first time. It's the moving on, the letting go, the opening up, the knowing that behind me are town, life, work, money, cars, computers . . . and ahead of me are only more trail and trees and creeks and birds and cliffs and mountains.

My brain knows that I can walk from that spot, using only forest trails, to Mount Hood, to countless other quiet, wild places—and that's a part of it. But it's my heart where the little moment happens: a kind of release and relaxation, a simple knowing that from here on, it's just me, or us, and the woods, and I can go wherever I feel, because I have everything I need right here with me.

Mountains have stirred my heart since I was a kid, and it's because they are filled with those little moments: walking over a ridge to see a great view, coming around a corner to surprise a deer on the path, catching a glimpse of an eagle or a big fish, or just sitting down for some peace next to a stream. Of course, it doesn't have to be in the mountains; much of Portland's magic lies in places like Macleay Park, where you leave "the city," in the metaphorical sense, and enter "the woods," where trout swim in the creek, massive trees grow all around, and a bird sanctuary lies just up the hill. It's there in the wooded ravine around Marquam Trail, which was at one time to be filled with apartments but instead remains a quiet, shady way to reach the highest place in the city.

My original, superficial reason for writing this book, way back in 2000, was so I could walk into Powell's, buy a latte, point at a book on the shelf, and say, "I wrote that." In other words, it was mostly ego. (Believe me, it wasn't the money.) There was something deeper, though. I have always wanted to visit interesting places, meet interesting people, and do interesting things, then tell people about them. Part of that is still ego, sure, but a bigger part is that I just think life is cool, and I want to share that coolness with people. I think hiking is particularly cool, even when I hate it—because, after all, don't you feel a little more satisfaction walking to the top of, say, Larch Mountain than driving up there? Especially if you start by the banks of the Columbia and walk to the top of a Cascades peak? The work, if you can do it, enhances the payoff. You get a connection with the whole mountain.

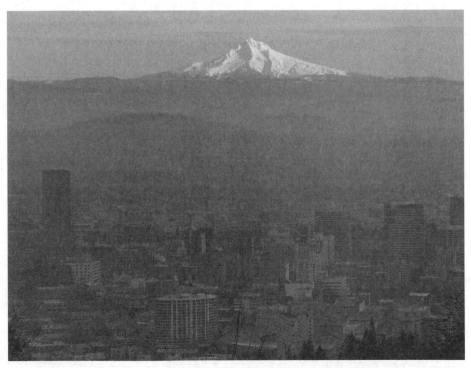

Mount Hood and Portland viewed from the Pittock Mansion (see Hike 54, page 284)

Over the years, the deeper reason for writing this book has really come to the sur-face. Tens of thousands of people have bought it, which amazes and humbles me, and more than a few have told me they like it. Ego again, sure, but also something else: They (you) are having those little moments, too! To think I drove all the ridiculous way to Whetstone Mountain to that somewhat boring hike—ah, but to get that mind-boggling view—and then somebody else read about it, made the same drive, and got the same view . . . well, it makes me feel warm and fuzzy. People often thank me for writing the book, and all I can think to say is, "Thanks for enjoying it."

And that's when they ask me The Question: "What's your favorite hike?" (Every-body asks it, and if you do too, it's not a problem.) And I, being a wordy writer (have you noticed?) always say, "Well, that depends." Depends, in my case, almost entirely on what month it is. I often think of Catherine Creek, Coyote Wall, and The Labyrinth, hikes that in April and May are awash in flowery, sunny, breezy, birdsongy little moments . . . and that in July or August would probably kill you with heat and boredom.

My "favorite" also depends on what mood I'm in. Sometimes I want a big adven-ture like Trapper Creek Wilderness, maybe even an overnight, and sometimes I just want to stroll along the Salmon River for a couple of miles, to gaze at the big trees and look for salmon.

I have written this book, five times now, with one intention: to help my fellow humans get out to some cool spots so they can experience those little moments. (It still isn't about the money. Well, not much.) I wrote the book as if you're actually going to carry it along with you, so I can point stuff out along the way and give you some things to think about while you're doing the dull stuff. I'll tell you why Ramona Falls is called that (it's a sweet story), where the Throne of the Forest King sits, and why there are cables around stumps high above the Clackamas River. I assume you want to know these things.

What I also assume is that, like most people I talk to, you may want to know what my favorite hike is. Like I said, that depends, so here, by way of introduction to the book, is my personal hiking calendar. I don't stick to this, or anything else in life, very strictly, but I bet that if you follow it you'll have a fine year of hiking, and there's a decent chance we'll bump into each other.

I get through winter the way most outdoorsy Portlanders do: I'll go up the Macleay or Marquam Trail to stretch my legs, to Tryon Creek to look for trillium, and maybe out to Angels Rest for a sunset. Otherwise it's snowshoes, coffee, and planning for better weather. For this edition, I've even included a list of good snowshoeing hikes, and if you want a list of breakfast places, I've got that in another book.

What I really look for, usually on **portlandhikers.org,** is the first picture of a grass widow. What's a grass widow? Well, objectively speaking, it's a small, unassuming,

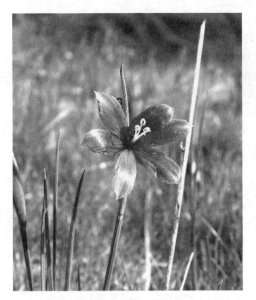

Behold the humble grass widow, harbinger of spring.

mostly purple flower, barely 6 inches tall. But to the local hiker's heart, it's The Beginning of It All, the first spring wildflower that blooms where such flowers bloom. Most often, the grass widow is first seen in March at Catherine Creek, and its appearance means that we can now leave rainy old Portland, drive an hour east, and listen to the meadowlarks while we look for the hundreds of types of flowers that will soon drape the slopes at Coyote Wall and Tom McCall Preserve.

That show goes until May, and in the meantime, the few dry days offer a chance to go to Silver Falls State Park, where you can walk 7 miles, see 10 full-tilt waterfalls, and sip a hot drink by a fireplace before and/or after you go. It's also time to start getting into shape, and for that there is Hamilton Mountain, itself a flowery scene by April, when flowers on the Oregon side of the Gorge have yet to bloom but the Washington side is catching rays. I also use, as a conditioner and a reminder of why I live here, the loop from Wahkeena Falls over to Multnomah Falls. You might like it as well, if you're into stuff like creeks and waterfalls and springs and views and soft-serve ice cream.

Other April favorites? The plunging waters of Eagle Creek or Falls Creek; walking the Salmonberry River canyon before the trackside plants leaf out; or the irises out at the end of Cape Falcon.

By May, in theory, I'm getting in pretty good shape, and the sun is starting to win its annual battle against the clouds. Barely. But May means one big thing in my hiking life: Dog Mountain. It's physically big, but psychologically bigger. The flower show up there from mid-May to mid-June wipes me out every year, and whenever I tell people the balsamroot is a "sea of yellow," it's an understatement. Really, if you do one hike this year, go up Dog Mountain in late May or so. Well, first do some other hikes to prepare.

By June the bloom is spreading and the clouds are clearing. June can be maddening, though; you want to get up high, but most years the snow still blankets those trails. June is about transition and midelevation: too late for spring flowers, too early for Mount Hood . . . just right for being around 2,000–3,000 feet for the first blast of summer. My June favorites are Silver Star Mountain for the flowers, Salmon Butte for the rhododendrons, Kings and Elk Mountains to see what shape I'm really in, or Saddle Mountain for both the flowers and a meal at Camp 18.

In July I play two little games called "Beat the Heat" and "Follow the Mosquitoes." See, for the first month after the snow melts, the mosquitoes will make you hate life. And July tends to be pretty warm. So I wait for word that the little varmints are gone from various shady forests, and then I move in to hike. This leads me to lower-elevation places like Breitenbush, Opal Creek, and Lewis River, or the ever-cool coast, where July means the big bloom at Cascade Head, and July 16 the opening of the upper trailhead there.

August is what it's all about around here. The snow and mosquitoes are gone everywhere, and my hiker's life is all about getting as high as possible. For me, this means it's Mount Hood Time: McNeil Point barely edges out Vista Ridge, Paradise Park, and Lookout Mountain as a favorite, but anything in the "Around Mount Hood" section will be a day well spent. And now we get to watch Vista Ridge recover from a tremendous fire.

For a lot of hikers, September is the best month. The weather is cooling, the crowds are gone, and there will just start to be some fall colors somewhere. I like Cooper Spur this time of year, because at about 8,000 feet you can just barely sense winter coming over the ridge. September is also your last shot at the high stuff, so it's a good time to hit Bull of the Woods for that big view as well.

For this hiker, October is the big show. You're in shape, you've got your hiking crowd of friends, you can still do any hike in the book, and there's a sweet sadness as the season closes, plus a sense of rush to get it all in before the snow blows. For highlights, it's all about two things: salmon and fall colors. October is when the ocean-run fish make it into the Salmon River and the Wilson River, and when the vine maples at Trapper Creek or Ape Canyon will blow your mind.

After a year like that, frankly, I'm more interested in watching college football or English soccer for November and December than I am in hiking. And I know that I just listed at least a third of the book as a favorite, but what can I say? The whole book is favorites! I've done close to 100 different hikes around here, and these are the 60 I believe anyone will enjoy.

So please do enjoy them. And take care of them. And remember: If you have one of those moments where you hate hiking, just keep truckin', and you'll soon get to one of those other little, but glorious, moments in between.

60 Hikes by Category

See **paulgerald.com/hike-list** *for an online version of this chart.*

Hike Categories

- distance (mi)
- difficulty*
- months open**
- best time**
- kid-friendly
- backpacking
- running

* Difficulty: **E** = easy, **M** = moderate, **S** = strenuous
** Numbers correspond to months (3 = March, etc.).

REGION Hike Number/Hike Name	page	distance (mi)	difficulty	months open	best time	kid-friendly	backpacking	running
IN THE COLUMBIA RIVER GORGE								
1 Angels Rest and Devils Rest	16	4.6/7.5	M–S	all	clear days	sort of		
2 Beacon Rock State Park	21	1.8/8	E–S	all	4–5	✓		
3 Cape Horn	26	2.6–6.3	E–M	all	4–5/10	✓		
4 Catherine Creek	31	Up to 4.1	E–M	all	3–6	✓		
5 Chinidere Mountain	36	4	M	7–10	8–9	✓	✓	
6 Coyote Wall and The Labyrinth	41	4.6/5.2	M	all	4–5			
7 Dog Mountain	46	6.9	S	all	5–6			
8 Eagle Creek	50	4/12	E–M	all	3–5/9–10	sort of	✓	
9 Larch Mountain	55	7.1–13.6	M–S	6–11	8			
10 Table Mountain	61	8.5	S	4–11	5/10			
11 Tom McCall Preserve	66	2.5–6	E–M	all	4–5	✓		
12 Triple Falls	70	4.5	M	all	4/10	✓		
13 Wahkeena Falls to Multnomah Falls	74	4.2	M	all	anytime			
AROUND MOUNT ST. HELENS								
14 Ape Canyon	82	11.6	M	6–10	9–10			✓
15 Bluff Mountain Trail	87	13.2	S	6–10	7/10			
16 Falls Creek Falls	91	3.4/6.1	E–M	5–11	5–6	✓	✓	
17 Lava Canyon	95	1–6	E–S	6–10	6/10			
18 Lewis River	100	5.2	E	4–11	6/10	✓		✓
19 Silver Star Mountain: Ed's Trail	104	4.8	M	6–10	7/10	✓		

REGION Hike Number/Hike Name	page	distance (mi)	difficulty	months open	best time	kid-friendly	backpacking	running
AROUND MOUNT ST. HELENS (*continued*)								
20 Siouxon Creek	108	Up to 10.8	E–S	3–11	6/10	✓	✓	✓
21 South Fork Toutle River	112	11.2	S	6–10	8–9		✓	
22 Trapper Creek Wilderness	116	Up to 14.5	E–S	5–11	9–10		✓	
UP THE CLACKAMAS RIVER								
23 Bagby Hot Springs	124	3–3.6	E	3–11	3–10	✓	✓	✓
24 Bull of the Woods	128	2.2/7	E–S	6–10	8–9	✓	✓	
25 Clackamas River	132	7.2/7.8	M	all	5/10	✓	✓	✓
26 Roaring River Wilderness	137	1.4–12.6	E–S	7–10	8–9	✓	✓	
27 Whetstone Mountain	142	4.8	M	6–10	6/10			
UP THE SANTIAM RIVER								
28 Battle Ax Mountain	148	5.1/6.5	S	6–10	8–9		✓	
29 Breitenbush Hot Springs Area	153	1–8	E–S	4–11	9–10	✓	✓	
30 Opal Creek Wilderness	158	7–13	E–M	4–11	7–10	✓	✓	✓
AROUND MOUNT HOOD								
31 Barlow Pass	166	5–10	M	7–10	8–9		✓	
32 Cooper Spur	170	7.5	S	7–10	8–9		✓	
33 Elk Meadows	175	2–12	M–S	7–10	8–9	✓	✓	
34 Lookout Mountain	180	3/9.6	E–S	7–10	8–9	✓		
35 Lost Lake	185	3.3–16	E–S	6–10	8–9	✓	✓	✓
36 McNeil Point	190	12	E–S	7–10	8–9		✓	
37 Mirror Lake	195	2.8/7	E–S	6–10	8–9	✓		
38 Ramona Falls	199	7.1/15.4	E	5–10	7–9	✓	✓	✓
39 Salmon River	204	5.2/6.6	E–S	all	10	✓	✓	✓
40 Tamanawas Falls	209	3.4	E	6–11	7–9	✓		
41 Timberline Lodge	213	1–13	E–S	7–10	8–9	✓	✓	
42 Trillium Lake	219	2	E	6–10	8–9	✓		✓
43 Twin Lakes	223	4/8.5	M	6–10	8–9	✓	✓	✓
44 Vista Ridge	228	4.4–11	M	7–10	8–9		✓	
45 Wildwood Recreation Site	234	1.75/10.6	E–S	all	8–10	✓		
46 Zigzag Mountain	238	6.8/9.4	E–S	6–10	8–9	✓	✓	✓

REGION Hike Number/Hike Name	page	distance (mi)	difficulty	months open	best time	kid-friendly	backpacking	running
THE COAST AND COAST RANGE								
47 Cape Lookout State Park	244	3.6–4.8	M	all	3–4/7–9	✓		
48 Cascade Head	249	2.5–5.4	M	all/7–12	7–9			
49 Kings Mountain and Elk Mountain	254	5.2–13.4	M–S	all	5–6			
50 Oswald West State Park	260	2.5–9	E–S	all	clear days	✓		
51 Saddle Mountain	266	5.2	S	all	6–7			
52 Salmonberry River	270	Up to 12+	E–M	all	3/11	✓	✓	
53 Wilson River	276	Up to 20.6	E–S	all	3–4/10	✓		✓
PORTLAND AND THE WILLAMETTE VALLEY								
54 Macleay Trail	284	2.2/4.5	E–M	all	clear days	✓		✓
55 Marquam Trail to Council Crest	289	3.7	F–M	all	clear days	✓		
56 Sauvie Island	294	3/7	E	all/4–9	4–5/10	✓		✓
57 Silver Falls State Park	300	Up to 7	E–M	all	3–4/9–10	✓		
58 Tryon Creek State Natural Area	305	3	E	all	4	✓		✓
59 Washington Park and Hoyt Arboretum	309	4	E	all	3/10	✓		✓
60 Willamette River Greenway	313	Up to 12.2	E–M	all	anytime	✓		✓

Hike Categories (*continued*)

- wheelchair/stroller-friendly
- big views
- waterfalls
- snowshoeing
- swimming
- good for shuttles
- camping at trailhead

REGION Hike Number/Hike Name	page	wheelchair/ stroller-friendly	big views	waterfalls	snowshoeing	swimming	good for shuttles	camping at trailhead
IN THE COLUMBIA RIVER GORGE								
Angels Rest and Devils Rest	16		✓	✓			✓	
Beacon Rock State Park	21	✓	✓	✓				✓
Cape Horn	26		✓					
Catherine Creek	31	✓	✓					
Chinidere Mountain	36		✓			✓	✓	✓
Coyote Wall and The Labyrinth	41	✓	✓					
Dog Mountain	46		✓					
Eagle Creek	50			✓				✓
Larch Mountain	55	✓	✓	✓			✓	
Table Mountain	61		✓					
Tom McCall Preserve	66		✓					
Triple Falls	70			✓				
13 Wahkeena Falls to Multnomah Falls	74	✓		✓				
AROUND MOUNT ST. HELENS								
14 Ape Canyon	82		✓					
15 Bluff Mountain Trail	87		✓					
16 Falls Creek Falls	91			✓				
17 Lava Canyon	95	✓		✓				
18 Lewis River	100			✓		✓		✓
19 Silver Star Mountain: Ed's Trail	104		✓					
20 Siouxon Creek	108			✓		✓		
21 South Fork Toutle River	112		✓					
22 Trapper Creek Wilderness	116		✓					

REGION Hike Number/Hike Name	page	wheelchair/ stroller-friendly	big views	waterfalls	snowshoeing	swimming	good for shuttles	camping at trailhead
THE COAST AND COAST RANGE (*continued*)								
49 Kings Mountain and Elk Mountain	254		✓			✓	✓	
50 Oswald West State Park	260		✓				✓	✓
51 Saddle Mountain	266		✓					✓
52 Salmonberry River	270						✓	
53 Wilson River	276					✓	✓	✓
PORTLAND AND THE WILLAMETTE VALLEY								
54 Macleay Trail	284	✓						
55 Marquam Trail to Council Crest	289		✓					
56 Sauvie Island	294							
57 Silver Falls State Park	300			✓				✓
58 Tryon Creek State Natural Area	305	✓						
59 Washington Park and Hoyt Arboretum	309	✓						
60 Willamette River Greenway	313	✓					✓	

Introduction

Welcome to *60 Hikes Within 60 Miles: Portland.* If you're new to hiking or even if you're a seasoned trailsmith, take a few minutes to read the following pages. We explain how this book is organized and how to use it.

How to Use This Guidebook

Overview Map, Map Key, and Map Legend

The overview map on the inside front cover shows the primary trailheads for all 60 hikes. The numbers on the overview map pair with the key on the facing page. A legend explaining the map symbols used throughout the book appears on the inside back cover.

Regional Maps

The book is divided into regions, and prefacing each regional section is an overview map. The regional maps provide more detail than the overview map, bringing you closer to the hikes.

Trail Maps

In addition to the overview map on the inside cover, a detailed map of each hike's route appears with its profile. On each of these maps, symbols indicate the trailhead, the complete route, significant features, facilities, and topographic landmarks such as creeks, overlooks, and peaks.

To produce the highly accurate maps in this book, I used a handheld GPS unit to gather data while hiking each route, then sent that data to Menasha Ridge Press's expert cartographers. Be aware, though, that your GPS device is no substitute for sound, sensible navigation that takes into account the conditions that you observe while hiking.

Further, despite the high quality of the maps in this guidebook, I strongly recommend that you always carry an additional map, such as the ones noted in "Maps" in each hike's Key At-a-Glance Information.

Elevation Profiles

Each hike contains a detailed elevation profile that corresponds directly to the trail map. This graphical element provides a quick look at the trail from the side, enabling you to visualize how the trail rises and falls. On the diagram's vertical axis, or height scale, the number of feet indicated between each tick mark lets you visualize the climb. To avoid making flat hikes look steep and steep hikes appear flat, varying height scales provide an accurate image of each hike's climbing challenge. Elevation profiles for loop hikes show total distance; those for out-and-back hikes show only one-way distance.

GPS Trailhead Coordinates

As noted in "Trail Maps," on the previous page, I used a handheld GPS unit to obtain geographic data and sent the information to the cartographers at Menasha Ridge. Provided for each hike profile, the GPS coordinates—the intersection of latitude (north) and longitude (west)—will orient you from the trailhead. In some cases, you can park within viewing distance of a trailhead. Other hiking routes require a short walk to the trailhead from a parking area.

The latitude–longitude grid system is likely quite familiar to you, but here's a refresher, pertinent to visualizing the coordinates:

Imaginary lines of latitude—called *parallels* and approximately 69 miles apart from each other—run horizontally around the globe. The equator is established to be 0°, and each parallel is indicated by degrees from the equator: up to 90°N at the North Pole, and down to 90°S at the South Pole.

Imaginary lines of longitude—called *meridians*—run perpendicular to lines of latitude and are likewise indicated by degrees. Starting from 0° at the Prime Meridian in Greenwich, England, they continue to the east and west until they meet 180° later at the International Date Line in the Pacific Ocean. At the equator,

longitude lines also are approximately 69 miles apart, but that distance narrows as the meridians converge toward the North and South Poles.

In this book, latitude and longitude are expressed in degree–decimal minute format. For example, the coordinates for Hike 1, Angels Rest (page 16), are as follows:

N45° 33.613' W122° 10.365'

To convert GPS coordinates given in degrees, minutes, and seconds to degrees and decimal minutes, divide the seconds by 60. For more on GPS technology, visit **usgs.gov.**

Hike Profiles

Each hike contains seven key items: an In Brief description of the trail, a Key At-a-Glance Information box, directions to the trail, GPS coordinates, a trail map, an elevation profile, and a trail description. Many hikes also include notes on things to see and do nearby.

In Brief

A "taste of the trail." Think of this section as a snapshot focused on the historical landmarks, beautiful vistas, and other sights you may encounter on the hike.

Key At-a-Glance Information

This gives you a quick idea of the statistics and specifics of each hike:

LENGTH How long the trail is from start to finish. There may be options to shorten or extend the hikes, but the mileage corresponds to the described hike. Use the Description as a guide to customizing the hike for your ability or time constraints.

CONFIGURATION Defines the type of route—for example, an out-and-back (which takes you in and out the same way), a point-to-point (or one-way route), a figure-eight, or a balloon.

DIFFICULTY The degree of effort an average hiker should expect on a given hike. For simplicity, the trails are rated as *easy, moderate,* or *strenuous*.

SCENERY Rates the overall environs of the hike and what to expect in terms of plant life, wildlife, natural wonders, and historical features.

EXPOSURE A quick check of how much sun you can expect on your shoulders during the hike.

TRAFFIC Indicates how busy the trail might be on an average day, and if you might be able to find solitude out there. Trail traffic, of course, varies from day to day and season to season.

TRAIL SURFACE Indicates whether the path is paved, rocky, smooth, or composed of a mixture of elements.

HIKING TIME How long it took me to hike the trail. I like to dawdle, and I can easily fritter away time eating or admiring wildflowers. On average, I cover 2 miles an hour (more mileage hiking downhill, less on steady ascents, particularly during hot weather). If you're an experienced hiker in great shape, you'll finish the hikes with time to spare, but if you're a beginner or you like to stop to take in the views, allow for a little extra.

DRIVING DISTANCE How far each hike is from Pioneer Courthouse Square in downtown Portland. Not that you'd want to start from here necessarily, but the numbers should give you a good estimate of travel times to the trailheads from where you live. Driving times are provided as well.

SEASON The time of year when a particular hike is accessible. In most cases, the determining factor is snow. Except where specific hours are noted, hikes are accessible daily, sunrise–sunset.

BEST TIME If you want to save a hike for when it's at its best, this is the time to shoot for.

BACKPACKING OPTIONS Feel like spending the night out? Here's a quick glance; more details are in the text.

ACCESS Notes any fees or permits needed to hike the trail.

A number of trailheads in this book require a **Northwest Forest Pass.** All of the outdoors shops listed in Appendixes A and B sell the pass, which costs $5 for one day and $30 for one year; you can also buy it at **discovernw.org/store.**

Other passes are available, such as the Interagency Senior Pass and various national passes, so make sure to get the one that best meets your needs. Visit **tinyurl.com/usfsregion6passesand permits** for more information.

WHEELCHAIR ACCESS Some trails have a small paved section.

MAPS Which supplementary map is the best or easiest for a particular hike. See Appendix B (page 321) for map resources.

FACILITIES Restrooms, phones, water, and other niceties available at the trailhead or nearby.

INFO Listed here are phone numbers and/or websites for checking trail conditions and gleaning other basic information.

SPECIAL COMMENTS Provides you with those little extra details that don't fit into any of the above categories. These may include insider information or special considerations about the trail, access, or warnings, along with ideas for enhancing your hiking experience.

GPS Information and Directions

Trailhead latitude and longitude can be used in addition to the Directions if you enter the data into your GPS unit before you set out. See page 2 for more information. Where pertinent, highway exit numbers are included in the Directions.

Description

The heart of each hike, summarizing the trail's essence and highlighting any special traits the hike has to offer. The route is clearly outlined, including any landmarks, side trips, and possible alternate routes along the way. Ultimately, the Description will help you choose which hikes are best for you.

Nearby Activities

Not every hike has this listing, but for hikes that do, look here for information about places of interest in the vicinity of the trail. In my case, many of these have to do with food.

Weather

For most folks, the hiking season around Portland starts in March or April, when flowers bloom and temperatures start to rise. Unfortunately, that's the least stable of seasons where the weather is concerned. Forecasts are notoriously off the mark during spring, so if you aren't absolutely, positively sure it will be clear, plan for 50-something degrees and drizzling into June.

Snow is a different matter: The higher-elevation hikes in this book generally won't be completely clear until July. Also note that in the Columbia River Gorge, wind is a constant reality, so even on a sunny June day, a hike such as the one to Dog Mountain (Hike 7) can have you reaching for a hat and gloves. By mid-to-late June, and all the way into October, you'll see mostly sunny skies, mild temperatures, and happy hikers. Then winter comes, and for all intents and purposes it rains until spring. We try to think of it as "waterfall loading."

Water

How much is enough? Well, one simple physiological fact should convince you to err on the side of excess when deciding how much water to pack: A hiker walking steadily in 90° heat needs about

AVERAGE DAILY HIGH TEMPERATURE BY MONTH: PORTLAND					
JAN	**FEB**	**MAR**	**APR**	**MAY**	**JUN**
47°F	51°F	56°F	61°F	67°F	73°F
JUL	**AUG**	**SEP**	**OCT**	**NOV**	**DEC**
80°F	80°F	75°F	63°F	52°F	45°F
AVERAGE DAILY PRECIPITATION BY MONTH: PORTLAND					
JAN	**FEB**	**MAR**	**APR**	**MAY**	**JUN**
6.14"	4.79"	4.50"	3.40"	2.55"	1.69"
JUL	**AUG**	**SEP**	**OCT**	**NOV**	**DEC**
0.59"	0.71"	1.54"	3.42"	6.74"	6.94"

Source: **weather.com**

10 quarts of fluid per day—that's 2.5 gallons. A good rule of thumb is to hydrate before your hike, carry (and drink) 6 ounces of water for every mile you plan to hike, and hydrate again after the hike. For most people, the pleasures of hiking make carrying water a relatively minor price to pay to remain safe and healthy, so pack more water than you anticipate needing, even for short hikes.

If you find yourself tempted to drink "found water," proceed with extreme caution. Many ponds and lakes you'll encounter are fairly stagnant, and the water tastes terrible. Drinking such water presents inherent risks for thirsty trekkers. Giardia parasites contaminate many water sources and cause the intestinal ailment giardiasis, which can last for weeks after onset. For more information, visit **cdc.gov/parasites/giardia.**

Effective treatment is essential before you use any water source you've found along the trail. Boiling water for 2–3 minutes is always a safe measure for camping, but dayhikers can consider iodine tablets, approved chemical mixes, filtration units rated for giardia, and ultraviolet filtration. Some of these methods (for example, filtration with an added carbon filter) remove bad tastes typical in stagnant water, while others add their own taste. Even if you've brought your own water, consider bringing along a means of water purification in case you've underestimated your consumption needs.

Clothing

Weather, unexpected trail conditions, fatigue, extended hiking duration, and wrong turns can individually or collectively turn a great outing into a very uncomfortable one at best. Some helpful guidelines:

➢ Choose silk, wool, or moisture-wicking synthetics for maximum comfort in all of your hiking attire—from hats to socks and in between. Cotton is fine if the weather remains dry and stable, but you won't be happy if that fabric gets wet.

➢ Always wear a hat, or at least tuck one into your daypack or hitch it to your belt. Hats offer sun and wind protection as well as warmth if it turns cold.

➢ Be ready to layer up or down as the day progresses and the mercury rises or falls. Today's outdoor wear makes layering easy, with such designs as jackets that convert to vests and zip-off or button-up legs.

➢ Biting bugs, poison oak, and thorny bushes found along many trails can generate short-term discomfort and long-term agony. A lightweight pair of pants and a long-sleeved shirt can go a long way toward shielding you from these annoyances.

➢ Wear hiking boots or sturdy hiking sandals with toe protection. Flip-flopping along a paved urban greenway is one thing, but you should never hike a trail in open sandals or casual sneakers. Your bones and arches need support, and your skin needs protection.

➢ Pair that footwear with good socks. If you prefer not to sheathe your feet when wearing hiking sandals, tuck the socks into your daypack—you may need them if temperatures plummet or if you hit rocky turf and pebbles begin to irritate your feet.

➢ Don't leave rainwear behind, even if the day dawns clear and sunny. Tuck into your daypack, or tie around your waist, a jacket that's breathable and either water-resistant or waterproof. Investigate different choices at your local outdoors retailer. If you're a frequent hiker, ideally you'll own rainwear in more than one weight, material, and style in order to protect you in all seasons in your regional microclimates.

The Ten Essentials

One of the first rules of hiking is to be prepared for anything. The simplest way to be prepared is to carry the "Ten Essentials." In addition to carrying the items listed below, you need to know how to use them, especially navigational aids. Always consider worst-case scenarios such as getting lost, hiking back in the dark, broken gear (for example, a broken hip strap on your pack or a water filter that gets plugged), twisting an ankle, or a brutal thunderstorm. These items don't cost a lot of money, don't take up much room in a pack, and don't weigh much—but they might just save your life.

➢ *Extra food:* trail mix, granola bars, or other high-energy snacks.

➢ *Extra clothes:* raingear, a change of socks, and, depending on the season, a warm hat and gloves.

➢ *Flashlight* with extra bulb and batteries.

➢ *Insect repellent.* For some areas and seasons, this is vital.

➢ *Maps and a high-quality compass.* Don't leave home without them, even if you know the terrain well from previous hikes. As previously noted, you should bring maps in addition to those in this book, and consult them before you hike. If you're GPS-savvy, bring that device, too, but don't rely on it as your sole navigational tool—battery life is limited, after all—and be sure to check its accuracy against that of your maps and compass.

➢ *Pocketknife and/or multitool.*

➢ *Sun protection:* sunglasses, lip balm, sunscreen (check the expiration date), and sun hat.

➢ *Water.* Again, bring more than you think you'll drink. Depending on your destination, you may want to bring a container and iodine or a filter for purifying water in case you run out.

➢ *Whistle.* It could become your best friend in an emergency.

➢ *Windproof matches and/or a lighter,* as well as a fire starter.

First-Aid Kit

In addition to the preceding items, the ones that follow may seem daunting to carry along for a dayhike. But any paramedic will tell you that the products listed here are just the basics. The reality of hiking is that you can be out for a week of backpacking and acquire only a mosquito bite . . . or you can hike for an hour, slip, and suffer a cut or broken bone. Fortunately, the items listed pack into a very small space. Convenient prepackaged kits are available at your pharmacy or online.

➤ Ace bandages or Spenco joint wraps
➤ Adhesive bandages
➤ Antibiotic ointment (such as Neosporin)
➤ Aspirin, acetaminophen (Tylenol), or ibuprofen (Advil)
➤ Athletic tape
➤ Blister kit (such as Moleskin or Spenco 2nd Skin)
➤ Butterfly-closure bandages
➤ Diphenhydramine (Benadryl), in case of allergic reactions
➤ Epinephrine in a prefilled syringe (EpiPen), typically available by prescription only, for people known to have severe allergic reactions to hiking mishaps such as bee stings
➤ Gauze (one roll and a half-dozen 4-by-4-inch pads)
➤ Hydrogen peroxide or iodine

Hiking with Children

No one is too young for a hike in the outdoors. Be mindful, though. Flat, short, and shaded trails are best with an infant. Toddlers who haven't quite mastered walking can still tag along, riding on an adult's back in a child carrier. Use common sense to judge a youngster's capacity to hike a particular trail, and be ready for the child to tire quickly and need to be carried.

When packing for the hike, remember the child's needs as well as your own. Make sure children are adequately clothed for the weather, have proper shoes, and are protected from the sun with sunscreen. Kids dehydrate quickly, so make sure you have plenty of fluids for everyone. Hikes suitable for children are noted in the 60 Hikes by Category chart on pages xvii–xix.

Finally, when hiking with kids, remember that the trip will be a compromise. A child's energy and enthusiasm alternate between bursts of speed and long stops to examine snails, sticks, dirt, and other attractions.

General Safety

While many hikers hit the trail full of enthusiasm and energy, others may find themselves feeling apprehensive about possible outdoor hazards. Although potentially dangerous situations can occur anywhere, your hike can be as safe and enjoyable as you had hoped, as long as you use sound judgment and prepare yourself before hitting the trail. Here are a few tips to make your trip safer and easier:

➤ *Hike with a buddy.* Not only is there safety in numbers, but a hiking companion can also help you if you twist an ankle on the trail or if you get lost, can assist in carrying food and water, and can be a partner in discovery. A buddy is good to bring along to both infrequently traveled or remote areas and to urban destinations.

➤ *If you're hiking alone, leave your hiking itinerary with someone you trust,* and let him or her know when you return.

➤ *Don't count on a mobile phone for your safety.* Reception may be spotty or non-existent on the trail, even on an urban walk—especially one embraced by towering trees.

➤ *Always carry food and water, even on short hikes.* Food will give you energy and sustain you in an emergency until help arrives. Bring more water than you think you'll need—we can't emphasize this enough. Hydrate throughout your hike and at regular intervals; don't wait until you feel thirsty. Treat water from streams or other sources before drinking it.

➤ *Ask questions.* Public-land employees are on hand to help. It's a lot easier to solicit advice before a problem occurs, and it will help you avoid a mishap away from civilization when it's too late to amend an error.

➤ *Stay on designated trails.* Most hikers get lost when they leave the path. Even on the most clearly marked trails, you usually reach a point where you have to stop and consider the direction in which to head. If you become disoriented, don't panic. As soon as you think you may be off-track, stop, assess your current direction, and then retrace your steps back to the point where you went awry. Using a map, compass, and this book—and keeping in mind what you've passed thus far—reorient yourself and trust your judgment about which way to continue. If you become absolutely unsure of how to continue, return to your vehicle the way you came in. Should you become completely lost and have no idea how to return to the trailhead, remaining in place along the trail and waiting for help is most often

the best option for adults and always the best option for children.

➤ *Always carry a whistle.* It may become a lifesaver if you get lost or hurt.

➤ *Be especially careful when crossing streams.* Whether you're fording the stream or crossing on a log, make every step count. If you have any doubt about maintaining your balance on a foot log, go ahead and ford the stream instead. When fording a stream, use a trekking pole or stout stick for balance and *face upstream as you cross.* If a stream seems too deep to ford, turn back. Whatever is on the other side isn't worth risking your life for.

➤ *Be careful at overlooks.* While these areas may provide spectacular views, they are potentially hazardous. Stay back from the edge of outcrops, and be absolutely sure of your footing.

➤ *Standing dead trees* and storm-damaged living trees pose a hazard to hikers and tent campers. Loose or broken limbs could fall at any time. When choosing a spot to rest, camp, or snack, *look up.*

➤ *Know the symptoms of heat exhaustion, or hyperthermia.* Lightheadedness and loss of energy are the first two indicators. If you feel these symptoms coming on, find some shade, drink your water, remove as many layers of clothing as practical, and stay put until you cool down. Marching through heat exhaustion leads to heat-stroke—which can be deadly. If you should be sweating and you're not, that's the signature warning sign. If you or a companion reaches this point, your hike is over: Do whatever you can to cool down, and seek medical help immediately.

➤ *Likewise, know the symptoms of subnormal body temperature, or hypothermia.* Shivering and forgetfulness are the two most common indicators of this stealthy killer. Hypothermia can occur at any elevation, even in the summer—especially if you're wearing lightweight cotton clothing. If symptoms develop, get to shelter, hot liquids, and dry clothes ASAP.

> *Most importantly, take along your brain.* A cool, calculating mind is the single most important asset on the trail. Think before you act. Watch your step. Plan ahead. Avoiding accidents before they happen is the best way to ensure a rewarding and relaxing hike.

Plant and Animal Hazards

Hikers should be aware of the following concerns regarding plant life and wildlife:

POISON OAK This deciduous plant **(below)** grows as a sparse ground cover, vine, or shrub; regardless of its form, poison oak always has three leaflets. It's easiest to spot in summer and early autumn, when the leaves flush bright-red. Beware of unknown bare-branched shrubs and vines in winter—the entire plant can cause a rash, no matter what the season.

Urushiol, the oil in the sap of the plant, is responsible for the rash. Reactions may start almost immediately or not appear until a week after exposure. Raised lines and/or blisters will appear, accompanied by a terrible itch. Try to refrain from scratching, though, because bacteria under your fingernails can cause an infection. Wash and dry the affected area thoroughly, applying calamine lotion to help dry out the rash. If the itching or blistering is severe, seek medical attention.

Most people come into contact with poison oak while bushwhacking or traveling off-trail, so stay on established trails whenever possible. If you do knowingly touch the plant, you must remove the oil within 15–20 minutes to avoid a reaction. Rinsing off the oil with cool water— hot water spreads it—is impractical on the trail, but some commercial products such as Tecnu are effective in removing urushiol from your skin. To keep from spreading the misery to someone else, wash not only any exposed parts of your body but also any oil-contaminated clothes, hiking gear, and pets.

SNAKES The most common snakes you'll encounter in and west of the Cascades are nonpoisonous garter snakes. The only venomous snakes in Oregon are

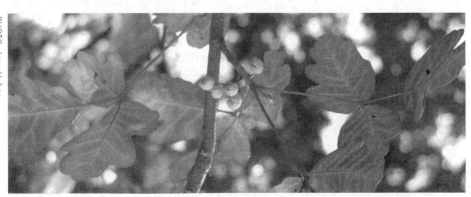

PHOTO: Jane Huber

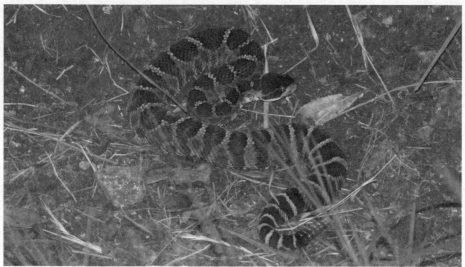

PHOTO: Jane Huber

rattlesnakes, but sightings of these pit vipers are generally infrequent, occurring most commonly in dry, rocky, or exposed zones during the warmest months of the year. The standard advice for hiking in rattlesnake territory is as follows:

➤ Don't put your hands or feet where you can't see them—say, at the top of a rock outcrop, or in tall grass or a log pile.

➤ Be extra-cautious in hot weather, when snakes are more active.

➤ Scan the trail continuously as you hike.

➤ Keep kids from running ahead on the trail. Bites to children are more severe than those to adults.

Should you encounter a rattlesnake, its body language will reveal its mood. A coiled rattler **(above)** is primed for a strike, while a relaxed rattler is more sanguine. If the snake is within striking distance, stand motionless and wait for it to calm down and move on. Taking small, slow steps backward is another smart

strategy. If you're out of immediate range, you can either skirt the snake or wait for it to move. Some people believe tapping the ground with a stick—from a safe distance, rather than in the snake's face—will encourage the snake to move on.

TICKS These arachnids like to hang out in the brush that grows along trails. I've noticed ticks mostly in the eastern Columbia River Gorge, but you should be tick-aware throughout the spring, summer, and fall. Ticks are ectoparasites, meaning they need a host for most of their life cycle in order to reproduce. The ticks that alight onto you while hiking will be very small, sometimes so tiny that you won't be able to spot them. All ticks need to attach for several hours before they can transmit disease.

A few precautions: Use insect repellent that contains DEET. Wear light-colored clothing, which will make it easy for you to spot ticks before they migrate to your skin. When your hike is done, inspect your hair, the back of your neck, your armpits, and your socks. During your posthike shower, take a moment to do a more complete body check. To remove a tick that is already embedded, use tweezers made especially for this purpose. Treat the bite with disinfectant solution.

Topographic Maps

The maps in this book have been produced with great care and, used with the hike text, will direct you to the trail and help you stay on-course. However, you'll find superior detail and valuable information in the U.S. Geological Survey's 7.5-minute series topographic maps. At **mytopo.com,** for example, you can view and print USGS topos of the entire United States free of charge. Online services such as **trails.com** charge annual fees for additional features such as shaded relief, which makes the topography stand out more. If you expect to print out many topo maps each year, it might be worth paying for such extras. The downside to USGS maps is that most are outdated, having been created 20–30 years ago; nevertheless, they provide excellent topographic detail.

Digital programs such as DeLorme's Topo North America enable you to review topo maps on your computer. Data gathered while hiking with a GPS unit can be downloaded into the software, letting you plot your own hikes.

Of course, **Google Earth** (**earth.google .com**) does away with topo maps and their inaccuracies . . . replacing them with satellite imagery and its inaccuracies. Regardless, what one lacks, the other augments. Google Earth is an excellent tool whether you have difficulty with topos or not.

If you're new to hiking, you might be wondering, "What's a topo map?" In short, it indicates not only linear distance but elevation as well, using contour lines. These lines spread across the map like dozens of intricate spiderwebs. Each line represents a particular elevation, and at the base of each topo is a contour's interval designation. If, for example, the contour interval is 20 feet, then the distance between each contour line is 20 feet. Follow five contour lines up on the same map, and the elevation has increased by 100 feet.

In addition to the sources listed previously and in Appendix B, you'll find topos at major universities, outdoors shops, and some public libraries, as well as online at **nationalmap.gov** and **store.usgs.gov.**

Trail Etiquette

Whether you're hiking in a city, county, state, or national park, always remember that great care and resources (from nature as well as from your tax dollars) have gone into creating these spaces. Treat the trail, wildlife, and fellow hikers with respect.

Here are a few general principles to keep in mind while you're on the trail:

➢ *Hike on open trails only.* Respect trail and road closures (ask if you're not sure), avoid possible trespassing on private land, and obtain all permits and authorization as required. Also, leave gates as you found them or as marked.

➢ *Be sensitive to the ground beneath you.* This also means staying on the existing trail and not blazing any new trails. Pack out what you pack in. **Leave No Trace** ethics make hiking and camping more fun for others (see **lnt.org** for more information).

➢ *Never spook animals.* An unannounced approach, a sudden movement, or a loud noise can startle them. A surprised snake or skunk can be dangerous to you, others, and itself. Give animals extra room and time to adjust to your presence.

➢ *Plan ahead.* Know your equipment, your ability, and the area in which you are hiking—and prepare accordingly. Be self-sufficient at all times; carry necessary supplies for changes in weather or other conditions. A well-executed trip is satisfying to you and to others.

➢ *Be courteous to other hikers, bikers, and equestrians you encounter on the trails.* Hikers and bikers should yield to equestrians, bikers should yield to hikers, and, whenever safe, everyone should yield to uphill hikers, bikers, or equestrians.

When you encounter equestrians, it's very helpful to move off-trail to the downhill side and greet the rider. This helps the horse understand that you aren't a threat.

Dollar Lake at Mount Hood (see Hike 44, page 228)

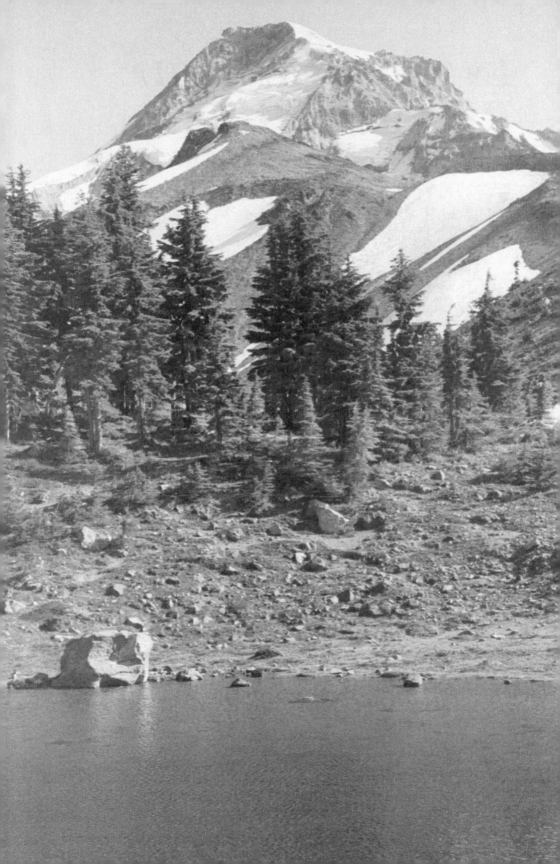

IN THE COLUMBIA RIVER GORGE

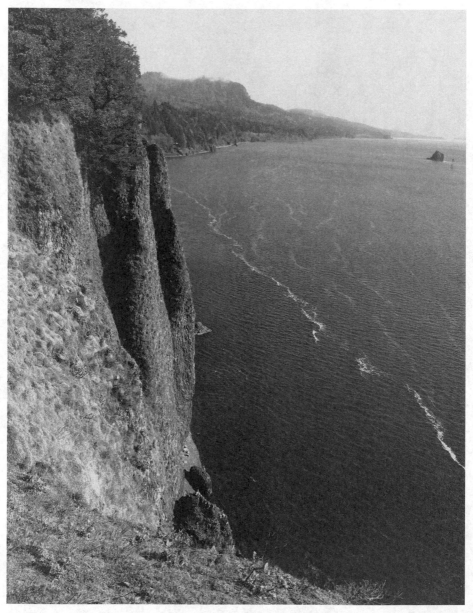

Cliff-top views of the Columbia River, like this one from the lower Cape Horn Trail (see Hike 3), are abundant in the Gorge.

In the Columbia River Gorge (Hikes 1–13)

1 Angels Rest and Devils Rest

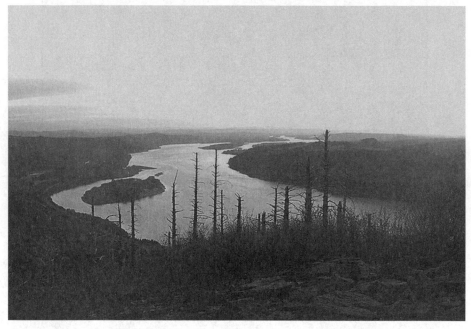

Looking down the Columbia River from Angels Rest —a nice view for sunset, by the way. Just bring a light to get back down.

In Brief

There's a reason for all the parking at this trailhead: It's one of the more accessible hikes in the region, with a gentle grade to a spectacular lookout point above the Columbia River. It also connects with Wahkeena Trail, making longer loops or one-way hikes with shuttles possible.

Description

As you drive out I-84, you can actually see Angels Rest, a flat-topped rock outcropping sticking out over the road at the end of a ridge. What looks like a building on top is in fact a clump of trees. And if it looks like it's way up there, just remember that if you take your time on the way up, you'll have plenty of breath left to be taken away by the view up top.

LENGTH 4.6 miles round-trip to Angels Rest, 7.5 miles one-way to Devils Rest

CONFIGURATION Out-and-back or optional point-to-point to Devils Rest with shuttle

DIFFICULTY Moderate to Angels Rest because of altitude gain and a little rock-scrambling at top; tougher to Devils Rest because of length and elevation

SCENERY Forest; waterfall, creek crossing, panorama from Angels Rest

EXPOSURE Mostly shady; one section at the top lies along a narrow, rocky ridge with steep drops.

TRAFFIC Very heavy—on a nice weekend day, this trail will have more dogs on it than many trails have hikers.

TRAIL SURFACE Packed dirt with some roots; rocks

HIKING TIME 2.5 hours to Angels Rest, 5 hours to Devils Rest

DRIVING DISTANCE 28 miles (30 minutes) from Pioneer Courthouse Square

SEASON Year-round, but often gets snow in winter

BEST TIME Any clear day

BACKPACKING OPTIONS One decent campsite just past Angels Rest

ACCESS No fees or permits

WHEELCHAIR ACCESS None, but nearby Bridal Veil Falls State Park (503-695-2261, **tinyurl.com/bridalveilfallssp**) has some accessible trails.

MAPS Green Trails *Map 428 (Bridal Veil)* or *Map 428S (Columbia River Gorge–West)*

FACILITIES Restrooms and water 0.5 mile west at Bridal Veil Falls State Park

INFO Columbia River Gorge National Scenic Area, 541-308-1700, **www.fs.usda .gov/crgnsa**

SPECIAL COMMENTS Dogs must be on a leash not exceeding 6 feet.

Angels Rest Trail #415 starts off easy enough, then hits a rocky climb that's steep only for a few moments, leading to an early reward: a rare view from above a waterfall, in this case the 100-foot Coopey Falls, named for Charles Coopey, a Portland tailor who owned land here. A short way past this, the trail crosses a wooden bridge over Coopey Creek and then starts climbing again.

After about a mile, you'll start switchbacking through an area that burned in 1991; note the blackened trunks of some of the bigger trees. Mostly just the underbrush and smaller trees burned, which opened up the forest floor to the sun and let wildflowers come in to take your mind off the climb. Follow a series of small switchbacks into more-open country, getting a view of the rocky face of Angels Rest as you go. When the trail traverses 100 yards of rockslide, you're almost done.

Just past the slide, the trail reenters the woods briefly, then you turn left out onto the final ridge. This last stretch of the trail might make you think twice about bringing small children: It gets a little narrow, with cliffs to the east falling away a few hundred feet, and in one spot you'll have to scramble up about 10 feet of rock. When the trail to Devils Rest goes back and to the right on the ridgetop, continue straight.

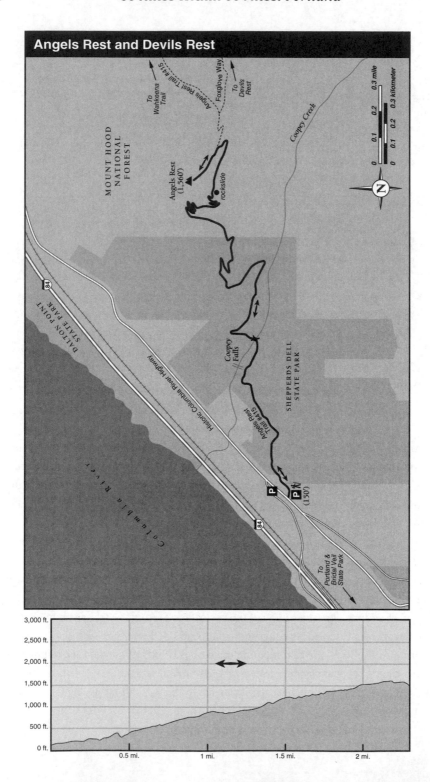

Angels Rest and Devils Rest

The reward for your effort is a view to rival any other in the Gorge—especially for the relative ease with which you got here. To the east you can see Beacon Rock and the high walls on either side of the river. To the west you can see Vista House (built in 1916 as a pioneer memorial and rest stop for travelers, now an interpretive center, museum, and gift shop) and the hills falling away toward Portland and the Willamette Valley. The Columbia River, right below you, seems close enough that if you got a running start you could jump into it. You might see some windsurfers out there; on one trip, I watched a floatplane practicing touch-and-go landings on this stretch of the river.

You can also see two other hikes from this book: Right next to Beacon Rock is the step-shaped Hamilton Mountain (see next hike), and the big flat-topped mountain looming behind that is Table Mountain (Hike 10, page 61). There's even a nice bench to sit on out here. Around to the left of the summit, a notch in some rocks offers shelter from frequently high winds. All in all, it's hard to imagine a better place to have lunch.

If you're up for more hiking, you can turn this into a longer out-and-back or do a one-way hike with another car parked farther east. To do either, as you walk back down the ridge, veer left (east) at the junction instead of continuing straight, which is where you came from. After a few minutes you'll come to another junction; go left for Wahkeena Trail or continue straight 1 mile up Foxglove Way to reach Devils Rest.

If you turn left, you'll soon pass a nice campsite and then come to Wahkeena Spring in 2.6 miles; 0.1 mile later, you'll intersect Wahkeena Trail #420. Here, you can turn left (downhill) and follow Wahkeena Creek 1.6 miles to the picnic area at Wahkeena Falls, or you can go straight and, in 1.2 miles, intersect Larch Mountain Trail (see Hike 9, page 55). Go down the latter 1.8 miles and you'll be at Multnomah Falls. I've provided a more detailed description of this trail section in the Wahkeena Falls to Multnomah Falls profile (Hike 13, page 74).

If you go up to Devils Rest, you might have a hard time finding the official spot, because there's no sign leading to it. When the trail crests and starts back downhill, look for a side trail to the left; the summit is about 50 yards that way. Once there, however, you may wonder why you came, as there's really no view. I don't know why Devils Rest would be higher than Angels Rest, but at least the angels have a view.

You can go beyond Devils Rest (catching a decent view just past it on the trail) and continue down to the same junction mentioned above on the Wahkeena Falls–Multnomah Falls loop, thus completing your one-way hike. All it really adds is exercise, though.

Nearby Activities

Vista House, and the road that leads to it, are both worth a visit (40700 E. Historic Columbia River Hwy., Corbett, OR 97019). To get here, simply drive back toward Portland on the Historic Columbia River Highway rather than on I-84. Follow this pre-1920 road past a few other waterfalls and then up the hill to Crown Point, where you can step into Vista House and take in a postcard view and historic displays about the building of the road. More information: 503-695-2230, **vistahouse.com.**

After your visit, keep going west on that road, past Vista House, and in a couple of miles you'll see a sign down a steep hill back to I-84.

GPS Information and Directions

Angels Rest Trailhead **N45° 33.613' W122° 10.365'**
Devils Rest **N45° 33.734' W122° 7.704'**

Take I-84 from Portland, driving 21 miles east of I-205 to Exit 28/Bridal Veil. Bearing right off the exit, drive less than a mile and park in the parking area at the intersection with the Historic Columbia River Highway; a second parking lot is down the road, to the right. The signed trailhead is on the old highway, between the two parking lots.

2 Beacon Rock State Park

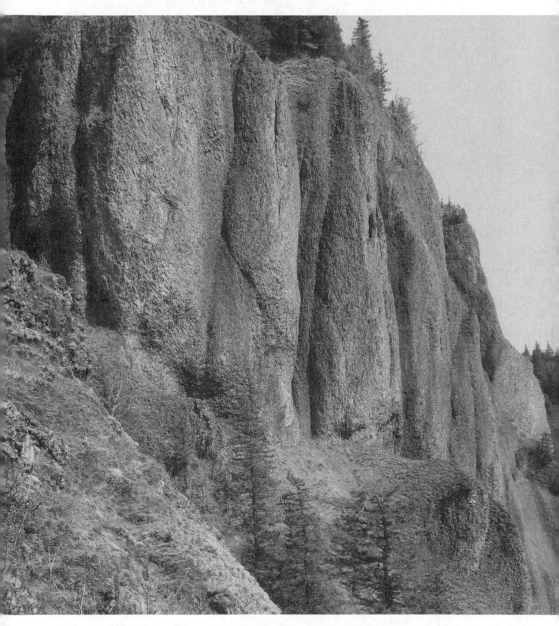

When you see these cliffs on the Hamilton Mountain Trail, you're almost there. Just be careful of your footing.

LENGTH 1.8 miles round-trip to top of Beacon Rock, 8 miles one-way to Hamilton Mountain

CONFIGURATION Out-and-back, optional loop

DIFFICULTY Beacon Rock, easy–moderate; Hamilton Mountain, strenuous

SCENERY Overlooks of the Columbia, waterfalls, and spring wildflowers

EXPOSURE Hamilton Mountain is mostly shady, with one rocky section near cliff tops; Beacon Rock is on the side of a cliff but has handrails.

TRAFFIC Heavy on weekends, moderate otherwise

TRAIL SURFACE Packed dirt with rocks, some pavement

HIKING TIME 1 hour for Beacon Rock, 4.5 hours for Hamilton Mountain

DRIVING DISTANCE 51 miles (1 hour, 10 minutes) from Pioneer Courthouse Square

SEASON Daily, year-round, 8 a.m.–sunset; call for trail conditions in winter.

BEST TIME April and May

BACKPACKING OPTIONS None

ACCESS A **Washington State Discover Pass** ($10/day, $30/year) is required and can be bought at the park or online at **discoverpass.wa.gov.**

WHEELCHAIR ACCESS Nearby on Hadley Trail; 1-mile loop at the Doetsch Day Use Area

MAPS Green Trails *Map 428 (Bridal Veil)* or *Map 432S (Columbia River Gorge–West);* free map at park headquarters and at website below

FACILITIES Water and restrooms at both trailheads

INFO Beacon Rock State Park, 509-427-8265, **parks.wa.gov/474**

SPECIAL COMMENTS Dogs must be on a leash not exceeding 8 feet.

In Brief

One of the most recognized symbols of the Columbia River Gorge, Beacon Rock is also a fascinating, if short, hiking experience—and it's not even all this Washington State Park has to offer. There's also a rigorous climb to the scenic Hamilton Mountain, with a couple of amazing waterfalls along the way.

Description

Beacon Rock

Beacon Rock got its name—well, its white man's name—on Halloween 1805, when William Clark described it in his journal. For the Corps of Discovery and the people who then lived along the Columbia River, Beacon Rock meant two important things: the last of the rapids on the Columbia and the beginning of tidal influence on the river. Today, it means a unique hiking experience to its summit, and the state park around it means a chance to take in more nice views of the Columbia River.

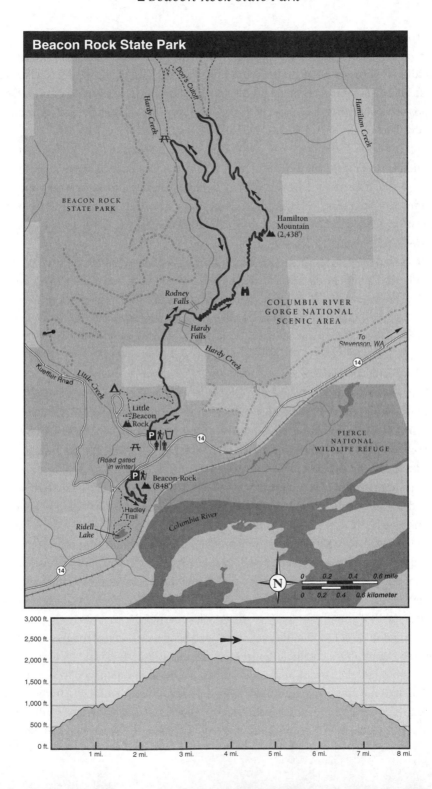

To climb Beacon Rock, which ascends nearly 600 feet in less than a mile, start at a sign on the south side of WA 14, and get ready to give thanks to a man named Henry J. Biddle. It was he who bought the rock (which is what's left of the inside of an ancient volcano) in 1914 to save it from being blasted to pieces for jetty material. He said his purpose was simply to build the trail you're about to hike, and he never charged hikers a penny. Eventually, his family donated the land to the state.

The trail is something of an engineering wonder, beginning with the fact that the builders couldn't scout the route: They had to just build a section, then figure out where to take it next. The finished product is 4,500 feet long and 4 feet wide, and includes 52 switchbacks, 100 concrete slabs, and, originally, 22 wooden bridges. Some of the original work remains, such as wrought-iron handrails at some switchbacks and steel eyebolts in the rock wall.

To get to the top, just persevere and, if heights bother you, don't look down. It's virtually all rails and bridges and platforms until you're just below the summit, where you'll have a view east to Bonneville Dam, north to Hamilton Mountain, and straight down the other side to the boat docks of the state park. Keep an eye out for rock climbers, and don't throw anything from the top.

Hamilton Mountain

For a more challenging and rewarding hike, drive—or walk, if the gate is closed—up the road across WA 14 to the campground and the Hamilton Mountain Trailhead. From here, you'll climb gently through forest until you reach a bench to take a break; the power lines you're under here aren't all that scenic, but you do get a view ahead to the summit of Hamilton Mountain. At 0.5 mile, continue straight at a trail leading left to the campground and a rock formation called Little Beacon Rock; 0.4 mile later, you'll come to a trail leading down and to the right 100 yards to two viewpoints overlooking Hardy Falls. A minute past that on the main trail, you'll see a sign that says HAMILTON MOUNTAIN; oddly enough, it points downhill.

For a sight to remember, and a soak to cool you down (if you'd like), walk a couple hundred yards to the left and check out Rodney Falls (also known as the Pool of Winds), which almost explodes out of a bowl in the rock face. You can get right in its spray, if you don't mind essentially wading the last part of the trail.

If you don't feel like climbing anymore, turn back here—it gets tougher quickly. To get to Hamilton Mountain, follow the signed trail as it descends to, then crosses, Hardy Creek and then heads up the hill. After 0.2 mile of climbing, you'll come to a trail junction with two wonderful options: difficult and more difficult. To the left is the return portion of a possible loop hike, but keep right (taking the more difficult way), and after 0.3 mile of sturdy climbing you'll reach a spectacular rock lookout.

There's nothing wrong with turning back here, but do be careful as you walk around on these rocks—in some spots it's more than 200 feet straight down.

If you want the real views, keep climbing. In just a few minutes you'll see side trails on the right leading to meadows on top of the ridge. (You can take one of the side trails to get a view of the river.) Along the main trail, you'll pass two fantastic viewpoints of the mountain's rocky face while gaining 700 feet in just over a mile, bringing you to a mountaintop junction. The view south is somewhat blocked by brush, but you can see up to Table Mountain (Hike 10, page 61) to the northeast, Mount Adams just east of that, and Mount St. Helens to the northwest. You should also be able to make out Dog and Wind Mountains up the river, Eagle Creek and the Benson Plateau across it, and the town of Cascade Locks.

To add some new scenery and make your hike a loop, continue 0.9 mile north along the dramatic north ridge of Hamilton, turn left onto an old road, and go 100 yards to Don's Cutoff Trail. This scenic but uneventful side trip—named for Don Cannard, cofounder of the Chinook Trails Association—leads down to Hardy Creek Trail, which at this point looks like a road. Turn left, follow the trail downhill past a picnic table, and after another mile you'll be back at the junction mentioned above, just east of Rodney Falls. Turn right and you'll reach the Hamilton Mountain Trailhead in 1.6 miles.

Nearby Activities

The **Columbia Gorge Interpretive Center Museum** (990 SW Rock Creek Dr., Stevenson, WA 98648), 10 miles east of the park on WA 14, features historical displays ranging from the geological (descriptions of the formation of the Gorge) to the mechanical (examples of steam engines used on railroads a bit more recently). More information: 800-991-2338 or 509-427-8211, **columbiagorge.org.**

GPS Information and Directions

Beacon Rock Trailhead **N45° 37.723' W122° 1.297'**
Hamilton Mountain Trailhead **N45° 37.929' W122° 1.207'**

Take I-84 from Portland, driving 37 miles east of I-205 to Exit 44/Cascade Locks. As soon as you enter the town, take your first right to get on Bridge of the Gods, following a sign for Stevenson, Washington. Pay a $1 toll on the bridge and, at the far end, turn left (west) on WA 14. Proceed 6.9 miles to Beacon Rock State Park (34841 WA 14, Skamania, WA 98648). To hike up Beacon Rock, park on the left; to go toward Hamilton Mountain, turn right on the campground access road and drive 0.4 mile to the trailhead. The gate to the upper trailhead is closed in winter, but the trail is open; you'll just have to park on the south side of WA 14 and walk up the access road.

3 Cape Horn

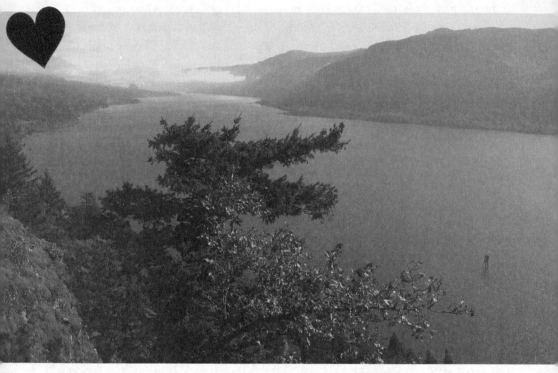

You'll actually be standing on a train tunnel when you get this view looking up the Columbia. This photo was taken on the lower portion of Cape Horn Trail.

In Brief

This is one of the newest trails in the Columbia River Gorge, and it's easy to see why it has become so popular. You can enjoy spectacular views of the Columbia from high up on the hill or just 200 feet above a riverside railroad, and in between you have a pleasant walk through forest and rolling-hill countryside reminiscent of a stroll in Europe.

Description

This trail has been sort of emerging for years: from off-limits private property to conservation struggle to informal trails to finally full-on U.S. Forest Service design and maintenance. (You can get all the history at **gorgefriends.org.**) Now that it's official, with tunnels under the highway and everything, it's really two hikes put together: an upper

LENGTH 2.6 miles round-trip for the upper section, 4 miles round-trip for the lower section, 6.3 miles for the entire loop (when it's open)

CONFIGURATION Loop or out-and-back

DIFFICULTY Easy–moderate

SCENERY Forest, countryside, cliff-top viewpoints of the Columbia River

EXPOSURE Shaded, with several points on unrailed cliff tops

TRAFFIC Moderate on spring and summer weekends

TRAIL SURFACE Packed dirt, gravel, rocks

HIKING TIME 2 hours for either section, 3.5 hours for the whole thing

DRIVING DISTANCE 33 miles (40 minutes) from Pioneer Courthouse Square

SEASON Upper loop open year-round, with possible snow and ice in winter; lower loop closed February 1–July 15

BEST TIME April and May for wildflowers, October for fall colors

BACKPACKING OPTIONS None

ACCESS No fees or permits

WHEELCHAIR ACCESS None

MAPS Green Trails *Map 428S (Columbia River Gorge–West);* online map at **cape horntrail.org**

FACILITIES Outhouse at trailhead

INFO Columbia River Gorge National Scenic Area, 541-308-1700, **www.fs.usda .gov/crgnsa**

SPECIAL COMMENTS Several sections, especially on the lower loop, are sketchy if you're afraid of heights. For the best photos of Gorge views, do this hike in the afternoon, when the sun will be behind you.

section of either 2.6 or 5.2 miles to viewpoints high above the river, and a lower section of about 4 miles that skirts the edge of cliffs just above the river and visits a waterfall— but is closed February 1–July 15 every year to protect nesting peregrine falcons.

When the lower portion is open, you can hike the whole loop in 6.3 miles. I should point out, if only for fun, that opinions vary wildly on how long this loop actually is: The Forest Service says 6 miles, the Cape Horn Conservancy says 7 miles, the Portland Hikers Field Guide says 6.8 miles, and Friends of the Columbia Gorge says 8 miles. My GPS said 6.3 miles, and my internal measuring device agreed.

The trail starts right across the road from the trailhead and follows a wide gravel path in a thick forest, which in October has great fall colors, mainly from bigleaf maples. The first mile crosses a small creek and then gains 650 feet in a series of mellow switchbacks with not much to see, though it's interesting to look for the old sections of volunteer-built trail, now blocked with logs and branches. Just for mileposts, at 0.9 mile ignore a trail leading to the right, and at 1.1 miles you'll pass almost under a set of power lines.

At 1.2 miles you come to a funny sign offering a choice between V I E W P O I N T and H O R S E S. Turns out it's because the viewpoint is on a narrow, rocky ledge that's unsafe for our four-legged fellows. For hikers, the trail goes left here. Don't be

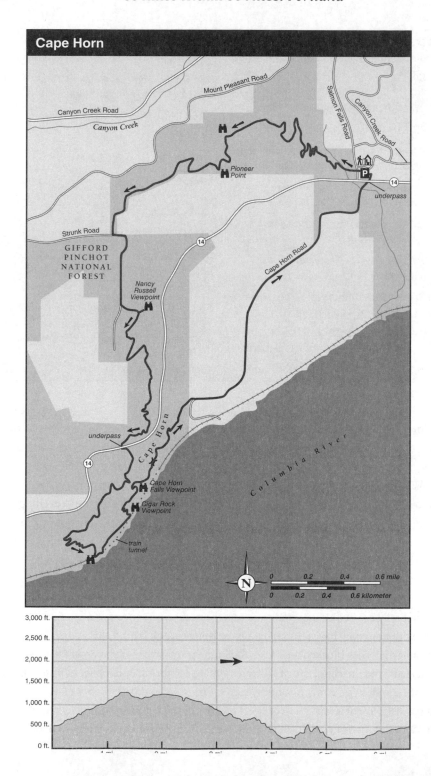

Cape Horn

a horse—go check out the view of the Gorge. Three of these viewpoints appear in the next few minutes; the last of these makes a good turnaround spot if it's spring and the lower section of trail is closed. If not, keep going.

At this point you've gone 1.3 miles with 800 feet of elevation gain, and you're done climbing for now. The trail crosses the viewless summit, drops for just over 0.5 mile, briefly joins an old road in the woods, and then at 2.1 miles crosses paved Strunk Road. The next 0.5 mile or so really reminds me of walking in England or Italy: rambling along country lanes past fields and houses and horses, with wooded hillsides in the background.

Now walking along a gravel road, look for the trail heading left, just as you reach the second clump of trees. The next big highlight is a new viewpoint built to honor Nancy Russell of the Friends of the Columbia Gorge, who did much of the work to save this place from development. In fact, the first time I hiked Cape Horn years ago, a big house stood here. The Friends bought it, tore it down, and put this up.

The viewpoint is at the 2.6-mile mark, so when the lower trail is closed, you might as well turn around here; that's the 5.2-mile stretch. But when you can do the whole loop, keep on truckin'. The trail now drops a few hundred feet in half a mile to a new tunnel under WA 14—so much better than the death-defying dash of the old days!

Just past the tunnel, things really get steep, as you lose more than 400 feet in 0.5 mile, and some of it is on scree, which I call The Stones of Tedium. At the bottom of the hill, now at the 4.2-mile mark, an unsigned junction turns out to be another horse-versus-viewpoint decision. Again, don't be a horse: Go right and follow the trail to the coolest viewpoints of the whole loop.

(*Note:* As I was working on the fifth edition of this book in the fall of 2013, this lower section of the trail was undergoing some reroutes. Even if what I describe here is gone, the trail will be clearly marked and essentially the same.)

Here, you're actually walking on top of a railroad tunnel, some 250 feet directly above the river. And what views—right above the tracks, with towering rock formations right by the river and the forested slopes of Oregon across the way. Too bad the Forest Service is considering moving much of this section of trail; I hope you get there before they do so.

After 0.25 mile of climbing and (perhaps) more Stones of Tedium, the trail crosses a bridge, another feature of the new trail. Used to be that the trail passed behind Cape Horn Falls, which was fun in the spring and summer, not so much in the winter.

Another steep drop brings you, after 0.4 mile, to the only semi-unfortunate aspect of this hike, which is that the last 1.3 miles are mostly on a road. Nothing to be done, since both sides are private property and there's no room for another trailhead. So just enjoy the country-road rambling. Right before the end, you'll use another tunnel to cross under WA 14, putting you back where you started.

If you just want to do the lower section when it's open, simply start at the trailhead and do these last few paragraphs in reverse, back to the Nancy Russell Viewpoint.

GPS Information and Directions

N45° 35.359' W122° 10.711'

From Portland, take I-205 across the Columbia River into Washington and take Exit 27/ WA 14–Camas. Follow WA 14 for 20 miles and turn left onto Salmon Falls Road; then make an immediate right onto Canyon Creek Road and another right into the parking lot. You can even take a Skamania County bus here during the week; the stop is called Salmon Falls.

4 Catherine Creek

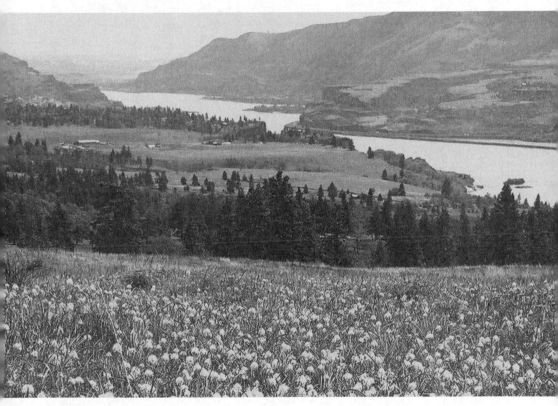

Camas on the Catherine Creek upper loop. This shot was taken from the little knoll by the pond in mid-April.

In Brief

For about 10 months of the year there's really no reason to go to Catherine Creek, but in April and May there's no better place to be, for Catherine Creek at that time is wildflower heaven, with close to 100 species in bloom.

Description

In a typical hiking year, I have some hikes that I usually do before Catherine Creek, but my personal hiking season really starts when the grass widow blooms at Catherine Creek in late March. It gets serious when the camas blooms in early April; my personal

LENGTH Up to 4.1 miles	**ACCESS** No fees or permits
CONFIGURATION Loop	**WHEELCHAIR ACCESS** A series of loops below the parking area offers access to flowers, birds, views of the Columbia River, and a waterfall on Catherine Creek.
DIFFICULTY Easy–moderate	
SCENERY Wide-open vistas, a geological curiosity, and (in spring) flowers, flowers everywhere!	**MAPS** Green Trails *Map 432S (Columbia River Gorge–East)*
EXPOSURE Out in the open most of the way; optional trip to a cliff top	**FACILITIES** Portable restroom at the trailhead February–May; no drinkable water
TRAFFIC Heavy on weekends in late spring and early summer, light otherwise	**INFO** Columbia River Gorge National Scenic Area, 541-308-1700, **www.fs.usda .gov/crgnsa**
TRAIL SURFACE Dirt and some rock, plus a small paved section	
HIKING TIME 30 minutes–4 hours	**SPECIAL COMMENTS** Dogs must be leashed. As this book was going to press, a new trail system was being planned and is scheduled to be implemented in 2014. Minor changes to the trails described here are possible, so check the contacts above for the latest. The trail plan is reflected on the Green Trails map referenced above.
DRIVING DISTANCE 72 miles (1 hour, 30 minutes) from Pioneer Courthouse Square	
SEASON Year-round	
BEST TIME Late March–early June	
BACKPACKING OPTIONS None	

Easter Sunday tradition is to pack a lunch, hike up the hill to a certain spot, spread out my food, take in the view, and listen to the meadowlarks. Then I go back to (usually) rainy old Portland.

There really isn't much to this hike, physically speaking. In fact, you could knock out the paved and wheelchair-accessible section below the road in about 15 minutes. It's really all about the flowers and the wide-open vistas uncommon elsewhere in our local hiking world.

From the road, walk through a gate and choose a path that tends to the right, toward a small canyon just up the hill. If you're like me, you'll stop within a few feet and start admiring flowers. One enthusiast has counted as many as 82 species in bloom here on an April day, with such fantastic names as chocolate lily, common bastard toad flax, rough wallflower, Columbia Gorge lupine, least hop clover, poet's shooting star, rigid fiddleneck, great hound's tongue, slender popcornflower, small-flowered blue-eyed Mary, and chickweed monkeyflower. (No, I didn't make these names up.)

Follow a gravel road into the canyon and up the creek. Watch out for poison oak; it's everywhere—beware an "old growth" stand of it on the right as you near the creek. After 0.25 mile, cross the creek on a bouncy plank bridge and, 100 yards later, you'll

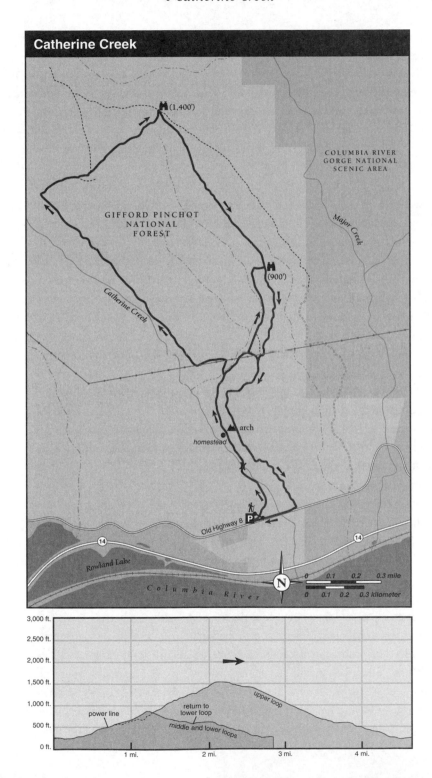

Catherine Creek

arrive at an old homestead. Above you now is a geological curiosity: a natural arch we'll visit later.

Past the homestead, staying to the right, ascend a slight rise into a meadow. In May, under some of the bushes, you'll find dense thickets of irises. When you reach the power lines, a total of 0.8 mile from your car, you'll have your first decision to make. You can go left and take a trail that parallels Catherine Creek before climbing into the high country, or you can continue straight and make another decision in a minute, which is what I recommend.

At the second junction, moments later, you have three options: a lower loop, an upper loop, and a trip to the high country. For the lower loop, follow a trail to the right and then along the top of a little ridge, and your hike will be 2 miles. I'll describe that section in a bit, because you really should do at least part of the upper loop.

For the upper loop, follow the trail left and up the draw until you see a faint, signed road, headed right and up the hill; follow it up into the meadows, then either head down toward the lower loop or find a trail east and across the meadows to eventually reach an overlook of Major Creek. (Some of this area burned in 2013, so you can see how it's coming back.)

For the high country, from this second junction, keep heading up the draw until the trail climbs into the meadows; then go down and back toward the car or take a trail that goes up to the tree line, where it turns to the west, crosses another line of trees, and enters yet another huge meadow. Here, if you look up and to the right, you'll see a clump of trees that shelters a tiny spring. Just below that, a berm gathers the spring water into a surprising pond. And on that berm someone could have quite a fine Easter picnic, with the Columbia River laid out at his feet, flowers all around, and Mount Hood across the way.

From that point, the trail continues west, reaches an overlook of Catherine Creek, and then drops back to the place where you made your first decision on this hike, down below the power lines.

OK, now for the lower loop, which is also the way down from the upper loop, or high country. Wherever you're starting, follow a trail that eventually hugs the top of the ridge above Catherine Creek. Following this, you'll get a view into the canyon where the homestead is, and then you'll be at the top of the arch. A fence now blocks access to the arch, which you used to be able to get on top of or even walk down through.

Keep descending the hill, following the trail near the cliff's edge. You'll cross a little draw filled with purple camas (in April), with creek access on your right, and a few minutes later you'll be at the road—and probably as close to power lines as you'll ever be in your life. Turn right and a little rock scramble will put you on the road's shoulder. Cross the creek again and see the parking lot, just up the hill.

Connection to Coyote Wall

But wait—there's more! Catherine Creek has a neighboring hike to the west called Coyote Wall (Hike 6, page 41), with a neat area called The Labyrinth in between. The two hikes share a (formerly) secret door to one another—I shall now give the secret away.

From the Catherine Creek Trailhead, go left on another old road, which climbs gently through marshy areas and over small hills. After 0.25 mile, it arrives at an uphill turn back to the right, near the top of a cliff. For many years, a big dead tree has lain here, and if you go behind that tree, you'll see a small trail heading down to the west, along the face of the cliff. Didn't see *that* before, did you?

This little trail hugs a steep, rocky hillside for a short time, then drops into a grassy bowl, where it intersects yet another old road heading steeply uphill. Follow this road as it climbs, then swings to the left and becomes a trail. You'll pass a series of rock pits that Native Americans used as vision-quest sites—don't disturb them!— as the trail keeps winding west, up through the oaks. I call it a "faith trail," because it seems to be going nowhere. Trust me, it isn't.

The path eventually leads through several meadows some 700 feet above Rowland Lake, then past a freaky tree known as the Coyote Tree (complete with bones hanging in it), and finally down into a mess of trails, all of which lead into an area called The Labyrinth. Combining these two hikes as an out-and-back or as a point-to-point with an easy car shuttle is one of my absolute favorites, and an April tradition.

An upper loop also connects these two areas. To do that from this end, look for an old road heading up the creek just before the creek crossing in the main loop. Climb that road for 1,000 feet of elevation, then follow jeep tracks to the west until you intersect the upper reaches of the Coyote Wall hike.

GPS Information and Directions

N45° 42.630' W121° 21.727'

Take I-84 from Portland, driving 62.8 miles east of I-205 to Exit 64, the third exit for Hood River, Oregon. Turn left at the end of the ramp, following the signs for White Salmon, Washington. Pay a $1 toll to cross the Columbia River, then turn right on WA 14. Travel 5.9 miles and turn left onto Old Highway 8. The parking area is 1.5 miles ahead, on the left.

5 Chinidere Mountain

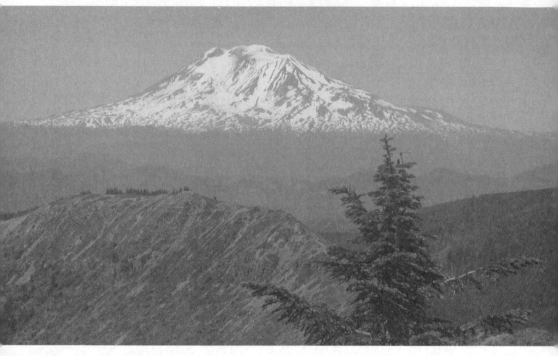

View of Mount Hood from Chinidere Mountain

In Brief

Unless you're spending the night, you might spend more time in the car than on the trail for this one. But the view from the top of Chinidere Mountain is more than worth the drive, and Wahtum Lake is a fine destination as well. Still, consider making this part of a longer trip to Lost Lake or the Hood River Valley.

Description

If you're using a view-for-effort scale to measure your hikes, Chinidere Mountain ranks 11 out of 10—once you get there. It's a 2-hour drive from Portland, but the roads are all paved, and you'll be rewarded with a fairly easy hike, a beautiful mountain lake with camping and fishing, and a view that stretches hundreds of miles.

LENGTH 4 miles	**ACCESS** Northwest Forest Pass required (see page 3). A Mount Hood National Forest wilderness permit (available free at the trailhead and national-forest boundaries) is also required May 15–October 15.
CONFIGURATION Loop	
DIFFICULTY Mostly easy, then moderate right below the peak	
SCENERY Old-growth forest, a deep mountain lake, and a panoramic view	**WHEELCHAIR ACCESS** None
EXPOSURE Mostly shady except on top	**MAPS** Green Trails *Map 429 (Bonneville Dam)* or *Map 428S (Columbia River Gorge–West)*
TRAFFIC Light	
TRAIL SURFACE Packed dirt, roots, rocks	**FACILITIES** Outhouse at trailhead
HIKING TIME 2.5 hours	**INFO** Hood River Ranger District, 541-352-6002, **www.fs.usda.gov/mthood**; Pacific Crest Trail Association, **pcta.org**
DRIVING DISTANCE 87 miles (2 hours) from Pioneer Courthouse Square	
SEASON Snow-free July–mid-October	
BEST TIME August and September	**SPECIAL COMMENTS** Wahtum Lake is at the very top of Eagle Creek Trail, so consider doing a fantastic one-way, downhill 14-miler with a car shuttle.
BACKPACKING OPTIONS Two good areas on the lake	

If you're wondering, *Chinidere* is pronounced **SHIN**-uh-deer, and it's named for the last chief of the local Wasco tribe. And *Wahtum* is a local Native American word meaning "pond" or "body of water." So you're looking through the trees here at "Lake Lake."

From the trailhead, walk through the campground—not down the road near the outhouse—and follow a trail called the Wahtum Express, which includes 250 wooden stairs. (You can skip this by following a parallel horse trail to the right, if you wish.) At the bottom of the Express, turn left and walk 100 feet down to a big tree with two Pacific Crest Trail (PCT) signs on it. You'll be right by the lake, with a picnic area in front of you—and also in the middle of several nice lakeshore campsites. Turn right here, heading north on the PCT toward Canada.

The trail meanders along at first, near the lake, weaving through a lovely forest of hemlocks interspersed with bunchberry, thimbleberry, vanilla leaf, columbine, huckleberry, and salmonberry. Look along the near shore for a small island with about four trees on it. There's also, around 0.5 mile up, some impressive trail construction to let water pass. Tiny springs and other mossy, flower-covered babbling brooks will keep you entertained and charmed.

After about 1 flat mile, you'll come into more-open forest, with beargrass that blooms in July, and you'll start climbing gradually on some classic Oregon PCT: wide

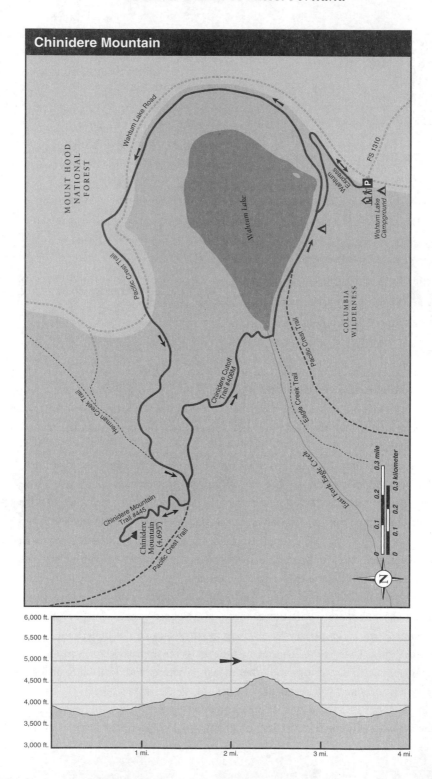

Chinidere Mountain

MOUNT HOOD NATIONAL FOREST

Wahtum Lake Road

Pacific Crest Trail

Wahtum Lake

Wahtum Express

FS 1310

Wahtum Lake Campground

Chinidere Cutoff Trail #406M

Eagle Creek Trail

Pacific Crest Trail

COLUMBIA WILDERNESS

Herman Creek Trail

Chinidere Mountain Trail #445

Chinidere Mountain (4,695')

Pacific Crest Trail

East Fork Eagle Creek

0.3 mile

0.3 kilometer

0.2

0.1

0

0.2

0.1

0

Z

trails over soft ground covered in pine needles and traversing thick forest. At a total of 1.75 miles, you'll cross a creek that dries up by midsummer, and at 1.9 miles (now having climbed only 400 feet) you'll intersect Herman Creek Trail, which leads all the way down to the outskirts of Cascade Locks.

A tenth of a mile later, you'll see Chinidere Cutoff Trail #406M plunging down to the left; we'll take that one back. For now, go another 100 feet and leave the PCT, taking Chinidere Mountain Trail #445. Starting here, you'll put in the climbing you've been warming up for, picking up 400 feet in a third of a mile to eventually reach the rocky summit. You might want to watch for a side trail from one of the first switchbacks, heading out into the open; this path leads to a rocky scramble up the west side of the mountain, where you'll find some interesting rock benches made by industrious hikers.

At the top, after you've caught your breath, take time to enjoy the view. Mount Hood rises to the south. To the right of that is Mount Jefferson, and just to the left of "Jeff" is Olallie Butte.

To the east, beyond "Lake Lake," you can see the upper parts of Hood River Valley, and to the left of that is Dalles Mountain and the desert of central Oregon. The big peak with all the radio towers is Mount Defiance, the highest spot in the Gorge, and Mount Adams is to the left of that. The bald ridge directly between you and Adams is Tomlike Mountain (named for Chief Chinidere's son), and to the left of that is the Herman Creek drainage. Off in the distance are Mounts Rainier and St. Helens, and right in line with the latter is the broad, flat Benson Plateau. Immediately below you, to the west, is Eagle Creek Canyon (the East Fork drains Wahtum Lake straight away from your feet), and in the distance beyond that is Tanner Butte. On a really clear day on Chinidere, I once saw Saddle Mountain, which is about 10 miles this side of the coast!

While we're up here, how about a little introduction to the PCT, a 2,600-mile trail from Mexico to Canada? The northbound PCT, which stretches some 460 miles across Oregon, comes up the right (west) side of Mount Jefferson, then past the right side of Mount Hood, mostly in the trees. In its approach to Wahtum Lake, the PCT rounds an open ridge between you and Hood called Indian Mountain, and from Chinidere it heads north across the Benson Plateau and down, heinously, into Cascade Locks. But most thru-hikers take Eagle Creek Trail, since it's well graded and has about a dozen waterfalls; then they walk the few miles along the road into Cascade Locks. After crossing Bridge of the Gods, the trail passes the west side of Table Mountain (which looks like a big gash from Chinidere), then heads around the north side of it before making a swing east toward Indian Heaven, Adams, the Goat Rocks, and Rainier. So, from Mount Jefferson to Mount Rainier, you're effectively looking at about 280 miles of PCT—slightly more than 10 percent of it!

And by the way, the rusty cables atop Chinidere are from an old Forest Service fire lookout, and the pits are tent sites, not Indian vision-quest sites. Sorry they aren't anything more romantic.

Head back down to the PCT, turn left, and take Chinidere Cutoff Trail, which will seem more like Chinidere Dropoff Trail for its steep descent to the lake. You'll cross a creek or two along the way, depending on the season, and you'll even see a pipe along the trail that used to carry water down to some campsites on the north shore of the lake. When you reach these campsites, stay on the main trail to where it crosses East Fork Eagle Creek on an impressive (and fun) logjam.

Cross the creek on the logjam, and in 200 yards you'll hit the top of Eagle Creek National Recreation Trail, which was built before 1920 and connects Wahtum Lake with the Historic Columbia River Highway, 14 miles below. (A 12-mile round-trip hike on that trail is described on page 50.) Turn left onto this trail and follow it a couple hundred yards back to the PCT, which leads 0.25 mile past campsites, swimming holes, and even the occasional beach, back to the bottom of the Wahtum Express—whose 250 steps will seem much less appealing to you now, no doubt.

GPS Information and Directions

N45° 34.635' W121° 47.57'

Take I-84 from Portland, driving 60 miles east of I-205 to Exit 62, the first exit for Hood River. At the exit, turn right on Country Club Road. After 3 miles, turn left at a stop sign, onto Barrett Drive. After 1.3 miles, turn right on Tucker Road, which turns into Dee Highway. After 8.5 miles, turn right on Lost Lake Road. After 4.8 miles, turn right on Forest Service Road (FR) 13. Drive 4.4 miles farther, then make a right on FR 1310. Stay on the pavement, driving 6 miles to find parking, on the right—if the pavement ends, you've passed the parking area.

6 Coyote Wall and The Labyrinth

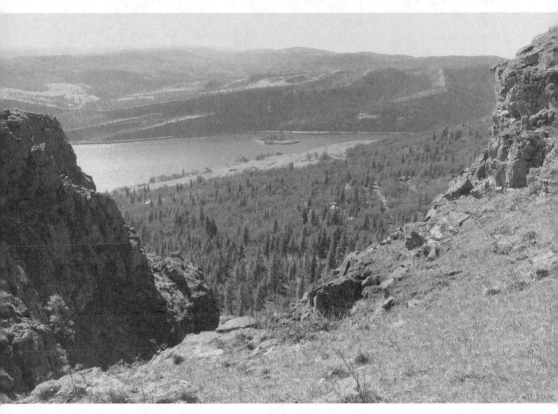

The Columbia River as seen through a notch in Coyote Wall

In Brief

Let's say it's springtime, at least according to the calendar, but Portland is socked-in and wet. Go east, young hiker!—to the high and dry lands of the Columbia River Gorge, where flowers bloom, birds croon, and Coyote Wall looms.

Description

Standing at the trailhead, looking up at Coyote Wall, you might feel a bit intimidated. Fear not, for the way is gradual and the work very rewarding. Just walk around the

LENGTH 4.6 miles just to the top of the wall, 5.2 miles to include The Labyrinth; any number of other possibilities

CONFIGURATION Out-and-back with optional side loops

DIFFICULTY Moderate

SCENERY Cliff-top vistas, wide-open country, spring wildflowers

EXPOSURE Along a cliff at times, and out in the open almost the whole way

TRAFFIC Heavy on spring weekends, moderate otherwise

TRAIL SURFACE Dirt; can be slick when wet

HIKING TIME 3–5 hours

DRIVING DISTANCE 69 miles (1 hour, 15 minutes) from Pioneer Courthouse Square

SEASON Year-round

BEST TIME April and May

BACKPACKING OPTIONS None

ACCESS No fees or permits

WHEELCHAIR ACCESS First 0.5 mile on an old paved road that extends beyond the trail

MAPS Green Trails *Map 432S (Columbia River Gorge–East)*

FACILITIES Restroom at the trailhead

INFO Columbia River Gorge National Scenic Area, 541-308-1700, **www.fs.usda .gov/crgnsa**

SPECIAL COMMENTS Dogs must be leashed January–June. Coyote Wall and The Labyrinth have been subject to a large-scale planning process for several years, which, by the time you get here, may have resulted in significant changes. Call ahead or check the website above or **wta.org** to get the latest information.

gate and follow the old road along Locke Lake, and eventually around the base of the wall itself. Turn left at the first cairn leading uphill, and immediately you're faced with numerous trailheads. Mountain bikers zip through here in every direction, but our path is always the one to the left and uphill.

The main trail travels to the left and, after a switchback to the right, leaves an old jeep path for a trail that continues left, headed for a small group of pines. Follow this trail to the edge of the wall—though rarely too close to be of concern. Just less than a mile up from the old road, the trail leaves the wall and you reach a fence, where you have to make a choice: go up the wall, cut over to The Labyrinth, do both of those, or wander around in the middle.

If you're going up, stay to the left and follow a switchbacking trail that's more scenic (and less destructive to the environment and your attitude) than the super-steep jeep road—this is Trail CO1 on Green Trails' *Map 432S.* After 1.3 miles of steep and steady climbing, through a sea of springtime flowers with views behind you to the Columbia and Mount Hood, you'll reach a junction with several old roads at the head of the wall, close to an area with plenty of big logs to rest on. From here, you can catch your breath and then head back down, or you can follow trails on the Green Trails map

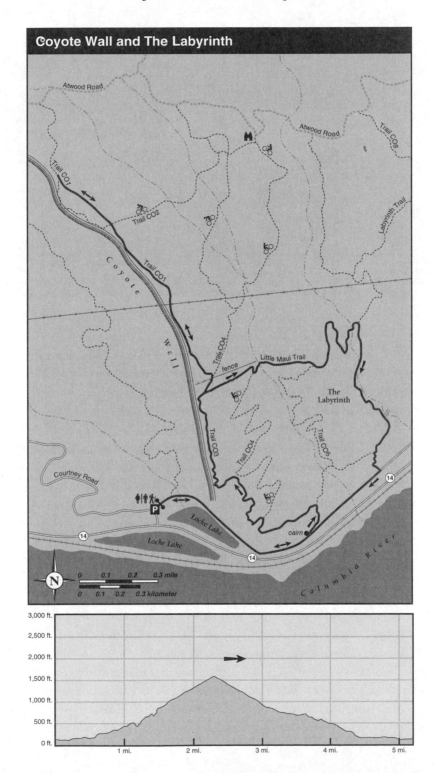

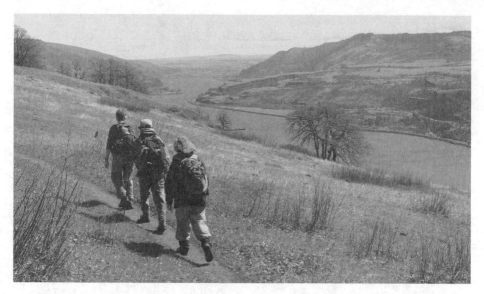

Headed toward The Labyrinth on the high trail heading over from Coyote Wall

to go west on Atwood Road toward Bourdoin Mountain or east another 1.3 miles to a three-way junction that I'll describe below.

Back at the fence, if you want to just head over to The Labyrinth, follow a trail leading east and dipping slightly downhill. (On the Green Trails map, this is labeled Little Maui Trail.) I will, again, just say, "Go wandering around in The Labyrinth. It's really cool." True to its name, this area can get confusing, with trails weaving between basalt pillars and through pocket meadows. The bottom line, though, is that if you keep heading downhill and to the right, you'll emerge on the abandoned highway very near where you first left it to head up Coyote Wall.

The Labyrinth is filled with hidden wonders: waterfalls, a small cave, small buttes to climb, and hidden meadows filled with flowers. So take your time, have faith, and enjoy yourself.

Now for that middle path, which is still evolving but, for my money, is the way to go if the climbing so far hasn't worn you out. It will take you way up the hill and back down through The Labyrinth; it's called Trail CO4 on the Green Trails map.

This is the middle, climbing path at the fence junction. Follow this track as it comes into an old road, then take a signed diversion around some private property, and after a mile that climbs 400 feet from the fence, you'll be back on the jeep road and pass between two giant oak trees to a viewpoint at what looks like the site of an old house. (In fact, you'll be able to see a house off to your left—don't go over there.)

Continue a moment to unsigned Atwood Road, and turn right. Follow Atwood's winding path for 0.6 mile to a trail on the right, which in 2013 had no sign but on the Green Trails map is called CO8—don't take one of the other trails marked C L O S E D. CO8 wanders down and around, with great views down to Rowland Lake and the Columbia, and after 0.7 mile it comes to, yes, *another* unsigned junction! (This area really could use some updating, if it hasn't happened already.)

Go straight ahead at this junction, now on Labyrinth Trail and headed back to the west toward The Labyrinth, which you can see spread out below you. After just a minute, see if you can spot a tree on the right with a skull nailed to the trunk way up high; there used to be a lot more bones and other weirdness hanging on it, but it got cleaned up. Stick with this trail for another 0.25 mile and go left at a junction, headed for an obvious meadow. Over the next 0.9 mile you'll cross a creek, wander among cool rock formations, go in and out of meadows and oak forest, see a waterfall and a cave—all sorts of cool stuff. Then you'll pop out at the old, closed highway, where you turn right; here, you're 0.8 mile from your car.

I know this is some confusing stuff; I'm doing my best! There are a lot of trails, and the bottom line for me is, it's a cool area but obey the signs and don't trespass. The Green Trails map referenced earlier is quite helpful. And if, since this book was published, the U.S. Forest Service has built and signed trails in the area, you'll have an easier time finding your way around. But I also think you (we) will perhaps have lost some opportunity for adventure.

Nearby Activities

The town of **Bingen, Washington,** is worth a stop on the way home, especially for its slightly bizarre combination coffee shop–antiques store, called **Antiques and Oddities** (211 W. Steuben St., Bingen, WA 98605; 509-493-4242, **facebook.com/antiquesaando**).

GPS Information and Directions

N45° 41.998' W121° 24.202'

Take I-84 from Portland, driving 62.8 miles east of I-205 to Exit 64, the third exit for Hood River, Oregon. Turn left at the end of the ramp, following the signs for White Salmon, Washington. Pay a $1 toll to cross the Columbia River, then turn right on WA 14. Go 4.6 miles and turn left onto Courtney Road; the parking lot is on the right.

7 Dog Mountain

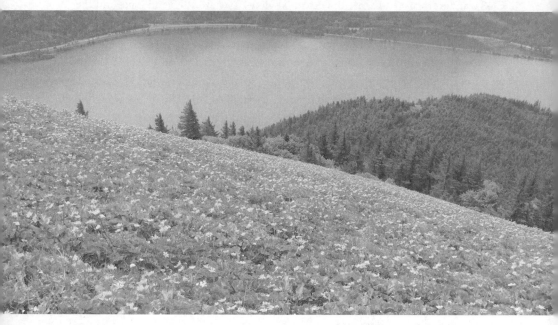

*One of the magnificent flower-filled meadows atop Dog Mountain,
3,000 feet above the Columbia*

In Brief

This is probably the most popular of the real hiking trails in the Columbia River
Gorge—"real" meaning it requires some real effort. But with an easy-access trailhead,
great views of the river, and sunshine and wildflowers at a time when it's usually still
raining in Portland, it's no wonder everybody on Earth comes here.

Description

It seems that every hiker around Portland has been up Dog Mountain, or at least heard
about it. Climbers use it as an early-season conditioner. Wildflower enthusiasts flock to
it in early summer. In spring, when it's still raining in Portland, it's often sunny here. But
most people take the main Dog Mountain Trail, which is therefore crowded, and which
was also designed, it seems, to punish the legs and lungs of those who would hike it. This
thing is steep! You can come down this way, if you want, but it's no bargain then, either.

LENGTH 6.9 miles	**BEST TIME** Mid-May–early June
CONFIGURATION Loop	**BACKPACKING OPTIONS** None
DIFFICULTY Strenuous	**ACCESS** Northwest Forest Pass (see page 3); $5/vehicle/day without pass
SCENERY Second-growth forest, wild-flowers, and a panoramic view of the Columbia River Gorge	
	WHEELCHAIR ACCESS None
EXPOSURE Alternately shady and open	**MAPS** Geo-Graphics *Trails of the Columbia Gorge* (available at Amazon and **Powells .com**); Green Trails *Map 430 (Hood River)* or *Map 428S (Columbia River Gorge–West)*
TRAFFIC Very heavy on weekends, especially in early summer; moderate otherwise	
	FACILITIES Restrooms at trailhead; no water
TRAIL SURFACE Packed dirt with rocks, some gravel	**INFO** Columbia River Gorge National Scenic Area, 541-308-1700, **www.fs.usda .gov/crgnsa**
HIKING TIME 4 hours	
DRIVING DISTANCE 56 miles (1 hour, 30 minutes) from Pioneer Courthouse Square	**SPECIAL COMMENTS** Start early in the day for this one, if only to make sure you get a parking spot.
SEASON Year-round, but occasional snow and ice on top	

From the parking lot, you have a choice to make, and it boils down to this: When hiking a loop of one steep trail and one *really* steep trail, which one would you rather go up, and which one down? Do you prefer the more gradual up or the more gradual down?

I prefer the gradual up (take my time, plus it's shadier) and the steep down (get it over with), so I'll describe that here. To do the opposite, walk up to the restroom and follow the main (crowded) trail, turning right at all junctions until you're out in the open at Puppy Point, just below the summit. Then aim for the top. To come down the other way, make two rights below the summit and stick with Augsperger Mountain Trail back to the trailhead, turning left at a junction in the woods about a mile down.

For the other way, from the trailhead, take the trail on the left, Augsperger Mountain Trail. It's 0.6 mile longer than Dog Mountain Trail, but whoever designed it had a much better grasp of the concept of "grade." That's not to say it's easy—it's 3.7 uphill miles, gaining 2,700 feet. But it's steady, whereas parts of the other trail are insane, and on this trail you'll spend more time in the meadows up top. So take this one as it contours left, with ever-improving views of the river and Wind Mountain. When you turn right and away from the river, you'll have gone 0.9 mile and gained 600 feet. Not so bad, right? Over the next 1.3 miles you'll gain 1,000 feet. That's when the switchbacks start—and remember, this is the easier way! The next 0.5 mile gains some 500 feet. Then you'll turn right at a junction toward Dog Mountain.

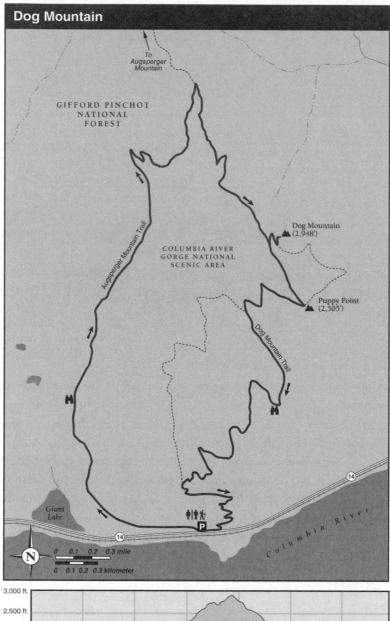

Dog Mountain

GIFFORD PINCHOT
NATIONAL
FOREST

To
Augsperger
Mountain

Augsperger Mountain Trail

COLUMBIA RIVER
GORGE NATIONAL
SCENIC AREA

Dog Mountain
(2,948')

Puppy Point
(2,505')

Dog Mountain Trail

Grant
Lake

14

Columbia River

N

0   0.1   0.2   0.3 mile

0   0.1 0.2 0.3 kilometer

14

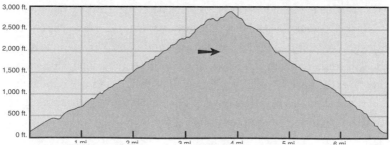

I'd like to take this moment to explain why Dog Mountain is called Dog Mountain. It's neither because of all the dogs on the trail, nor because the hike is a real bitch. It's because some pioneers in the area were forced to eat dog meat to avoid starvation. The town of Hood River was in fact first called Dog River, but the name was changed because nobody liked it. Imagine that.

Try to forget you know this so you can enjoy a few minutes of flat trail before you climb again and pop out into the sun. Now it's time to claim your reward for all that climbing. In May and June, the open slopes of Dog Mountain are awash in flowers, especially big yellow balsamroot, purple lupine, and red paintbrush; but year-round, the views here of the river and other mountains—including Mount Hood, which peeks over the far side—are sublime. Stroll through this area and know that virtually all your climbing is done. You'll intersect Dog Mountain Trail after 0.9 scenic mile; turn left and, just 0.1 mile up, you'll be at the top of a sloped meadow with everybody else and their dogs. I once counted 72 people on this summit.

The view here stretches from the high desert of central Oregon to Beacon Rock in the west—look how small it is! Way to the right is Mount St. Helens. Directly opposite is the 4,960-foot Mount Defiance, the one with the radio towers on top. The highest point in the gorge, it seems to taunt, "Yeah, right, you've climbed barely half of me."

To descend Dog Mountain, either follow the crowds down through the meadows to your left or take an alternate loop. From the summit, head left on a trail that soon ducks into the trees, some of which are surprisingly large. Keep an eye out for Mount Adams to the north. This trail rejoins the other branch of Dog Mountain Trail at a lookout called Puppy Point (2,505 feet). Then the bottom drops out and you lose 600 feet in the next 0.5 mile before a junction. You'll save 0.2 mile by going right, but it's worth it to head left for one last view of the river 0.6 mile down. Stay left at a junction 1 mile ahead, and after a final 0.5 mile you can finally rest your throbbing feet.

Nearby Activities

When you get back across to Cascade Locks, take a ride on the sternwheeler **Columbia Gorge,** which makes several scenic trips per day May–October. More information: 503-224-3900, **portlandspirit.com.**

GPS Information and Directions

N45°41.960' W121° 42.477'

Take I-84 from Portland, driving 37 miles east of I-205 to Exit 44/Cascade Locks. As soon as you enter the town, take your first right to get on Bridge of the Gods, following a sign for Stevenson, Washington. Pay a $1 toll on the bridge and, at the far end, turn right (east) onto WA 14. Proceed 12 miles to the trailhead, on the left.

8 Eagle Creek

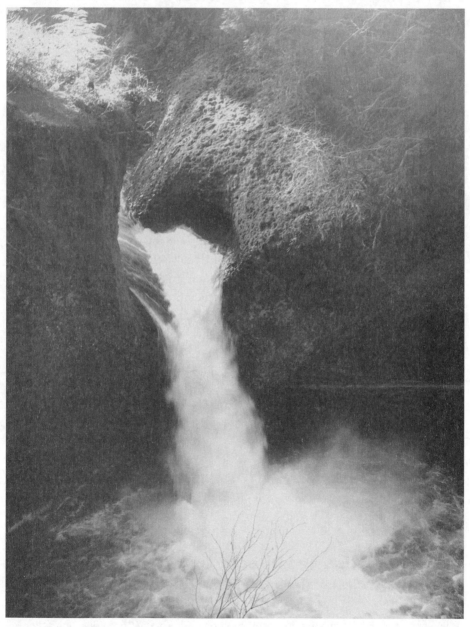

Punchbowl Falls

LENGTH 4 miles round-trip to Punchbowl Falls, 12 miles round-trip to Tunnel Falls

CONFIGURATION Out-and-back

DIFFICULTY Easy–moderate depending on how far you go

SCENERY Waterfalls, old-growth forest, spawning salmon in the fall

EXPOSURE Several sections of trail follow the tops of ledges and cliffs—only sometimes with cables to hold on to.

TRAFFIC Heavy all summer, moderate in spring and fall

TRAIL SURFACE Packed dirt and rocks

HIKING TIME 2.5 hours to Punchbowl Falls, 6 hours to Tunnel Falls

DRIVING DISTANCE 41 miles (45 minutes) from Pioneer Courthouse Square

SEASON Year-round, but muddy in winter and spring; you may also encounter snow and ice in winter.

BEST TIME March–May for big water flows, September and October for fall colors and fish

BACKPACKING OPTIONS Several sites starting a few miles up, plus access to more

ACCESS Northwest Forest Pass required (see page 3)

WHEELCHAIR ACCESS A road along (and bridge over) Eagle Creek near trailhead

MAPS Green Trails *Map 428S (Columbia River Gorge–West);* online map at **tinyurl .com/eaglecreektrail**

FACILITIES Restrooms at trailhead; no water

INFO Columbia River Gorge National Scenic Area, 541-308-1700, **www.fs.usda .gov/crgnsa**

SPECIAL COMMENTS This isn't a good trail for dogs, and you shouldn't hike it if you're afraid of heights—people have died here. Also, be aware that hikers have had their cars broken into at the trailhead.

In Brief

It seems everybody has hiked at least some of Eagle Creek; it's easily one of the classic and most popular hikes in Oregon. That's because this hike's easy to get to, easy to hike, and traverses a deep, forested canyon filled with waterfalls. With that in mind, start early, or go on a weekday, so you won't have to share the trail with the rest of Oregon.

Description

The magic of this hike, at certain times of the year, begins before you even hit the trail itself. Eagle Creek has a small run of fall chinook salmon—fish that spend their adult lives in the ocean, come more than 70 miles up the Columbia, swim the fish ladder at Bonneville Dam, and then arrive here to spawn. A small dam blocks their further

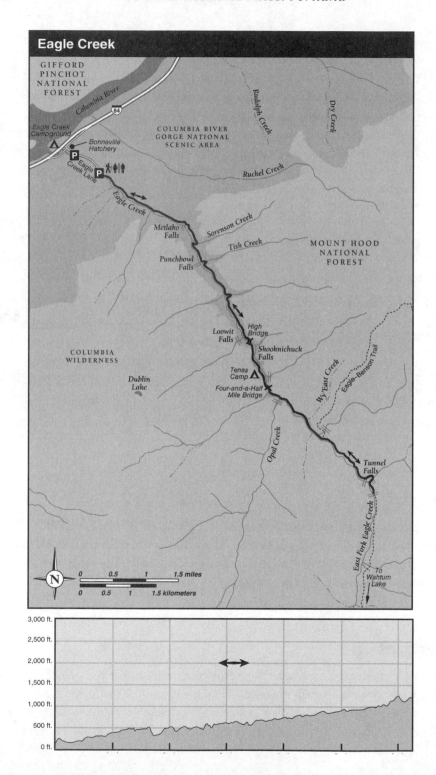

Eagle Creek

progress up Eagle Creek, but in October and November they spawn in little round pools cleared by volunteers to simulate conditions of a wild mountain stream.

The trail was built before 1920 to coincide with the opening of the Columbia River Highway. Although that historic roadway has been mostly gobbled up by I-84, the section from Bonneville Dam to Cascade Locks, which passes right by Eagle Creek, has been converted into a hiking and biking trail, as have a few other sections.

The construction of the Eagle Creek Trail was a heroic feat, all for the sake of recreation. The trail builders chipped the path into cliff faces, built High Bridge over a deep gorge, and blasted a tunnel behind a falls 6 miles up. It's work like this that inspired me to dedicate this book to the builders and maintainers of trails.

In the first mile, you'll get an idea of what you're in for: a deep canyon, waterfalls, and a lovely creek without too much elevation gain. At 1 mile, you come to the first of several places where you walk a ledge—in this case, but not all, with a cable to hang on to. If it's a summer weekend, things can get interesting here while you compete for cable space with dozens of other hikers. But the importance of being careful cannot be overstated: People have fallen to their deaths from this trail.

At 1.5 miles, you'll see a trail to a viewpoint of Metlako Falls (named for a Native American goddess of salmon), the first of many such sights. Just past the viewpoint is a bench, if you need a rest. At 1.8 miles is another bench; from here a side trail leads down to Punchbowl Falls, a must-see sight and the end of the line for a lot of people. Descend this trail 0.2 mile to reach Lower Punchbowl Falls; just above that is a large clearing that's often filled with swimmers and sunbathers. At the upstream end of the clearing is a lovely (and often photographed) view of the main Punchbowl Falls (see page 50).

If you turn back here, you'll have hiked 4 miles, but it's not much more work to go at least as far as High Bridge, another 1.2 miles up. If you continue, you'll get a bird's-eye view of Punchbowl Falls just 0.3 mile ahead; then the gorge narrows considerably. You'll see Loowit Falls on the right just before High Bridge, which is a spectacular site at 120 feet above the river in a narrow gorge. It's above here that you're allowed to camp, by the way.

If you turn around at the bridge, you'll have a 7-mile day. But before you turn back, put in another 0.3 mile to reach Tenas Camp and, 100 yards farther, enjoy a rare chance for creek access at the top of Skooknichuck Falls. Just past that are some very impressive Douglas-firs right on the trail.

Continuing up the trail, you'll soon cross what is officially known as Four-and-a-Half-Mile Bridge. Now, even the map acknowledges that this is exactly 4 miles from the trailhead, so what's with the name? Well, the fish hatchery back at the trailhead wasn't there when the trail was built (there was no need for it, because Bonneville

Dam didn't exist yet), so the trailhead used to be 0.5 mile farther north, at Eagle Creek Campground.

Just past the bridge, look on the right for a double waterfall—that's Opal Creek, but don't confuse it with the world-famous Opal Creek described elsewhere in this book (Hike 30, page 158). About 0.5 mile above that waterfall, a sign explains that the area you're now entering was burned in a 1902 fire; you can still see some charred stumps around. So all the trees you'll see in this area are less than 100 years old.

Hiking another 1.5 miles brings your total to 6 miles hiked, and you'll come into a deep gorge, where Tunnel Falls plunges 160 feet and the trail continues behind it through a 35-foot tunnel. Tunnel Falls is actually on East Fork Eagle Creek, which flows from Wahtum Lake. You could get to Wahtum Lake by hiking another 8 miles (and 2,500 feet) up this trail or by following the directions in the Chinidere Mountain profile on page 36.

To return to Eagle Creek and see one final, dramatic falls, hike on about 0.2 mile. This falls doesn't have an official name, but it does have an interesting crisscross feature in its upper section, leading many people to call it Crisscross Falls or Crossover Falls.

If you're backpacking, you'll find good camping at 7.5 Mile Camp (7 miles up) and at Wahtum Lake. Otherwise, if you head back at this point, you'll wind up having put in 12 miles—which should be enough for a day. Besides, you'll get to see everything again on your way back.

Nearby Activities

Stop at the **Bonneville Hatchery** on your way home (70543 NE Herman Loop, Cascade Falls, OR 97014; 541-374-8393; **tinyurl.com/bonnevillehatchery**). They have a fish ladder where, at certain times of year, you can see salmon and steelhead swimming up past the dam to spawn, and year-round ponds where you can view big trout and sturgeon. It's 1 mile west of Eagle Creek on I-84, and admission is free.

GPS Information and Directions

N45° 38.205' W121° 55.182'

Take I-84 from Portland, driving 34 miles east of I-205 to Exit 41/Eagle Creek. Go 0.2 mile, turn right, and drive 0.6 mile to the end of the road. If the parking area is crowded, you might have to park closer to the highway and hike that much farther.

9 Larch Mountain

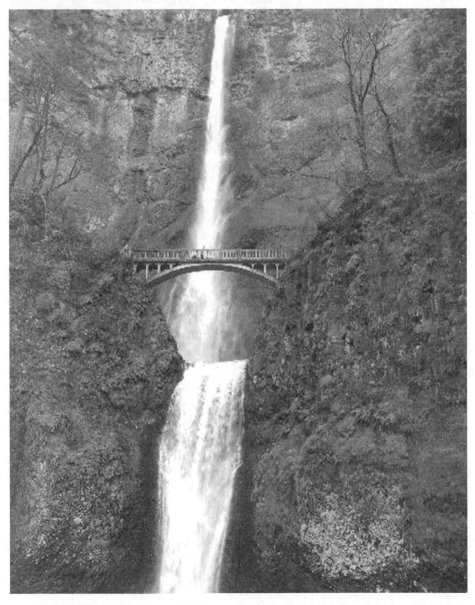

Benson Bridge and Multnomah Falls

LENGTH 6.8 miles one-way with shuttle, 13.6 miles round-trip, 7.1-mile optional middle loop	**SEASON** June–mid-November
	BEST TIME Late August (for amazing huckleberries)
CONFIGURATION Out-and-back, point-to-point, loop	**BACKPACKING OPTIONS** Poor
DIFFICULTY Moderate–strenuous	**ACCESS** No fees at Multnomah Falls or the middle trailhead; Northwest Forest Pass (see page 3) required at the upper trailhead
SCENERY Waterfalls, creeks in wooded canyons, colossal trees, solitude, a panoramic view	
EXPOSURE Mostly shady until summit	**WHEELCHAIR ACCESS** First 0.2 mile to Benson Bridge and some trails from the upper lot
TRAFFIC Always heavy on lower stretches and at the very top; low–moderate in between	
	MAPS National Geographic *Columbia River Gorge*, Green Trails *Map 428S (Columbia River Gorge–West)*
TRAIL SURFACE Pavement, packed dirt, some gravel	
HIKING TIME 5 hours one-way, 8 hours round-trip, 4 hours for upper loop	**FACILITIES** Full services at Multnomah Falls trailhead; restrooms atop Larch Mountain
DRIVING DISTANCE 31 miles (40 minutes) to lower trailhead or 36 miles (1 hour) to upper and middle trailheads from Pioneer Courthouse Square	**INFO** Columbia River Gorge National Scenic Area, 541-308-1700, **www.fs.usda .gov/crgnsa**

In Brief

Sure, you can drive almost to the top of Larch Mountain, but the trail between there and Multnomah Falls is one of the classic walks in Oregon—from the shores of the Columbia River to a high lookout in the Cascades, with old-growth forest on the way up and a view from the top that takes in everything from Portland to several volcanoes. A shorter loop hike encompasses the upper parts of the mountain only.

Description

Pick a clear day to get the best view, or think about timing your arrival at the top to coincide with sunset—you'll get to see Mount Hood bathed in pink light, and the lights of Portland are spectacular from the summit. Consider doing this one in late August, when the upper parts of the hill are awash in huckleberries.

You can actually see Larch Mountain as you drive out I-84; it's just to the left of Mount Hood and has a notch in the top. The top of that notch is where you're headed.

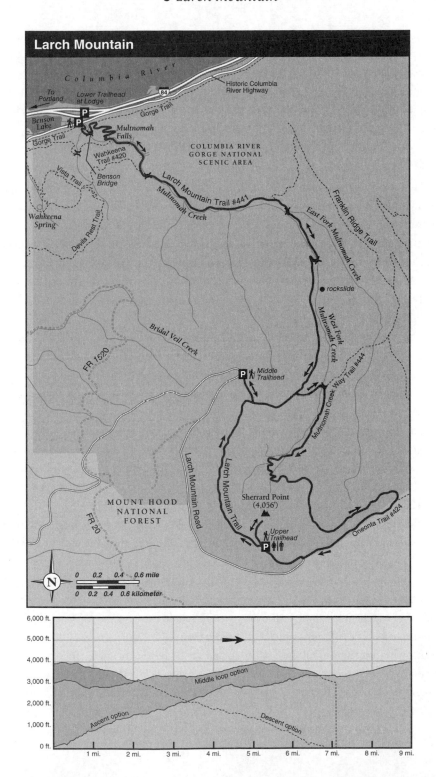

Larch Mountain

Columbia River

To Portland

Historic Columbia River Highway

84

Lower Trailhead at Lodge

Gorge Trail

Benson Lake

P P

Gorge Trail

Multnomah Falls

COLUMBIA RIVER GORGE NATIONAL SCENIC AREA

Wahkeena Trail #420

Larch Mountain Trail #441

Vista Trail

Benson Bridge

Multnomah Creek

Franklin Ridge Trail

Wahkeena Spring

Devils Rest Trail

East Fork Multnomah Creek

rockslide

Bridal Veil Creek

West Fork Multnomah Creek

FR 1520

Middle Trailhead

P

Multnomah Creek Way Trail #444

Larch Mountain Trail

Larch Mountain Road

MOUNT HOOD NATIONAL FOREST

FR 20

Sherrard Point (4,056')

Upper Trailhead

P

Oneonta Trail #424

N

0   0.2   0.4   0.6 mile

0   0.2   0.4   0.6 kilometer

6,000 ft.

5,000 ft.

4,000 ft.

3,000 ft.

Middle loop option

2,000 ft.

Ascent option

Descent option

1,000 ft.

0 ft.

1 mi.   2 mi.   3 mi.   4 mi.   5 mi.   6 mi.   7 mi.   8 mi.   9 mi.

As for the hike, I confess a bias in favor of walking up hills as opposed to walking down them. It seems easier to recover from losing your breath while climbing than to recuperate from pounding your knees and feet while you descend. Still, you've got three options here, all quite worthwhile. You can start at the top or at the bottom and put in 6.8 miles (assuming you have a second car for a shuttle), or you can start in the middle and do a loop that takes in the view but with less work. Or you can combine these.

Up from the Falls

Let's assume you put a second car at the top parking lot, and we'll start at the bottom, then include the upper loop on the way. From Multnomah Falls Lodge, walk with the crowds up the paved trail that leads over Benson Bridge. This covers 1 mile (climbing 600 feet) to reach a junction with a side trail leading to the viewing platform at the top of the falls. Continuing past that junction, you'll leave 90 percent of your comrades behind so that, for the next several miles, you may well have Larch Mountain Trail #441 to yourself. You'll also enter one of the few areas of old-growth forest in the Columbia River Gorge.

The trail was built in the early 1900s to coincide with the opening of the Columbia River Highway. One thing we should get straight is that there are probably no larch trees on Larch Mountain. The name stuck after old-time settlers confused the noble fir with the larch, which grows only east of the Cascade Range (although a few grow at Hoyt Arboretum; see Hike 59).

Staying on this trail, you'll cross Multnomah Creek and pass two lovely waterfalls in a lush canyon. At 1.6 miles, ignore Wahkeena Trail #420, on the right. At 2 miles you'll cross Multnomah Creek again, then at 3 miles traverse East Fork Multnomah Creek. Just 0.6 mile later, you'll cross a one-log footbridge over West Fork Multnomah Creek.

At 3.9 miles you'll cross a rockslide and then start climbing through an old-growth forest of western hemlock and Douglas-fir trees that get as thick as 5 and 6 feet in diameter and as old as 400 years. In late summer, this area abounds with huckleberries, and in autumn the red, yellow, and orange vine maple is astounding.

At 4.8 miles you'll come to a junction with Multnomah Creek Way Trail #444, and you'll have the option to simply stay on Larch Mountain Trail #441 (to reach the top in 2 miles) or to take Trail #444, to the left, a more scenic route to the top but one that's 0.7 mile longer. If the latter sounds OK, follow the trail 0.2 mile, cross Multnomah Creek, then turn right to follow Trail #444 and go 2.8 miles, through a marsh and up the ridge of Larch Mountain. The last bit of this is on the level bed of an old road, the remnant of decades of logging activity up here. Notice how the trees in that section aren't so big anymore?

When you come to Oneonta Trail #424 at the top of the ridge, turn right and follow it 0.9 mile slightly uphill to the shoulder of Larch Mountain Road. Walk up that for 0.25 mile to the parking area, then take a signed, paved trail to Sherrard Point for the big view. Along the way you'll pass a picnic area with tables and grills. It's 0.7 mile from where you enter the road to Sherrard Point—a total of 7.5 miles from the trailhead at Multnomah Falls.

Any way you go, make sure to go have a look around from Sherrard Point. (It's named for Thomas H. Sherrard, who ran the Mount Hood National Forest from 1907 to 1934 and helped develop the Bull Run water preserve.) If it's a clear day, you'll see Portland, Mount Hood, Mount Jefferson, Mount Adams, Mount St. Helens, and Mount Rainier. You'll also notice that you're at the top of a cliff on a semicircular ridge. That's because Larch Mountain is what remains of an ancient volcano, and what you're looking down into is the remnant of a crater.

The Upper Loop

Now, as for your other hiking options on Larch Mountain, you can either start at the top and descend to Multnomah Falls, following Larch Mountain Trail all the way down or taking the loop described (which uses Multnomah Creek Way Trail), or you can park at the middle trailhead (see Directions). The middle trailhead accesses the upper part of Larch Mountain, saving you from climbing 3,000 feet from the Columbia.

From the middle trailhead, follow the gated gravel road a short distance to intersect the Larch Mountain Trail, then either head right and walk 1.5 miles up to reach the top, or head left to descend 0.5 mile and take Multnomah Creek Way Trail #444 and the loop described earlier.

Nearby Activities

If you did the one-way car shuttle, stop on the way to or from Multnomah Falls at the **Portland Women's Forum State Scenic Viewpoint** (39210 E. Historic Columbia River Hwy., Corbett, OR 97019). Because it's a little farther west than the more famous Vista House (see page 20), it's a less-visited spot for viewing the Columbia River Gorge. More information: 800-551-6949, **oregonstateparks.org/park_164.php.**

The 1925 **Multnomah Falls Lodge** is well worth checking out, with its skylights and fireplace in the restaurant and its old-style stone-and-wood construction. The food isn't as good as the setting, but the Sunday brunch is massive. More information: 503-695-2376, **multnomahfallslodge.com.**

GPS Information and Directions

Upper Trailhead N45° 31.776' W122° 5.303'
Middle Trailhead N45° 32.97' W122° 5.516'
Lower Trailhead N45° 34.659' W122° 7.032'

To start at the lower trailhead, take I-84 from Portland, driving 24 miles east of I-205 to Exit 31/Multnomah Falls, the exit for the parking lot. Park and walk under the expressway to historic Multnomah Falls Lodge. For the middle and upper trailheads, take I-84, driving 15 miles east of I-205, and take Exit 22/Corbett. At the exit, turn right onto NE Corbett Hill Road. After 1.5 miles, turn left onto East Historic Columbia River Highway. Drive 2 miles, then veer right onto Larch Mountain Road. The upper trailhead is in the parking lot at the end of the road, 14 miles up. The middle trailhead is 11.5 miles ahead, on the left, after Larch Mountain Road heads right and a gravel road takes off to the left.

10 Table Mountain

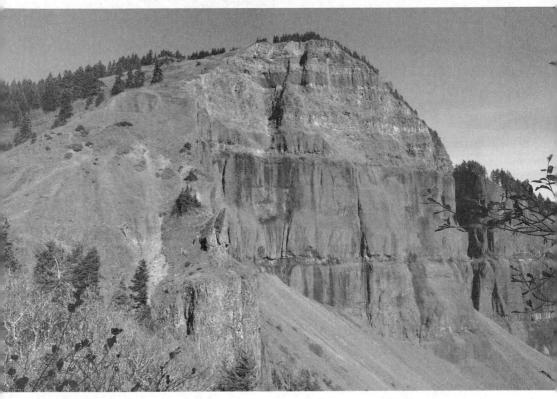

If you do the whole hike, you can have lunch at the very top of these 800-foot cliffs looking out over the Columbia.

In Brief

This leg-buster of a climb has a great reward on top: one of the best panoramas in the whole Columbia River Gorge, including a bird's-eye view of Bonneville Dam, from a lunch spot atop 800-foot cliffs. And there are hot springs at the trailhead!

Description

You have two options for where to start this hike. Using the "official" trailhead on WA 14 at North Bonneville makes it a tromp of about 14 miles, though it does visit a lake and an additional viewpoint along the way. If that's what you're after, take the

LENGTH 8.5 miles	**SEASON** April–November
CONFIGURATION Balloon	**BEST TIME** May for flowers, October for fall colors
DIFFICULTY Strenuous	
SCENERY A tumbling stream, five volcanoes, some of the steepest trail around, and a bird's-eye view of the Columbia River Gorge	**BACKPACKING OPTIONS** One poor site
	ACCESS No fees or permits
	WHEELCHAIR ACCESS None
EXPOSURE Mostly shady but with rocky slopes to climb and descend; open rock at the top; extreme cliff-top exposure in places	**MAPS** Green Trails *Map 429 (Bonneville Dam)* or *Map 428S (Columbia River Gorge–West),* though only the PCT appears on the former
TRAFFIC Moderate on nice-weather weekends, light otherwise	**FACILITIES** Trailhead for longer hike has toilets; the other one has no facilities other than those at a nearby resort.
TRAIL SURFACE Grass, packed dirt with rocks, then just (sometimes loose) rocks	
HIKING TIME 7 hours	**INFO** Columbia River Gorge National Scenic Area, 541-308-1700, **www.fs.usda .gov/crgnsa**
DRIVING DISTANCE 45 miles (50 minutes) from Pioneer Courthouse Square	

trail 0.6 mile from WA 14 up to the PCT and turn left, following the PCT 1.9 miles to Gillette Lake, then 1.3 miles to Greenleaf Overlook, then 1.7 miles to the top of the ridge, where the other route comes in.

As for that other route, which I highly recommend, it's almost 6 round-trip miles shorter and starts at a hot-springs resort. Please note that the resort has become weary of hikers stomping around with their muddy boots—treat the place with respect so they'll let us keep parking here.

To begin the hike, from the left-hand parking lot, head for the far west end of the pavement and look for an old road ascending the hill. Climb it 100 yards to a T-intersection, then look for a little trail headed into a bank of blackberries. It's usually just a little to the left of where you hit the T.

Follow that trail as it winds up through a young forest choked with vine maple, and pass a tiny lake on the right after 0.5 mile. Just past that, top out over a ridge and, 0.2 mile later, cross a tiny creek on a plank bridge.

A few steps later, take a moment to look up toward Table Mountain beyond the meadow on your right—yes, that's where we're headed. See if you can also spot a "rabbit ears" rock formation up there; that's Papoose and Sacajawea Rocks. Just past this area, turn right at a road junction, go 100 yards on that road, turn left onto another road, and then, after taking a swooping switchback to the right, continue straight,

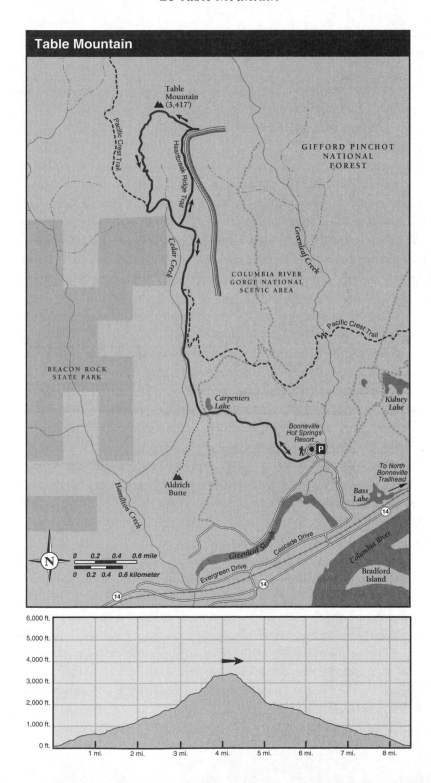

through yet another junction. This section is unsigned, so if all that gets confusing, remember this: Your goal here is to climb on an old jeep road, with the meadow below you and on your right.

Climb up from that meadow, in which lies the tough-to-spot Carpenters Lake, and just less than 0.5 mile up (about 1.5 miles since the trailhead), cross the ridge to climb along Cedar Creek, which is lined almost exclusively with alder, Douglas-fir, and vine maple. Go figure.

When you've gone a total of 2.3 miles—that is, about a mile past the meadow—you'll arrive at what looks like a campground area at an intersection with the PCT. (This is the spot that's 5.5 miles from the North Bonneville Trailhead.) Turn left on the PCT, which goes left from the road and climbs a moderate grade through a more interesting forest. You'll notice a few Douglas-firs of decent size, but this whole area has been logged, much of it more than once. After about 0.4 mile on the PCT, you'll encounter a kiosk. Welcome to Heartbreak Ridge, a trail seemingly designed by elk, improved by masochists, and hiked by fools . . . like you and me.

You'll soon see how the trail got its name. If I had to rank the steepest sections of trail in this whole book, this stretch would easily make the top three. If you want stats, it's a 1,600-foot climb over the 1.3 miles from here to the summit, but there's actually a smidgen of *downhill* in there! So take your time and have faith—it's worth it.

After 0.5 mile—and 700 feet of elevation gain—you'll come to a rocky outcrop with a nice view back to Hamilton Mountain (see Hike 2), whose summit you're now above. This is a popular break spot, as it marks a (temporary) reprieve from the climbing. Just 0.1 mile later, you reach a tiny saddle with a big-time view of Table's rocky face, then you'll descend briefly (darn it) and make your way to the base of a talus. Climb straight up that slope (lovely!), finding footing wherever you can, and at the top, catch the trail heading back into the woods. There, you'll find a junction with a most ambitious sign, saying it's 0.28 mile to the Gorge Overlook—boldly confident, I'd say, considering a hundredth of a mile is all of 53 feet.

When you get to the top and catch your breath, you'll find that trails actually crisscross the broad summit. Head left and through a patch of trees for views of Mount St. Helens, Mount Rainier, Dog Mountain, the Columbia, and Mount Adams. Go right, toward the Columbia River, for a spectacular view that ranges from Mount Defiance to Mount Hood and the western Gorge. As you look at Hood and Bonneville Dam, note two obvious drainages on the far side: The one on the left is Eagle Creek (see Hike 8), and on the right is Tanner Creek.

Beware that the final portions of this trail take you literally a foot away from a drop of 800 feet, and there's no protection. Those cliffs are part of Table Mountain's fascinating geological history. As you look out toward the Columbia, you might realize that the southern half of Table Mountain actually slid into the river, leaving behind the cliffs and narrowing the Columbia to just a hundred yards at the most (at the point where Bridge of the Gods crosses). This slide, spanning more than 10 square miles, occurred about 550 years ago—basically yesterday in geologic time. It first created a natural dam that blocked the river, and then it created the Cascades of the Columbia, which were submerged when Bonneville Dam went in.

Now look up at Mount Hood. On the left, you can see a ridge leading up to a bump just below the snow line—that's Cooper Spur (Hike 32, page 170). For a real adventure, hike up that one and look for Table Mountain!

To finish the loop, go back to the junction at the top of the boulder field. Here, you have a choice: go back down the way you came, or follow the sign saying PCT 1.1 MILES and head west. This steep, rocky scramble along the spine of the ridge eventually drops you back, exhausted, onto the PCT. Turn left here, and in 0.4 mile you'll be back at the Heartbreak Ridge junction. Then just retrace your steps to your car, making sure you don't miss the unsigned left turn onto the trail, back at the gravel roads near the meadow.

Nearby Activities

Now, about **Bonneville Hot Springs Resort & Spa** (1252 E. Cascade Dr., North Bonneville, WA 98639). It's a giant, lush place with a restaurant; hotel rooms (not cheap); and a day spa with hot tubs, massage, skin treatments, and so on. Your basic soak starts at $20. More information: 509-427-7767, **bonnevilleresort.com.**

GPS Information and Directions

Bonneville Hot Springs Resort N45° 39.333' W121° 57.591'
North Bonneville Trailhead N45° 39.027' 121° 55.972'

Take I-84 from Portland, driving 37 miles east of I-205 to Exit 44/Cascade Locks. As soon as you enter the town, take the first right to get on Bridge of the Gods, following a sign for Stevenson, Washington. Pay a $1 toll to cross the bridge and, at the far end, turn left (west) onto WA 14. The North Bonneville Trailhead is 1.5 miles ahead on the right—this is the starting point for the longer hike and also has the only public restroom in the area. For the shorter hike, continue another 1.2 miles on WA 14 and turn right, crossing under the railroad tracks onto Cascade Drive. Just beyond the tracks, turn right to stay on Cascade Drive. The entrance to Bonneville Hot Springs Resort is 0.9 mile ahead; enter here and park in the left-hand lot.

11 Tom McCall Preserve

In Brief

Tom McCall Preserve at Rowena is in a different world from most of the hikes in this book. It's a glimpse into central Oregon, a land of wide-open vistas, grass blowing in the nearly constant wind, and semiarid forests of oak and ponderosa pine. It also boasts panoramic vistas of the Columbia and Mounts Adams and Hood, and more than 300 species of plants, some of them unique to the Columbia River Gorge.

Description

OK, so this one is more than 60 miles from Portland, even as the crow flies. But it's truly worth the extra bit of easy driving, especially in the spring and early summer. At those times of the year, there is a kind of rain shroud somewhere between Cascade Locks and Hood River; while it's still pouring in Portland, places like the McCall Preserve are bathed in sunlight and carpeted in a few dozen kinds of wildflowers all blooming at once.

Start with McCall Point Trail and get your exercise out of the way. The trail, which climbs about 1,000 feet in 1.5 miles, starts out nearly flat and on an old wagon road, winding through the kind of open space that is so rare in the western part of the state. The trees you eventually encounter are oaks, most of them Oregon white oak, and some as much as 800 years old. After 0.5 mile, leave the road for a trail that ascends slightly when it gains the edge of the ridge, with ever-more-impressive views out to the east. Keep an eye out for Mount Adams as its summit comes into view across the river.

The second half of the trail is a little steeper, and after a rain it might be slick and muddy, so add shoes with good traction to your clothing list. But soon enough you'll come to McCall Point, an open hilltop with a sprawling view from Mount Hood to Mount Adams; you're actually about halfway between the two peaks, each of which is roughly 35 miles away. Looking west, you can see into the Columbia River Gorge; just to the left of it, the high peak with the towers on top is Mount Defiance, the highest point in the gorge.

Now, you summit-hounds out there might stand at McCall Point and notice there's some more trail going south, through a notch, and then climbing again. I walked about a mile down (and then up) that trail, through some very peaceful

LENGTH McCall Point Trail, 6 miles round-trip; Rowena Plateau Loop, 2.5 miles one-way	open year-round, McCall Point open May–November
CONFIGURATION Balloon to Rowena Plateau, out-and-back to McCall Point	**BEST TIME** April and May
	BACKPACKING OPTIONS No camping allowed
DIFFICULTY Rowena Plateau, easy; McCall Point, moderate due to the climb	**ACCESS** No fees or permits
SCENERY Wildflowers, the Columbia River below, two volcanoes, old oak trees	**WHEELCHAIR ACCESS** None
	MAPS Green Trails *Map 432S (Columbia River Gorge–East)*
EXPOSURE Wide open most of the time	**FACILITIES** None
TRAFFIC Moderate when flowers are out, light otherwise	**INFO** Columbia River Gorge National Scenic Area, 541-308-1700, **www.usda.gov /crgnsa;** The Nature Conservancy, 503-802-8100, **tinyurl.com/tommcallpreserve**
TRAIL SURFACE Packed dirt	
HIKING TIME 1 hour for Rowena Plateau Loop, 2 hours to McCall Point	**SPECIAL COMMENTS** Consider wearing long pants—ticks, poison oak, and rattle-snakes are all found in the area. Dogs are prohibited on both trails.
DRIVING DISTANCE 76 miles (1 hour, 30 minutes) from Pioneer Courthouse Square	
SEASON Rowena Plateau Loop	

oak stands, but technically speaking it didn't go anywhere special before it got pinched between a fence and the edge of a cliff. My advice is to have yourself a picnic at McCall Point and don't worry about that other trail.

Now, for the Plateau Loop. Back at the highway, use the steps over the fence to start on a wide path that actually drops 100 feet in elevation, traversing flower and grass country to loop around a pond. Early in the year, there will be numerous other little ponds and wet areas, each supporting their own microhabitats. The small canyon below you on your left is called Rowena Dell.

When a sign reading T R A I L indicates a right turn, you'll notice a trail that continues straight out into the grasslands. There is another pond out there among the trees, in addition to other viewpoints out over the river. But the most dramatic view is on the official trail to your right. After that trail has passed the pond, it turns right again. A small trail to the left leads to the top of a cliff that is not for the acrophobes among us: It's a sheer drop of 500 feet from where you stand—without a railing, so keep an eye on the kids—down to the railroad tracks and the river. The town across the river is Lyle, Washington, which lies on a gravel bar formed by catastrophic floods more than 10,000 years ago.

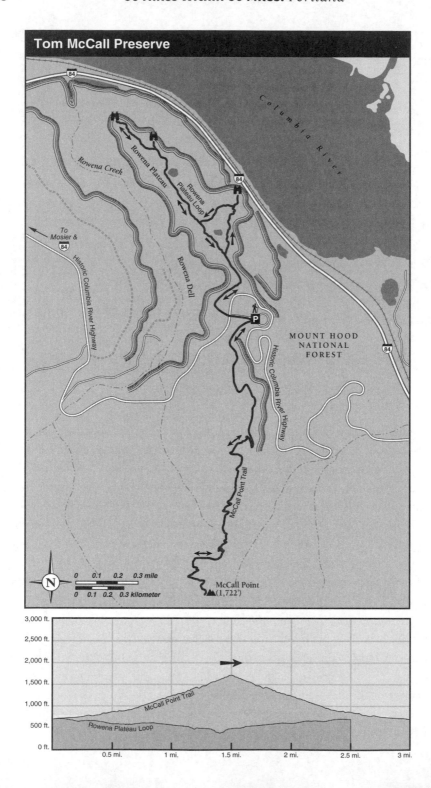

To return to the North Bonneville, follow the trail back around the pond and turn left (uphill) at the sign. Or wander farther to your right, toward the viewpoint of Lyle, to keep exploring.

Nearby Activities

As long as you're this far east, keep going to The Dalles to visit the **Columbia Gorge Discovery Center** (5000 Discovery Dr., The Dalles, OR 97058), where displays range from an exhibit about the Columbia River during the last ice age to an interactive installation about the Lewis and Clark expedition. More information: 541-296-8600, **gorgediscovery.org.**

GPS Information and Directions

N45° 40.964' W121° 18.034'

Take I-84 from Portland, driving 62 miles east of I-205 to Exit 69/Mosier. Turn right and follow Historic Columbia River Highway (US 30) 6.5 miles through Mosier to Rowena Crest Viewpoint. McCall Point Trail begins at a sign at the end of the stone wall. The Plateau Loop begins across the highway, where a set of steps leads over a fence.

12 Triple Falls

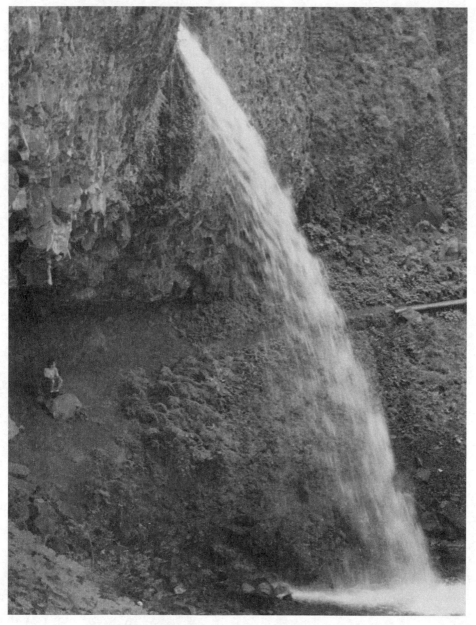

Hanging out behind Ponytail Falls

LENGTH 4.5 miles round-trip

CONFIGURATION Out-and-back or loop

DIFFICULTY Moderate

SCENERY Four waterfalls, a spectacular gorge, a view of the Columbia River

EXPOSURE In the forest all the way

TRAFFIC Moderate on summer weekends, light otherwise

TRAIL SURFACE Gravel and packed dirt; roots, rocks

HIKING TIME 3 hours

DRIVING DISTANCE 33 miles (40 minutes) from Pioneer Courthouse Square

SEASON Year-round but gets muddy in winter and spring

BEST TIME April for water flow and flowers, October for colors

BACKPACKING OPTIONS None

ACCESS No fees or permits

WHEELCHAIR ACCESS None

MAPS Green Trails *Map 428 (Bridal Veil)* or *Map 428S (Columbia River Gorge–West)*

FACILITIES None at trailhead; water and restrooms 0.5 mile east at Ainsworth State Park (503-695-2261, **tinyurl.com /ainsworthsp**)

INFO Columbia River Gorge National Scenic Area, 541-308-1700, **www.fs.usda .gov/crgnsa**

In Brief

A unique waterfall lies at the end of this moderate hike, but you don't have to go that far to see some fine Columbia River Gorge scenery. You can, in fact, just drive by the trailhead and admire Horsetail Falls.

Description

If all you do is slow down while driving by Horsetail Falls, you'll be pleased. But at least cross the parking area to pick some blackberries over by the railroad tracks; they're ripe in late summer. The great thing about this trail is that the farther you go, the better it gets, and you never have to work very hard at all.

From Horsetail Falls, follow the gravel trail behind the sign describing some of the animals that live in the area. At 0.2 mile, stay right at a trail junction. A few hundred yards later, you'll come around a bend and see Upper Horsetail Falls, also known as Ponytail Falls. A popular turnaround spot because it's so near the car, these falls are also a hit with kids, who with supervision can get under them and catch some spray. The falls seem to shoot out of a basalt cliff face, and the area behind them is a grotto through which the trail passes. If you get under them, some smaller streams will trickle down onto your head. Just don't get directly under the main stream of water—even this relatively small waterfall is extremely powerful.

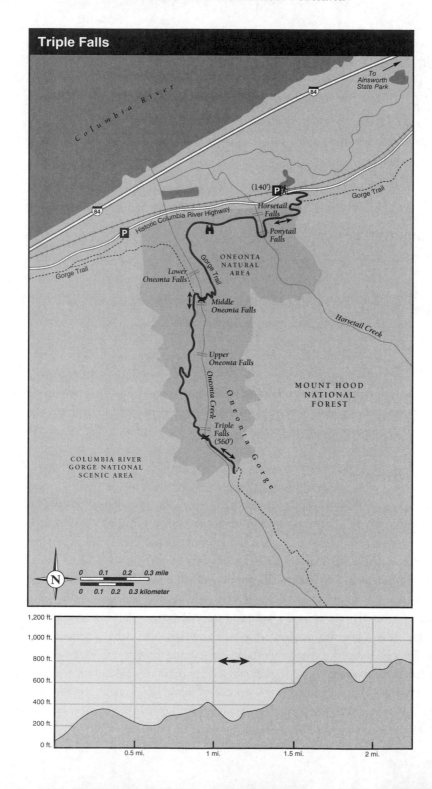

To keep going, simply follow the trail as it contours around the gorge wall. It soon comes to a brushy area on the right, through which several trails lead out to cliff-top viewpoints over the Columbia River. You can make a side loop out there and work your way back to the main trail as it turns away from the river. A network of trails crisscrosses this tiny area, but they all lead to the same place, so you won't get lost.

A mile past Ponytail Falls, after you pass under a mossy "weeping" rock face, you'll descend to a bridge spanning the spectacular Oneonta Gorge. A geological and biological wonder, Oneonta alone is worth a visit; from here, you're looking down into it, with waterfalls above and below you. Just across the bridge, and after a little climbing, is another junction—here, you can loop back to the highway by going right (you'll have to walk nearly 0.5 mile along the road, however, to get back to your car), or you can turn left and head up toward Triple Falls. The trail is rocky in places, and there's a little more elevation gain, but nice views of the narrow gorge will help keep you moving.

About a mile up you'll see Triple Falls. It's actually just one creek (Oneonta), but it divides into three just before it goes over the edge. So take your pictures from here, then walk another minute or two to a wooden bridge across the wide stream just above the falls. Across the bridge are some nice rocks for picnicking, and just upstream are some pools the kids can jump into, if you've managed to get them this far.

Nearby Activities

You can get about 0.5 mile into **Oneonta Gorge** and see a 50-foot waterfall, but not without getting wet. Even in late summer, adults will find themselves wading in waist-high water or climbing rocks to avoid it. As of 2014, the entrance was also choked by a massive logjam that's tricky to climb over. Put on your swimsuit (along with some shoes you don't mind soaking), be careful, and explore this official U.S. Forest Service Botanical Area.

GPS Information and Directions

N45° 35.420' W122° 4.065'

Take I-84 from Portland, driving 21 miles east of I-205 to Exit 28/Bridal Veil. Turn left onto Historic Columbia River Highway and continue 5.2 miles to the signed parking area at Horsetail Falls.

13 Wahkeena Falls to Multnomah Falls

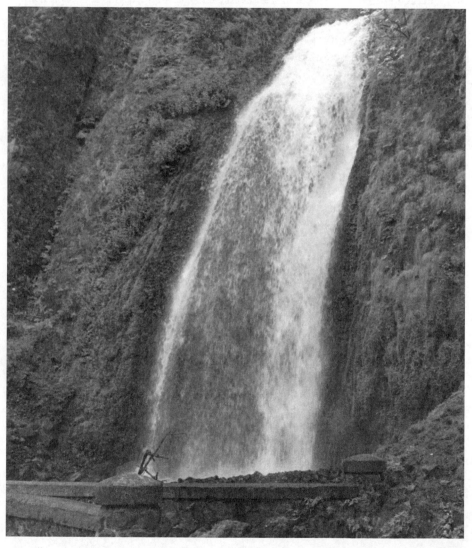

You'll probably get a nice little spray when the trail crosses the creek halfway up Wahkeena Falls.

LENGTH 4.2 miles	possibly icy in spots during winter and spring
CONFIGURATION Loop	
DIFFICULTY Moderate	**BEST TIME** Whenever you can get out here!
SCENERY Waterfalls, canyons, river views, flowers, a spring, big trees	**BACKPACKING OPTIONS** A couple of sites along the trail toward Angels Rest
EXPOSURE In the forest all the way, nothing dangerous	**ACCESS** No fees or permits
TRAFFIC Heavy, especially on weekends and around Multnomah Falls; moderate on weekdays	**WHEELCHAIR ACCESS** The first section of trail heading up from either falls is paved—but kind of steep.
TRAIL SURFACE Pavement, gravel, packed dirt with some rocky sections	**MAPS** Green Trails *Map 428 (Bridal Veil)* or *Map 428S (Columbia River Gorge–West)*
HIKING TIME 3 hours	**FACILITIES** Full services at Multnomah Falls Lodge
DRIVING DISTANCE 31 miles (35 minutes) from Pioneer Courthouse Square	**INFO** Columbia River Gorge National Scenic Area, 541-308-1700, **www.fs.usda .gov/crgnra**
SEASON Year-round, but muddy and	

In Brief

Just off I-84 and bookmarked by two waterfalls, this excursion is the ideal introduction to all the Columbia River Gorge has to offer, including great scenery, big crowds, and nice steep climbs. Word of warning: Parking is nearly impossible on summer weekends.

Description

When hiking friends come to visit Oregon, this is where I take them first. They get to see the scenic spectacle that is the Columbia River Gorge, they get to view the highest waterfall in Oregon, they get to see old-growth Douglas-firs, and they get their hearts pumping—from excitement and, at times, from effort.

You can hike either way on this trail and park at either falls; I prefer to park at Multnomah Falls and start the hike at Wahkeena Falls. I'll tell you why in just a bit.

To do this, walk 100 yards down the historic highway west of Multnomah Falls Lodge and take Return Trail #442, which parallels the road 0.6 mile to Wahkeena Falls. Along the way you'll pass under a giant boulder and be cooled by a mossy "weeping" rock wall.

Actually several falls in one, Wahkeena Falls encompasses everything from sheer drops to cascades to misty sprays. This falls, by the way, is fed primarily by a spring up

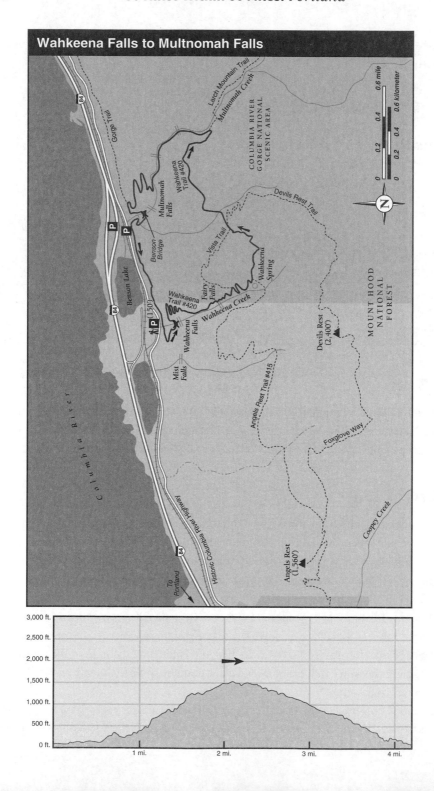

Wahkeena Falls to Multnomah Falls

on the ridge that you'll see later. To start the loop, follow the paved trail across the creek and then 0.2 mile up to a footbridge at the base of the upper falls. Take a nice deep breath of that cool, moist air—your workout is about to begin.

In the next 0.4 mile of paved switchbacks, you'll gain about 400 feet; such quick climbs are the trademark of Gorge hikes. When you get to the top, you'll find a new and very confusing sign from the Forest Service—to be clear, it indicates mileages to trail intersections, *not* the destinations themselves. Head right here, to Lemmon's Viewpoint, for a lookout on the Columbia; then start back up, leaving the pavement. You can rest a few minutes later on a bench at the lovely Fairy Falls, sort of a miniature version of Ramona Falls (Hike 38, page 199). You still have some climbing to do; it's just that now it's more gradual and you have the creek and some lovely old forest to take your mind off it. Fairly recent fires took out smaller growth, blackened the trunks of bigger trees, and opened the forest floor for berries and wildflowers to move in. Just above Fairy Falls, you'll encounter Vista Point Trail—turn right here, staying on Wahkeena Trail #420. After another 0.4 mile, you'll come to an intersection with Angels Rest Trail #415. The sign here, also confusing, was helpfully edited: Because it lacked the word *Trail* after *Vista Point*, *Devils Rest*, and *Larch Mountain*—again, the distances listed apply to those trails, not to the destinations—somebody came by and scratched T R A I L after each name. At any rate, you should at least take a 100-yard detour here on Angels Rest Trail to see Wahkeena Spring, where the creek emerges from the ground all at once in a magical (and tasty) scene. A few campsites sit a bit farther down this trail.

At the intersection of the Wahkeena and Angels Rest Trails, back near the spring, take Wahkeena Trail up the hill 0.4 mile to a four-way intersection. Ascending the hill from your left is Vista Point Trail—ignore it. Ascending the hill to your right is Devils Rest Trail, which climbs briefly and then heads over to what, frankly, is a disappointing viewpoint. So unless you just want some more exercise, continue straight on Wahkeena Trail.

This eastbound stretch on Wahkeena Trail soon descends and, in 0.9 mile, intersects Larch Mountain Trail #441, which connects Multnomah Falls with Larch Mountain (see Hike 9, page 55). For our purposes, turn left and head down the rock-filled Multnomah Creek. In the next mile, you'll pass several waterfalls in a gorge filled with ferns and large, old-growth Douglas-firs. This is an awesome section of trail!

A well-marked (and well-traveled) trail to the left leads 0.1 mile to the top of Multnomah Falls, where a wooden platform offers an ego-building view of the camera-toting throngs below. "Yeah," you can say later at the bottom, "I've been up there." This brings me to why I like to do the hike this way: From this point on, especially on a weekend, you'll be among hundreds of people. In my opinion, it's better (that is, faster) going downhill than uphill through such a mob. Multnomah Falls and Benson Bridge are just 1 mile on.

The highest falls in Oregon, at 542 feet, upper Multnomah Falls is quite a sight. Be sure to stop at the information office at the lodge to see pictures of the various floods and a massive rockfall that have occurred there.

Now, for the final reason I like to start this hike at Wahkeena Falls but park at Multnomah Falls Lodge: When you're all done, you can get yourself an ice-cream cone or an espresso, or cruise the gift shop, if you're into that, and your car is right there waiting for you.

Nearby Activities

The 1925 **Multnomah Falls Lodge** is well worth checking out, with its skylights and fireplace in the restaurant and its old-style stone-and-wood construction. The food isn't as good as the setting, but the Sunday brunch is massive. More information: 503-695-2376, **multnomahfallslodge.com**.

GPS Information and Directions

Wahkeena Falls Parking Area **N45° 34.517' W122° 7.681'**
Multnomah Falls Lodge **N45° 31.776' W122° 5.303'**

Take I-84 east 21 miles to Exit 28/Bridal Veil. Turn left onto Historic Columbia River Highway, and proceed 2 miles to the signed parking area at Wahkeena Falls or continue another 0.7 mile to Multnomah Falls Lodge.

*Just above Multnomah Falls, you'll see this falls in
a canyon filled with old-growth forest.*

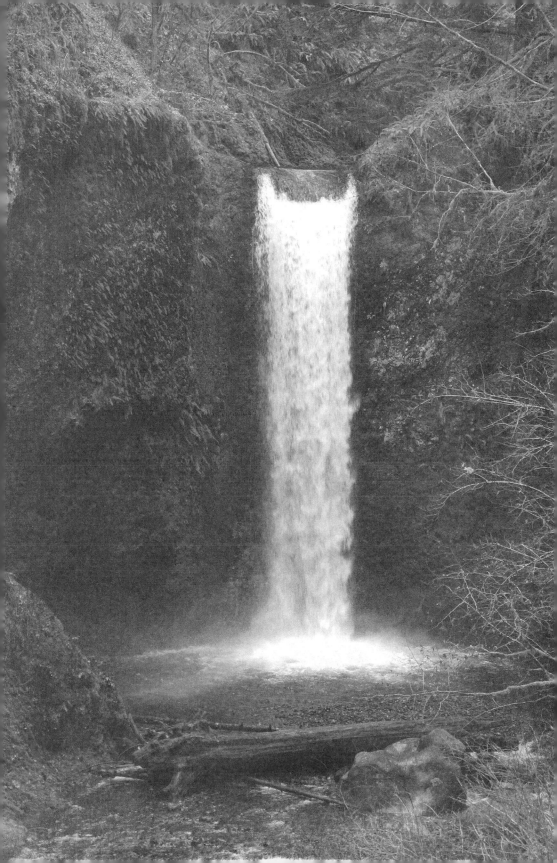

AROUND MOUNT ST. HELENS

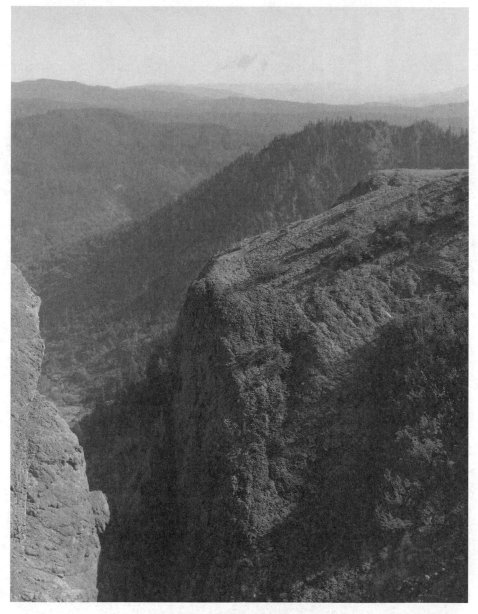

The head of Ape Canyon (Hike 14), with a great view of Mount Adams in the distance, lies at the top of an amazing hike through ancient forest.

Around Mount St. Helens (Hikes 14–22)

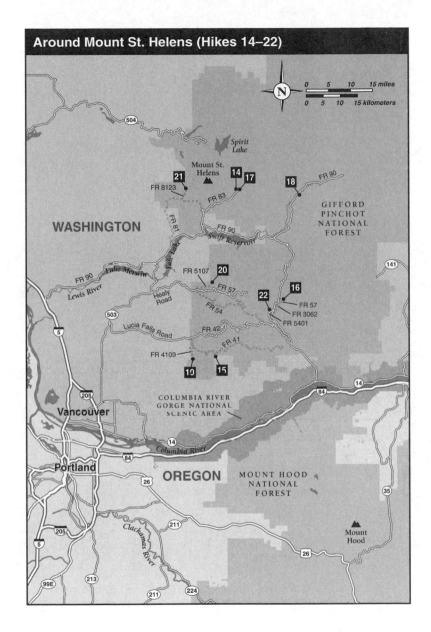

14 Ape Canyon

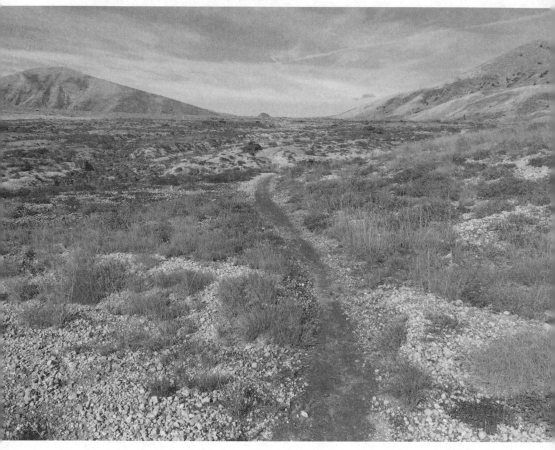

When you reach the Plains of Abraham on Loowit Trail, you'll have a waterfall behind you and Mount St. Helens in front of you.

In Brief

This trail visits two worlds not ordinarily seen: the upper reaches of a volcano and the edge of what they call the "blast zone." Without too much climbing, you can stand in a wonderful old-growth forest and be about 20 feet from an area that was completely obliterated in 1980. At the top, you'll enjoy a sweeping view highlighted by an amazing geological oddity, right at the base of the volcano.

LENGTH 11.6 miles round-trip	**BACKPACKING OPTIONS** Poor
CONFIGURATION Out-and-back	**ACCESS** Northwest Forest Pass required (see page 3)
DIFFICULTY Moderate	
SCENERY Old-growth forest, a volcanic mudflow, a narrow canyon	**WHEELCHAIR ACCESS** None, but some of the nearby Lava Canyon Trail is accessible.
EXPOSURE Shady and open areas on the way up, then wide-open at the top	**MAPS** U.S. Forest Service *Mount St. Helens National Volcanic Monument*
TRAFFIC Moderate on summer weekends, light otherwise	**FACILITIES** None at trailhead; restrooms at Lava Canyon Trailhead
TRAIL SURFACE Packed dirt with roots and rocks; rock at the top	**INFO** Mount St. Helens National Volcanic Monument, 360-449-7800, **www.fs.usda.gov/mountsthelens**
HIKING TIME 5.5 hours	
DRIVING DISTANCE 66 miles (1 hour, 35 minutes) from Pioneer Courthouse Square	**SPECIAL COMMENTS** In June, check ahead to make sure FR 83 is open and snow-free. This trail gets a fair amount of mountain bike traffic.
SEASON Late June–October	
BEST TIME September and October for fall colors	

Description

As soon as you start walking, stay straight at an unsigned junction, and you'll get your first glimpse of the contrasts ahead when you've walked only 500 feet on this trail. At this point you'll be at the top of a little bluff, looking out over a wide area of rocks. Those rocks used to be on the upper slopes of Mount St. Helens, but on May 18, 1980, they tumbled down the hill at about 45 miles per hour, part of a landslide triggered when most of Shoestring Glacier melted a moment after the volcano erupted. But the mudslide stayed generally within the boundaries of the Muddy River, so the forest you're standing in—even though it was within feet of the slide—was spared. You'll spend the next 5 miles climbing this ridge, but don't worry: You'll gain only a little more than 1,300 net feet along the way.

Before you leave this viewpoint, look down. You're standing on several layers of rock, the result of a 1980 lahar, or mudflow, that exposed the rock, giving scientists clues to the volcano's history of eruptions.

If you're on this trail in September or October, you'll be in the world of the vine maple; its red and orange explosion contrasts beautifully with the evergreen canopy. Keep an eye out for deer and elk as well. At 0.25 mile, look for an island of trees on the edge of the mudflow and, after 0.5 mile, enjoy your first view south (behind you) to

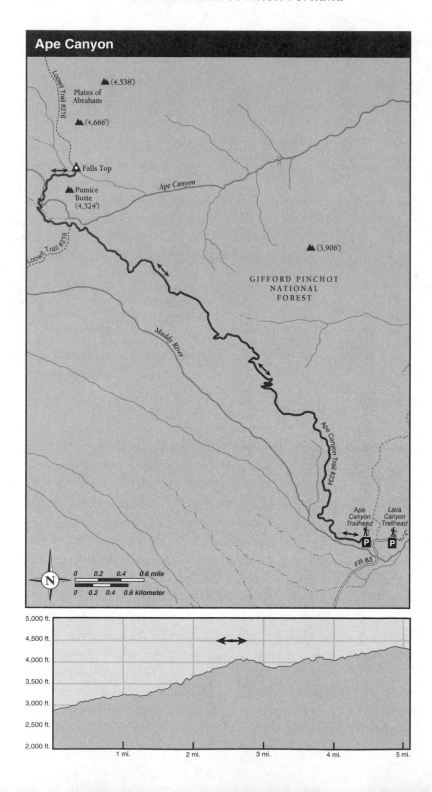

Ape Canyon

Mount Hood. Ahead, on the slopes of Mount St. Helens, you can see the canyon left behind by Shoestring Glacier.

At 1.2 miles, you'll reach a little ridge, then soon after make a switchback to the right and climb a bit more; you'll also notice some social trails heading out to brushy viewpoints facing east to Mount Adams. You'll enter an impressive forest around 1.5 miles up; get your first view of Mt. Adams at 1.7 miles; and, at 2 miles, start a series of switchbacks among old-growth hemlock and thick vine maple. Just past 3 miles, you'll actually lose some elevation before a viewpoint that takes in two-humped Mount Rainier off to your right. From here, you can also make out a large waterfall (mostly dry by late summer) on an eastern ridge of St. Helens—we'll be at the top of that soon!

At 4.4 miles, you'll be out in the open at the head of Ape Canyon proper—and in the "blast zone" itself. There you'll see trees that were killed by the superheated gases produced when the mountain blew in 1980, and to the north (ahead of you) you'll see the utter desolation the eruption created. (The volcano exploded in that direction.)

When you come to a lookout point on the right, you can scramble down a bit—be very careful—and look into the 300-foot slot at the head of Ape Canyon, which now stretches away to your right. It's also visible from a little farther up the trail, where, if you work it right, it makes a heck of a foreground for a picture of Mount Adams.

Just 0.2 mile farther up, Ape Canyon Trail #234 ends at an intersection with Loowit Trail #216, which goes all the way around Mount St. Helens. Walking up to a saddle on the left will get you a nice view south toward Mount Hood and the way you've come up, as well as a weather station and some rocks to sit on.

Back on the trail, stay to the right at the junction, now on Loowit Trail #216. Wind through another lahar as you go around Pumice Butte on your right, and 0.5 mile later you'll climb out of it to the east, where a series of rock cairns marks the trail's path onto the moonlike Plains of Abraham. When the trail dips to the cliff edge, you'll be at the top of that waterfall I told you about, with a sweeping view south.

Turning around here gets you the 11-mile hike advertised, but it's more than worth it to continue a bit onto the Plains of Abraham, which were also created by the 1980 eruption. Look for trees on the nearby hilltops that are lying down and pointing away from the mountain; they were blasted down when the mountain blew. The Plains themselves are fantastic, especially when the weather is clear and the mountain looms over you.

If you're wondering about the name Ape Canyon, it recalls a 1920s incident in which an apelike "Bigfoot"—decades later found to be a kid playing a prank—threw rocks at some miners in the area. The only connection between Ape Canyon and Ape Cave is in the name. The Mount St. Helens Apes, a local Boy Scout troop that took its name from the Ape Canyon legend, discovered Ape Cave.

Nearby Activities

On the way back down Forest Service Road (FR) 83, you'll pass a sign for **Ape Cave,** which is actually a long lava tube divided by an access ladder. Exploring the lower cave involves a 1.6-mile round-trip walk through a large cavern. Taking in the upper, 2.3-mile cave is trickier, requiring some rock scrambling here and there. Take two flashlights if you go.

GPS Information and Directions

N46° 9.926' W122° 5.537'

Take I-5 from Portland, driving 21 miles north of the Columbia River to Exit 21/Woodland, Washington. Turn right onto WA 503 (Lewis River Road), which after 31 miles (2 miles past the town of Cougar) turns into FR 90. Continue 3.3 miles, then turn left onto FR 83. The trailhead is 11.2 miles ahead on the left, just before the Lava Canyon Trailhead.

15 Bluff Mountain Trail

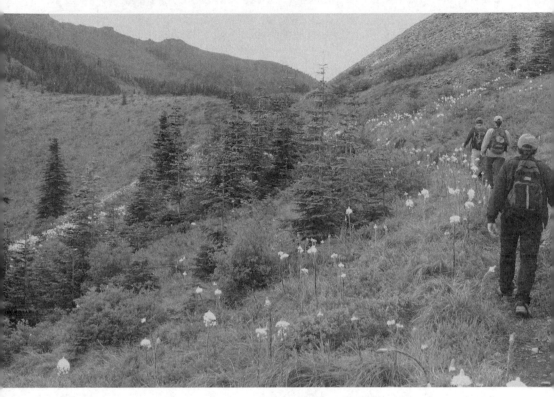

Hikers wind through beargrass on Bluff Mountain Trail. These flowers are among the many that bloom in July on Silver Star Mountain.

In Brief

There are several ways to reach the summit of Silver Star Mountain—this is the longest and toughest path to climb, and possibly the hardest to reach. But it is without question the most entertaining option, offering excellent views, heaps of flowers, and few hikers, giving it an almost expeditionary feel.

Description

Epic. That's the word that always comes to mind when I think of this hike. By the end of the (long, often hot) day, you'll feel like you've been on an adventure. And as you sit

LENGTH 13.2 miles round-trip	**BACKPACKING OPTIONS** Poor
CONFIGURATION Out-and-back	**ACCESS** No fees or permits
DIFFICULTY Strenuous	**WHEELCHAIR ACCESS** None
SCENERY Wide-open, flower-covered ridges; exposed mountainsides; waterfalls; a panoramic vista	**MAPS** Green Trails *Map 396 (Lookout Mountain, WA)* and *Map 428 (Bridal Veil, OR)*
EXPOSURE Open almost the whole way, occasionally on knife-edge ridges	**FACILITIES** None at the trailhead; restrooms and water at Sunset Falls Campground, on the way
TRAFFIC Light	**INFO** Mount Adams Ranger District, 509-395-3400, **www.fs.usda.gov/giffordpinchot**
TRAIL SURFACE Rocky	
HIKING TIME 7.5 hours	**SPECIAL COMMENTS** FR 41, while passable, is rife with potholes and other problems—which have gotten worse over the years. Also, the last sections of the trail often retain snow well into July. Avoid this hike on a hot day, as you'll be in the open about 95 percent of the time.
DRIVING DISTANCE 55 miles (1 hour, 45 minutes) from Pioneer Courthouse Square	
SEASON Late June–October	
BEST TIME July for flowers, October for fall colors	

atop Silver Star, with all the slackers who came up one of the easy ways, you can tell 'em you ain't done nothin' if you ain't done Bluff Mountain Trail.

Speaking of those "easy" ways, one of them, Ed's Trail, is described in the Silver Star Mountain profile (Hike 19, page 104). It's also a tedious drive, but the hike is easier than this one. The third option, via Grouse Vista, has the advantage of good road access but the disadvantage of being dull.

From the trailhead, Bluff Mountain Trail #172 starts on an old jeep road along a ridge that looks and feels like it's way up in the alpine country of Mount Hood. That's because it's wide-open and covered with flowers—but it's open because of a fire, not elevation. The 1902 Yacolt Burn was so intense that very few trees have grown back, though the 1960s saw some terracing and replanting.

Wander along this ridge, with views of other peaks and ridges swept clean by the fire, for 2.5 sunbaked miles, then descend into a notch where the road ends. Here, look for the trail taking off for the right (west) side of the ridge and passing under a series of dramatic cliffs (the north side of Bluff Mountain), with views of Little Baldy off to the right. You'll probably have to skip over a couple of small creeks, which will be welcome sights on hot summer days.

At 3.5 miles, the trail climbs westward into a patch of forest notable for thin but thickly packed trees that seem like clones of each other. Emerging from this forest at

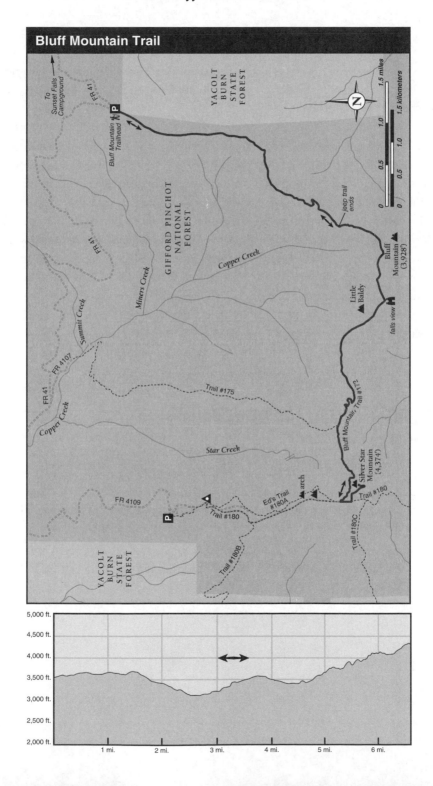

Bluff Mountain Trail

To Sunset Falls Campground

FR 41

P Bluff Mountain Trailhead

YACOLT BURN STATE FOREST

1.5 miles
1.5 kilometers
1.0
0.5
0

GIFFORD PINCHOT NATIONAL FOREST

Copper Creek

jeep trail ends

▲ Bluff Mountain (3,928')

Miners Creek

▲ Little Baldy

falls view

Summit Creek

FR 41

FR 4107

FR 41

Trail #175

Copper Creek

Bluff Mountain Trail #172

Star Creek

▲ Silver Star Mountain (4,374')

FR 4109

P

Ed's Trail #180A

arch

Trail #180

Trail #180

Trail #180C

Trail #180B

YACOLT BURN STATE FOREST

3.8 miles, you'll be greeted by a big view of your destination, the two-humped Silver Star Mountain, ahead. Having come this far and climbed through a forest to be greeted by this view, don't you feel like you're on an expedition? Silver Star looks bigger and more dramatic than other peaks, as its generally treeless east face rises beyond an impressive foreground.

Back out in the sun, continue south along the east side of Little Baldy, and in just under 5 miles you'll have a view of a big waterfall on Silver Star's flanks. At 5.3 miles, continue straight through an intersection with Trail #175, and you'll soon climb to the dramatic (perhaps nerve-wracking, for the acrophobic) ridges of Silver Star, which you wind along for almost a mile before descending into forest again just below the peak.

In these woods, your path intersects a road coming in from the right; this is the end of the Ed's Trail hike. Turn left on the road for a fairly steep climb—stay left again when the road splits—to a saddle between Silver Star's peaks. The higher one is on the left, and the view from here is as impressive as the one on the 6.6-mile hike you just did. On a clear day, you can see from the Three Sisters to Mount Rainier, and because you're on the highest peak in the immediate vicinity, there's a sense of being on a mountain throne.

The next rock to the south is Pyramid Rock. It's not impressive in and of itself, but in recent years there have been reports of at least one mountain goat hanging around there. So keep an eye out before returning the way you came.

GPS Information and Directions

N45° 46.803' W122° 10.010'

Take I-205 from Portland, driving 5 miles north of the Columbia River to take Exit 30B/ Orchards, Washington. Turn right on WA 500 East, which turns into WA 503 in 0.9 mile (follow signs for Battle Ground). Continue 14.7 miles on WA 503, then turn right onto NE Rock Creek Road, which turns into Lucia Falls Road. Drive 8.5 miles on this road, then make a right onto NE Sunset Falls Road and follow it 7.4 miles to Sunset Falls Campground. Turn right to go through the campground and across a bridge over the East Fork Lewis River, and then leave the pavement, driving 9 bumpy miles on Forest Service Road 41 to a big ridgetop parking area. The trailhead is on the right.

16 Falls Creek Falls

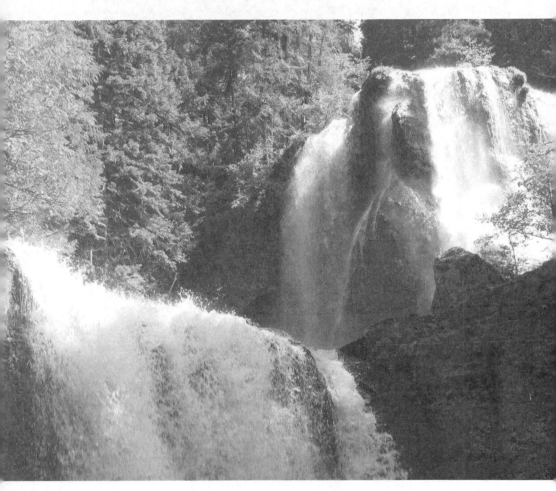

Two of the three tiers of Falls Creek Falls. This view is easy to reach, while the upper tier takes a little more work.

In Brief

Looking for an easy trail to a spectacular destination? This is it. This 1.7-mile ramble gains about 700 feet—which you will hardly notice on the way and will forget entirely when you reach one of the area's most impressive waterfalls. And if you're willing to put in a little more effort, you can visit the top of the falls.

LENGTH 3.4 miles round-trip to the Lower Falls, 6.1 miles if you also visit the Upper Falls	**DRIVING DISTANCE** 68 miles (1 hour, 20 minutes) from Pioneer Courthouse Square
CONFIGURATION Out-and-back or balloon	**SEASON** May–November; road gated December–April 1
DIFFICULTY Easy–moderate	**BEST TIME** May and June
SCENERY Shady forest, a serene stream, and a big-time waterfall	**BACKPACKING OPTIONS** One decent site at Upper Falls
EXPOSURE Some cliff edges (easily avoided) at the end of the trail	**ACCESS** No fees or permits
TRAFFIC Moderate on weekends, light otherwise	**WHEELCHAIR ACCESS** None
	MAPS Green Trails *Map 397 (Wind River)*
TRAIL SURFACE Packed dirt	**FACILITIES** Outhouse at the trailhead
HIKING TIME 2.5 hours to see the lower falls, 4 hours for the whole loop	**INFO** Mount Adams Ranger District, 509-395-3400, **www.fs.usda.gov/giffordpinchot**

Description

The trail starts out flat through forest that's less than 60 years old, passing among huckle-berry, Oregon grape, and Douglas-fir. Not much to see here, but at least you don't have to work hard. A hundred yards in, ignore Trail #152 on the left and continue up Trail #152A. (If you're doing the loop to the top of the falls, you'll see Trail #152 later.)

After 0.5 mile, you'll traverse meadows with a view of an interesting rock forma-tion to the left. Soon after this, you'll cross the creek on a suspension bridge over a narrow gorge; look for some cool round, water-formed rock faces.

At 0.6 mile, now in an older forest, you'll pass a couple of impressive root balls in an area that might get treacherous when wet; a good slip could send you tumbling down toward the creek. At 0.75 mile, you pass nearly under a big Douglas-fir; look for a dead one nearby with countless woodpecker holes.

After hiking 1 mile almost effortlessly, you'll reach another junction with Trail #152; this is where the loop to the Upper Falls takes off, but for now stay on the path you've been hiking. It may sound odd, but on this creek, the Lower Falls is much more impressive than the Upper Falls.

Over the next 0.5 mile, you'll pass a nice creekside picnic area on the right, cross a metal bridge over a lovely cascading creek, and pass under a big rock formation on the left. By this time you should be hearing, and seeing through the trees, the main Lower Falls.

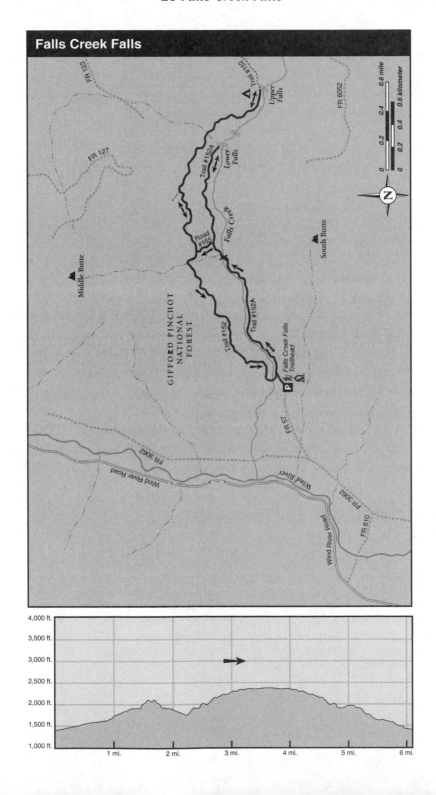

When you arrive at the falls, in an area of large boulders that provide plenty of seating, you'll see two levels of water plunging into a mossy bowl filled with maidenhair ferns. (In fact, a hidden, third level is even higher, making for a total drop of 200 feet.) The whole scene seems like something straight out of *The Lord of the Rings;* you expect to see archers on the hill, guarding their sacred pool. It's particularly impressive in early summer, when water flows are high.

Linger here awhile, then on your way back consider taking the upper loop, recently maintained and signed by the Washington Trails Association. Follow Trail #152 for a steep 0.25 mile through a draw to a junction. Turn right, following pointers for Road #165, and you'll climb another 0.5 mile—your last uphill for the day!

Right after the trail levels, look for a social trail leading right 50 yards or so to the top of some cliffs. Here, you'll get a view of the upper third of the big falls and down the canyon to some of the peaks of Trapper Creek Wilderness (See Hike 22, page 116).

Walk another 5 minutes and you're back at the creek, where a trail leads right and to another view. From this point, a sketchy path descends toward the top of the falls; it can be done, but be very careful, and keep dogs leashed and kids nearby. Even if you don't go down there, you'll notice that you can't see the lower viewpoint from here— you're seeing a whole new section of falls.

A tiny bit of hiking remains here, but it's just a few minutes to the Upper Falls. Though the falls is only about 6 feet high, maybe, it does have a nice campsite where you can overnight or picnic before heading back.

When you do head back, stay with Trail #152 all the way down, just to see some new terrain. It's unspectacular but also uncrowded. It will dump you out on the trail where you started, #152A, just above the trailhead.

GPS Information and Directions

N45° 54.339' W121° 56.385'

Take I-84 from Portland, driving 37 miles east of I-205 to Exit 44/Cascade Locks. As soon as you enter the town, make your first right to get on Bridge of the Gods, following a sign for Stevenson, Washington. Pay the $1 toll, cross the river, and turn right (east) onto WA 14. Go 5.9 miles and turn left, following a sign for Carson, Washington—this is Wind River Road. Drive 14.5 miles on Wind River Road, then turn right, staying on Wind River, and drive 0.8 mile. Make a right onto gravel Forest Service Road (FR) 3062. Drive 2 miles on this road and make a right onto FR 57, following a sign for Lower Falls Creek Falls Trail. The sprawling trailhead is 0.5 mile ahead, at the end of the road.

17 Lava Canyon

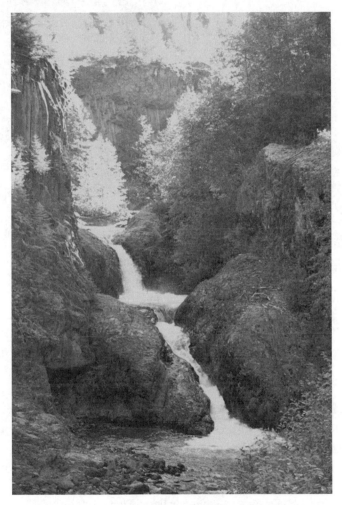

Some of the many waterfalls in Lava Canyon, which was scoured out by the 1980 eruption of Mount St. Helens

In Brief

An unparalleled look at geological forces at work, Lava Canyon is also a beautiful place to be, with numerous waterfalls, a dramatic bridge, some challenging hiking, and a short, barrier-free loop trail.

LENGTH 1–6 miles round-trip	**DRIVING DISTANCE** 85 miles (1 hour, 40 minutes) from Pioneer Courthouse Square
CONFIGURATION Out-and-back, loop	
DIFFICULTY Easy for the upper section, strenuous for the whole thing	**SEASON** June–October; check ahead in June to make sure the road is snow-free.
SCENERY Waterfalls, canyon, geological wonders, a suspension bridge	**BEST TIME** June for water flow, October for fall colors
EXPOSURE Mostly open, with several sections that are quite exposed. People have fallen to their deaths here, so if it's rained or snowed recently or you don't like heights, stick to the upper section.	**BACKPACKING OPTIONS** None
	ACCESS Northwest Forest Pass required (see page 3)
	WHEELCHAIR ACCESS Barrier-free trail in the upper section
TRAFFIC Very heavy on summer weekends, heavy during the week, moderate the rest of the season	**MAPS** U.S. Forest Service *Mount St. Helens National Monument*
TRAIL SURFACE Paved, boardwalk, gravel, and a ladder	**FACILITIES** Restrooms at trailhead; no water
HIKING TIME 30 minutes to do upper loop, 3 hours to do the whole thing	**INFO** Mount St. Helens National Volcanic Monument, 360-449-7800, **www.fs.usda .gov/mountsthelens**

Description

First, a little history, so you'll know what you're looking at here: In ancient times, a forest covered a deep valley. Then, 3,500 years ago, Mount St. Helens erupted, sending a massive mudflow down through the canyon, filling it with volcanic rock. Over the years, the river carved a path through the rock, forming a canyon with waterfalls, deep cuts, and towers of harder rock—Lava Canyon. Later mudflows covered all of that, and eventually forest grew back over the whole thing.

Then, on May 18, 1980, Mount St. Helens erupted again, melting 70 percent of its glaciers in an instant and sending millions of cubic feet of mud and rock blasting down the side of the mountain at about 45 miles an hour. That eruption cleaned out the forest and rock, exposing Lava Canyon for the first time in thousands of years. As you drove in, you got a glimpse of this 1980 mudflow (also known as a *lahar*); now go see what it gave us.

From the trailhead, take the paved path leading left, which, though officially barrier-free, would require some work to push a wheelchair through. You can see here that the trees around you survived the 1980 eruption, but everything below was wiped out. Also, look around for trees that have rocks embedded in them—that's how strong

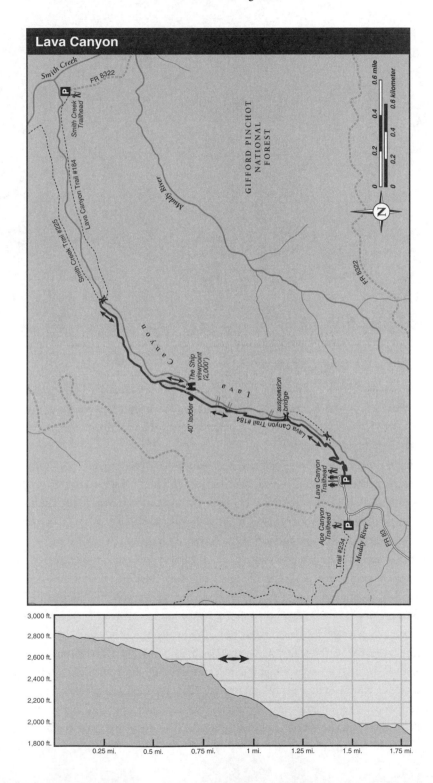

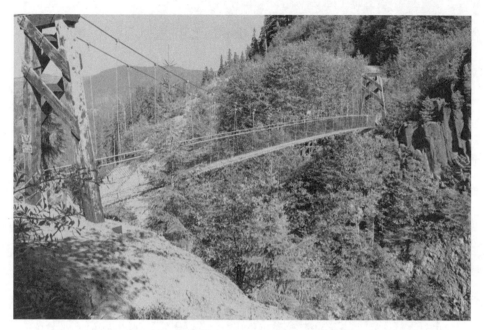

*Somewhat nerve-rattling but completely optional, this suspension bridge is part of
the upper (easy) loop at Lava Canyon.*

the mudflow was, and this point is some 5 miles from its origin. The pavement will
soon give way to boardwalk; two viewing platforms offer both information and dramatic views of the upper canyon.

Hike 0.4 mile to a junction with the loop trail. By now you've seen perhaps
15 warning signs telling you about various dangers and imploring you to stay on the
trail. My favorite such sign is at this junction: D A N G E R is written in seven languages—
and you have to get off the trail to read it! Anyway, be careful and stay on the trail.

For the longer loop, continue straight for now; 100 yards on, you'll have a nice view
of a waterfall and the swirling pools above it. In 0.2 mile you'll come to the suspension
bridge, which is only 3 feet wide and 125 feet long. Kids, dogs, and people afraid of
heights should not go beyond the suspension bridge, and everyone should be careful if it
has rained recently. If you'd like to do only a 1.3-mile loop, cross the bridge and follow
the trail back up to reach the first intersection after crossing another small bridge.

Otherwise, follow the trail down—and I do mean down—from the suspension
bridge. In the next section of trail, you'll descend steep slopes, walk along unguarded
ledges, cross a couple of creeks with no bridges (though one has a cable to hang onto),
and climb down a 30-foot metal ladder. So if it's been raining, or you have small kids,
or you're tired or nervous about heights, think twice before you go past the bridge.

After a steep 0.5-mile descent that passes several beautiful waterfalls and an area where the river flows through a chute just a few feet wide, the trail mellows somewhat. After you've hiked a total of 1.1 miles, you'll climb down the ladder (be careful if your shoes are wet!) and then cross a mossy stream. The rock formation on your right is known as The Ship; it was one of the formations left standing thousands of years ago when the river cut a new course through the ancient canyon. The top of The Ship was the floor of the valley before 1980. There's a little perspective, eh?

It's worth the effort to get to the top of The Ship. A couple hundred yards past the ladder, a trail on the right leads 0.2 mile up it; it's pretty steep and includes rock steps and yet another (smaller) ladder, but there are late-summer huckleberries up there, and it's a heck of a place for a picnic, with an excellent view back up the canyon.

At this point, you've seen the best of the hike, so it's a good spot to turn around. But if you'd like to keep going, Lava Canyon Trail #184 continues another 1.3 miles to the Smith Creek Trailhead, losing 350 feet in elevation on the way. A bridge over the creek just 0.4 mile below the Ship trail is worth visiting.

When you head back up the trail, cross the suspension bridge and take the loop hike back onto a pre-1980 lava flow. When you cross a small metal bridge, turn left and you're 0.4 mile from your car.

GPS Information and Directions

N46° 9.945' W122° 5.275'

Take I-5 from Portland, driving 21 miles north of the Columbia River to Exit 21/Woodland, Washington, then make a right onto WA 503 (Lewis River Road). Drive 23 miles, continuing straight to leave WA 503 for the 503 Spur. Ten miles ahead (3 miles past the town of Cougar), the 503 Spur turns into Forest Service Road (FR) 90. Drive 3.5 miles on FR 90, then turn left onto FR 83, following a sign for Ape Cave and Lava Canyon. The Lava Canyon Trailhead is 11.5 miles ahead, at the end of FR 83.

18 Lewis River

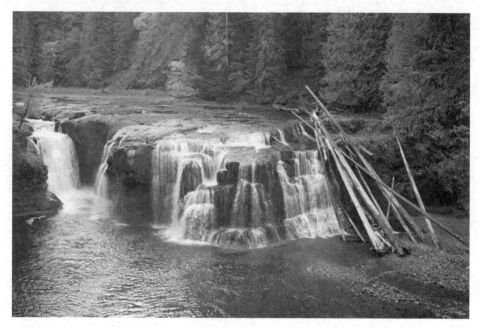

You don't even have to hike to view Lower Falls, which is right next to the trailhead and camping on the Lewis River.

In Brief

Here's a pleasant, mostly flat stroll along a beautiful river with three dramatic water-falls. Chances are they're unlike most falls you've ever seen. The long drive to the trailhead is worth it, especially if you get a campsite at the Lower Lewis River Falls Recreation Area and make a night of it.

Description

From the trailhead in the picnic area, follow a trail that starts just left of the restrooms. In 100 yards, turn right to reach several viewpoints above Lower Falls, one of the most dramatic falls around. The water looks like it's spilling off a shelf, and in fact it is—this is the edge of an ancient lava flow. Over the next stretch of trail, you're walking around the campground, so there are a lot of trails. Turning left will send you into the

LENGTH 5.2 miles round-trip	**SEASON** April–November; check ahead to see if the road is snow-free.
CONFIGURATION Out-and-back	
DIFFICULTY Easy	**BEST TIME** Early summer or fall
SCENERY Several waterfalls, a wild stream flowing through a wooded canyon, old-growth forest	**BACKPACKING OPTIONS** A few decent sites along the river
	ACCESS Northwest Forest Pass required (see page 3)
EXPOSURE Shady all the way	
TRAFFIC Heavy all summer long, especially on weekends	**WHEELCHAIR ACCESS** Campground loop only
	MAPS Green Trails *Map 365 (Lone Butte)*
TRAIL SURFACE Gravel at first, then packed dirt with some roots	**FACILITIES** Restrooms at trail-head; drinking water at campground May–October
HIKING TIME 3.5 hours	
DRIVING DISTANCE 92 miles (2 hours, 10 minutes) from Pioneer Courthouse Square	**INFO** Mount St. Helens National Volcanic Monument, 360-449-7800, www.fs.usda .gov/mountsthelens

campground, but turning right will offer several opportunities to get down to the river. Once you're safely above the falls, you'll find some nice swimming spots.

About 0.5 mile after you leave the campground area, look for the remains of Sheep Bridge over the Lewis. According to the 1965 U.S. Geological Survey map of the area, Lewis River Campground used to be on the far side of the river, so that bridge offered access from the campground to this trail, as well as for driving sheep to pasture. You may also spot a rusted-out "steam donkey," a piece of equipment that was once part of a logging operation.

Around 0.8 mile from the campground, you'll pass the top of a small waterfall, and then at 1.2 miles you'll pass a trail heading up the hill to Wright Meadow; this is a 0.5-mile scenic loop that you can do on the way back, if you like. Just past that trail, cross a bridge above larger Copper Creek Falls, which looks like a waterslide into the Lewis River—don't try it. Soon after that, the main trail arrives at Middle Falls, another shelf-like falls. A side trail leads down to the creek here, but be careful on the slippery rocks.

Back on the main trail, you'll soon pass under some enormous cliffs, then descend into an area with some seriously large trees. Western red cedars here reach close to 6 feet in diameter, and one Douglas-fir on the left must be 10 feet in diameter—definitely one of the biggest trees you'll see on any hike in this book. Just past this area you'll come to a campsite on the right, then cross Alec Creek and enter the amphitheater of Upper Falls, which makes an 80-foot plunge. Logs and rocks in the sun here

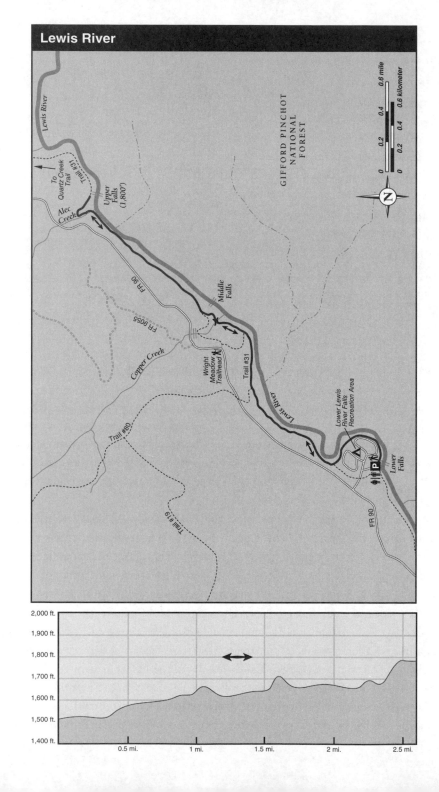

make for good picnicking or lounging. A trail to the left leads 0.2 mile up the hill to a platform at the top of Upper Falls, a worthwhile side trip. Another 0.2 mile up, there's a view of Taidnapam Falls in the rocky gorge above Upper Falls.

On the way back, just before Middle Falls, go ahead and take the Wright Meadow "scenic byway." Just take a right before Middle Falls, climb briefly to another waterfall along the trail that follows Copper Creek, then make a left at the fork (the road is to the right) and you'll be back on the main trail, 1.5 miles from your car.

Extending Up Quartz Creek

If you go another 0.7 mile past Taidnapam Falls—that would be 4 miles from this trailhead—you'll reach the end of Lewis River Trail at Forest Service Road (FR) 90. Beyond that, the Quartz Creek Trail begins, entering some of the grandest old-growth forest around. The Washington Trails Association has been working for two years to log this trail out, and by the time this book comes out it should be mostly done. Here's a brief description to tempt you to check it out:

The first 0.5 mile is along Quartz Creek and passes several nice picnic or camping spots. The trail then spends a mile climbing, then descending, to a ford of Straight Creek. This crossing will be sketchy during the early season, but there's a nice camp-site on the east side of the creek. After Straight Creek, the trail climbs through younger forest before entering, after a mile, some awesome old-growth.

Even longer backpacking loops are possible via this and the Quartz Butte Trail; for more information, check with the national-forest office.

GPS Information and Directions

N46° 9.293′ W121° 52.782′

Take I-5 from Portland, driving 21 miles north of the Columbia River to Exit 21/Woodland, Washington. Make a right onto WA 503 (Lewis River Road), which after 31 miles (2 miles past the town of Cougar) turns into FR 90. Continue 30 more miles on FR 90—you'll have to turn right just past the Pine Creek Information Center to stay on this road—to reach the Lower Lewis River Falls Recreation Area. Take the first right off the entrance road to reach the trailhead. You may notice that a mile before the campground on FR 90 there's a Lewis River trailhead, just past a bridge. You could start here if you like, but it adds 3 miles to the round-trip hike without the benefit of waterfalls.

19 Silver Star Mountain: Ed's Trail

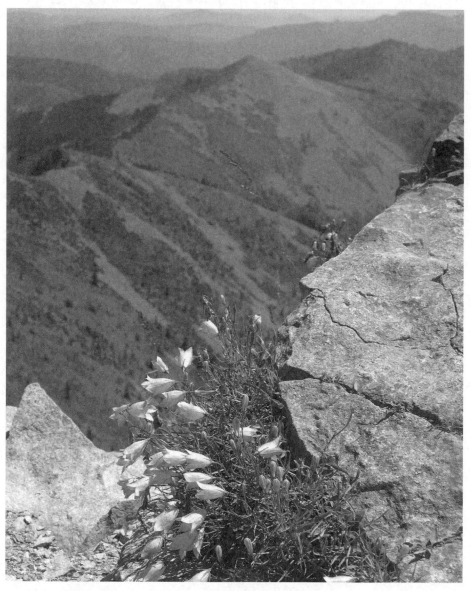

Looking east from Silver Star at Little Baldy

LENGTH 4.8 miles	**SEASON** June–October
CONFIGURATION Balloon	**BEST TIME** July for flowers, October for cool temps
DIFFICULTY Moderate	
SCENERY Wildflowers, open ridgetops, rocky crags, a natural arch, several volcanoes	**BACKPACKING OPTIONS** Poor
	ACCESS No fees or permits
	WHEELCHAIR ACCESS None
EXPOSURE In the sun the whole time, with occasional stretches along rocky cliff edges and a brief section of semi-climbing	**MAPS** Green Trails *Map 396 (Lookout Mountain)* and *Map 428 (Bridal Veil)*, though Ed's Trail isn't on either one
TRAFFIC Moderate on weekends, light otherwise	**FACILITIES** None at trailhead; available at a campground along the way
TRAIL SURFACE Dirt, rocks, some scrambling	**INFO** Mount Adams Ranger District, 509-395-3400, **www.fs.usda.gov/giffordpinchot**
HIKING TIME 3 hours	**SPECIAL COMMENTS** The road to this one is nowhere near smooth, but it passed my 1992 Nissan Sentra test.
DRIVING DISTANCE 56 miles (1 hour, 30 minutes) from Pioneer Courthouse Square	

In Brief

You may be reading the directions to this one and thinking, "What a drive!" And the road *is* rough. But when you're on Ed's Trail approaching Silver Star Mountain, you'll be thinking, "This is too beautiful and mountainous to be so close to town!" This flower-soaked traverse through rocky alpine country is worth all the hassles of getting here.

Description

Even the trailhead for this one is scenic, and other than a few short stretches here and there, every foot of the trail is, too. From the trailhead, look for the path heading to the right, past a brown hiker sign. Follow this pathway through several brushy switchbacks to an old jeep road, then head up that 150 yards to a wide gravel area with a nice view of Mount Hood through a notch in a ridge. Stop here, at the 0.5-mile point, and catch your breath.

Where the road swings back to the right and heads uphill, look for Ed's Trail #180A heading left, along the ridge. We'll come back on the road, but it's better to follow Ed for now. Ed was Edward Robertson, a cofounder of the Chinook Trail Association, which built and maintains this trail. Ed must have been a lover of flowers and open country, because his trail is an amazing piece of work: an ambling, gentle climb along a ridge that looks as if it's thousands of feet higher than it really is. That's because

Silver Star Mountain: Ed's Trail

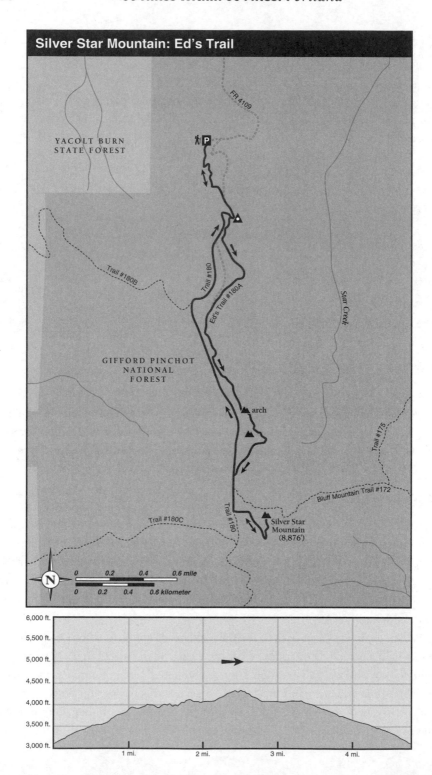

in 1902 fires razed the forest, and very few trees have grown back—though more than 100 varieties of wildflowers and flowering shrubs have. So it's like you're getting a look at the decorated skeletons of the mountains, complete with bony spurs, cliffs, and rock formations normally covered by forest.

Climb toward some of these exposed formations, ascending 0.7 mile before the trail flattens and starts a tour of the rocky ridgetop. At 1.5 miles, pass through a rock arch and beside a small, overhanging cave that offers just about the only shade around on a hot day. Soon the trail takes off up the ridge face, forcing you to almost climb in spots as you scramble up through the rocks to your first view of the two-humped Silver Star ahead. Dramatic, huh?

Now the trail descends through meadows and into the trees, then climbs again to a junction with the road you left behind. (This whole Ed's Trail was just a scenic, adventurous diversion.) Follow the road to the left, staying left at a junction a couple hundred yards up, and after 0.25 mile the road approaches a saddle between the two peaks. Head left for the big (shadeless) view at the official summit, and enjoy views of the Columbia River Gorge, Mount Defiance (with radio towers), the back of Dog Mountain, Larch Mountain, the Portland area, and everything from Mount Jefferson to Mount Rainier. Look also for Bluff Mountain Trail (Hike 15, page 87) along the narrow ridges to the east.

By the way, Silver Star Mountain got its name because, when seen from above, the ridges running out from the summit form a five-pointed star.

The next rock to the south is Pyramid Rock. It's not impressive in and of itself, but in recent years there have been reports of at least one mountain goat hanging around there. So keep an eye out.

On your way back to the car, enjoy some different scenery while avoiding a treacherous descent on Ed's Trail. Simply stay on the jeep road as it winds along the opposite side of the ridge. This will take you back to the far end of Ed's Trail, where you picked it up, and then you'll just retrace your steps to your car.

GPS Information and Directions

N45° 46.344' W122° 14.678'

Take I-205 from Portland, driving 5 miles north of the Columbia River to Exit 30B/Orchards, Washington. Make a right on WA 500 East, which turns into WA 503 in 0.9 mile (follow signs for Battle Ground). Continue 14.7 miles on WA 503, then make a right onto NE Rock Creek Road, which turns into Lucia Falls Road. Drive 8.5 miles on this road; then turn right onto NE Sunset Falls Road, follow it 2 miles, and make another right onto NE Dole Valley Road. Drive 2.4 miles on Dole Valley, then turn left onto Department of Natural Resources Road L-1100— you'll see "1100" on a tree and a sign for Tarbell Picnic Area. Continue straight on L-1100 for 2.2 miles, bear left (downhill) at 4.3 miles, and then, at 7.7 miles, turn right (uphill) onto Forest Service Road 4109. The trailhead is 2.6 miles up, at the end of this narrow, bumpy road.

20 Siouxon Creek

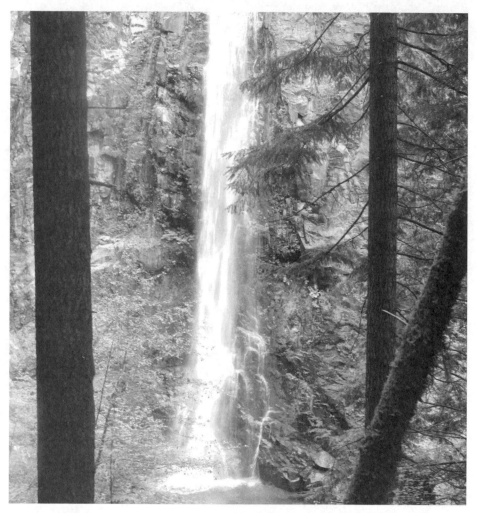

Wildcat Falls is your reward for a little effort (and a stream crossing) on this hike.

In Brief

An easy, pleasant stroll along a mountain stream, with old-growth forest and waterfalls all around, plus options that include a stream crossing and rugged climbing—what more could you want? Even the kids will like it; with supervision, they could go for a swim.

LENGTH Up to 10.8 miles round-trip along the creek, with side trips possible	**DRIVING DISTANCE** 55 miles (1 hour, 30 minutes) from Pioneer Courthouse Square
CONFIGURATION Out-and-back with optional loop	**SEASON** March–November; muddy in winter and spring, with occasional snow
DIFFICULTY Easy–moderate along the creek, strenuous to Siouxon Peak	**BEST TIME** Early summer or fall
SCENERY Old-growth forest, waterfalls, pools in the river, mountaintop viewpoint	**BACKPACKING OPTIONS** Several good sites along the creek
EXPOSURE Shady all the way, optional creek-wading, one set of slippery rocks	**ACCESS** No fees or permits
	WHEELCHAIR ACCESS None
TRAFFIC Moderate on summer weekends, light otherwise	**MAPS** Green Trails *Map 396 (Lookout Mountain)*
TRAIL SURFACE Packed dirt with some rocks and roots	**FACILITIES** None at trailhead; water on trail must be treated.
HIKING TIME 3–5 hours; more for the peak	**INFO** Mount St. Helens National Volcanic Monument, 360-449-7800, **www.fs.usda .gov/mountsthelens**

Description

The only spectacular thing about this hike is how easy and scenic it is. There are no panoramic viewpoints, no exotic geological features, and no serious hiking challenges—unless you want them. It's just a beautiful river in a peaceful, lush, tree-filled canyon, with waterfalls and campsites all over the place and not too many hikers.

In fact, two mysteries have long intrigued me about this hike: One is why more people don't seem to know about it, and the other is why most people stop at Chinook Falls when numerous beautiful spots lie farther up the creek and the most amazing falls of all (Wildcat) is just across it.

From the trailhead, you can choose from several paths into the woods. Take any one and turn right when you reach the main trail, Siouxon Creek Trail #130. You'll walk downhill briefly, cross West Creek on a log bridge, and then stroll over a small ridge to Siouxon Creek—and the first of many good campsites. At 0.9 mile you'll see, on the right, Horseshoe Ridge Trail #140, which makes a 7-mile, rugged, solitary loop back to this trail. After 1.4 miles, your trail crosses Horseshoe Creek, so named because it drains a horseshoe-shaped ridge, of which you're crossing the open mouth. There will be a waterfall above and below you here; to get a view of the lower one, and visit a fine campsite, take a side trail to the left just after the bridge.

Over the next 0.3 mile you'll climb slightly to a viewpoint of Siouxon Falls, which could almost be called a really big rapids as opposed to a classic falls. Then the trail

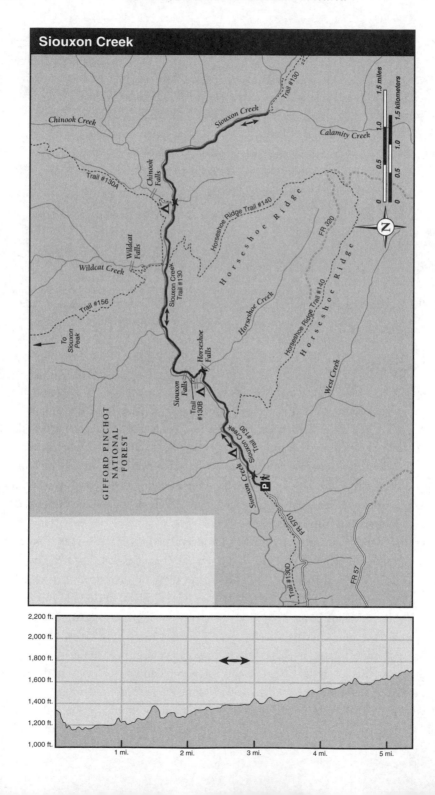

traverses flat ground for 0.5 mile, some 200 feet above the creek, before dropping to its side for another 0.5 mile. This is where some swimming might happen—just know that any dip will be brief, unless you're part polar bear.

At the 3-mile mark, you'll see two side trails in quick succession. The first, unmarked and on the left, leads down to the creek—this is one way to reach Wildcat Falls, but it involves a tricky crossing of Siouxon Creek that will be difficult for most people until late summer, at least. There's an easier way a little farther up. The second trail you'll see, heading up and to the right, is the second appearance of Horseshoe Ridge Trail.

Go another 0.7 mile and you'll come to an unnamed creek on the right; careful here, as the rocks tend to be slick. There's also a nice bridge over Siouxon Creek, which at this point flows through a narrow gorge. Cross the bridge and go 0.3 mile to the beautiful, 50-foot Chinook Falls on Chinook Creek. There's another good campsite along this trail.

Here, you could head back the way you came and, at just under 8 miles, call it a day. Or you could go visit Wildcat Falls by wading across Chinook Creek here and following an up-and-down trail to the left for 0.5 mile to Wildcat Creek. Go up that creek from a junction, and after 0.2 mile you'll arrive at the base of the 100-foot beauty. The views are even more dramatic farther up the trail. And if you're really looking for some exercise, go another 3.5 miles (and about 3,000 feet) up this trail to Siouxon Peak, following a route that's well marked on the Green Trails map.

At the very least, from the bridge near Chinook Falls, go a little farther up Siouxon Creek. I have no idea why no other guidebook recommends this, because it's just as beautiful up there, requires no more effort, and passes several more waterfalls. Another 1.7 miles of creekside trail end at a crossing of Calamity Creek (no bridge) and gain only another 250 feet. Beyond Calamity Creek the trail climbs away from Siouxon, ending some 2 dull miles later on a road near Observation Peak and Sister Rocks.

GPS Information and Directions

N45° 56.797' W122° 10.649'

Take I-205 from Portland, driving 5 miles north of the Columbia River to Exit 30B/Orchards, Washington. Make a right on WA 500, which turns into WA 503 in 0.9 mile (follow signs for Battle Ground). Continue 25 miles on WA 503, passing through the town of Amboy. Just past the Mount St. Helens National Volcanic Monument headquarters, make a right on NE Healy Road. Drive 9 miles—noting that Healy Road turns into Forest Service Road (FR) 54 at 2.4 miles—then turn left (uphill) on FR 57. After 1.2 miles on FR 57, turn left on FR 5701. The trailhead is 3.6 miles ahead, at the end of the road.

21 South Fork Toutle River

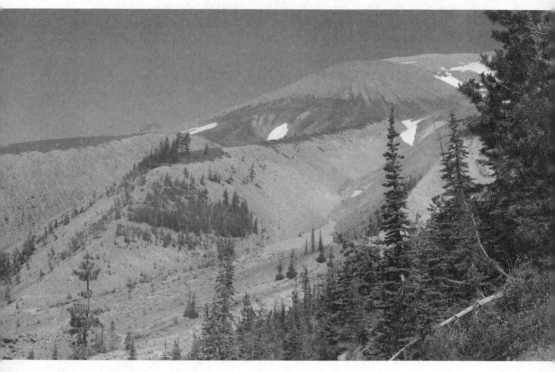

The great thing about this hike is its variety of scenery—for example, the alpine splendor on the slopes of Mount St. Helens.

In Brief

It's back! A mudslide (which you'll walk on) wiped out the trailhead years ago, but one of my favorite hikes is available again. Without driving all the way to the other side of Mount St. Helens, this is the most dramatic view you can get of the results of that mountain's 1980 eruption. You'll see where the mudflow was half a mile wide, as well as tour the majesty that survived the eruption.

Description

Back in 2003, this hike got a bit longer when the road beyond the Blue Lake Trailhead was washed out, cutting off a trailhead that was only 0.5 mile from Sheep Canyon.

LENGTH 11.2 miles	**SEASON** June–October; in June, check ahead to make sure the road is snow-free.
CONFIGURATION Balloon	
DIFFICULTY Strenuous	**BEST TIME** August and September
SCENERY Old-growth forest, waterfalls in canyons, flower-filled meadows, close-up view of Mount St. Helens and the aftermath of its eruption	**BACKPACKING OPTIONS** One nice site on the loop, others nearby on Loowit Trail
	ACCESS No fees or permits
EXPOSURE Alternately shady and sunny; one optional cliff-top viewpoint	**WHEELCHAIR ACCESS** None
TRAFFIC Light	**MAPS** USFS *Mount St. Helens National Monument;* Green Trails *Map 364 (Mount St. Helens)* or *Map 364S (Mount St. Helens NW)*
TRAIL SURFACE Rocky in places, packed dirt with roots, occasionally brushy with a poor tread; 1 bridgeless (small) stream crossing	
	FACILITIES None at trailhead; water on trail must be treated.
HIKING TIME 7–8 hours	**INFO** Mount St. Helens National Volcanic Monument, 360-449-7800, **www.fs.usda.gov/mountsthelens**
DRIVING DISTANCE 73 miles (1 hour, 30 minutes) from Pioneer Courthouse Square	

Then, in 2006, the Blue Lake Trailhead itself was destroyed, making this an even longer hike! For now, anyway, the mountain doesn't seem to be in a destructive mood, so let's go do this wonderful, varied walk.

From the trailhead, you'll start out on a path hacked through the most recent mudslide. There seem to be a few trails in here, but stick generally to the left, aiming for a low ridge you can see ahead. After 0.6 mile, look for a crossing of a tiny creek up against that ridge—ribbons marked a good crossing when I visited—then scramble up the other side to find the original trail in the woods, climbing gradually toward Blue Lake.

In just minutes, you'll pass well above the lake, visible through the trees to the right, then go slowly up and over a low ridge through a beautiful old forest. After a total of 2.1 miles, you'll start down and pass through a meadow and intersect Blue Lake Horse Trail #237 on the right, then drop 0.9 mile to arrive at Sheep Canyon Trail #240, coming up from the left (from the old, road-end trailhead that was cut off in 2003).

Here, you have a few options: For the easiest route to Sheep Canyon and the South Fork Toutle River, follow this trail straight ahead for 1.6 miles; but for the recommended loop, which will come back that way, turn right and immediately cross a lovely creek, along which is the route's only campsite. Past that, you climb gradually through a lovely forest and into spectacular alpine high country. You'll gain 850 feet in 1.3 miles to reach an intersection with Loowit Trail #216, which goes all the way

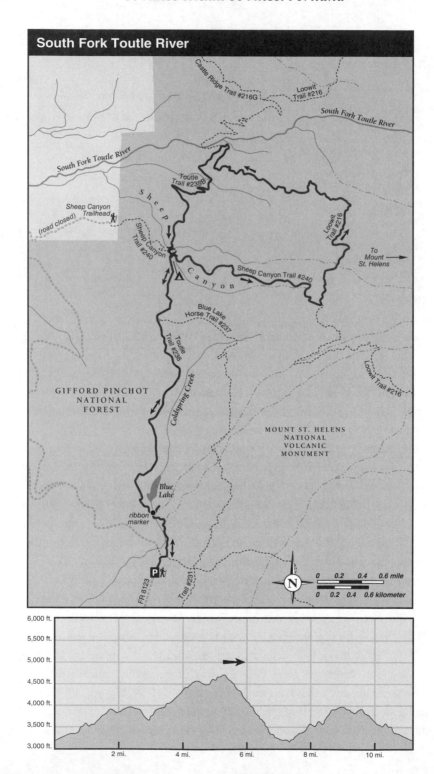

South Fork Toutle River

around Mount St. Helens. Turn left here, descend about 0.5 mile to traverse an ash-filled ravine with a wetland below you, then climb 0.5 mile through a wonderful sub-alpine area of firs and hemlocks. In July you'll find beargrass going wild; in August the place will be ablaze with flowers, especially blue lupine; and in fall the mountain ash and other plants will roar with color. And the views up here, at the foot of the mountain, are splendid. This is a fantastic stretch of trail.

Just over the hump of a small ridge, you'll come to a big viewpoint on a boulder. The South Fork Toutle, some 800 feet below you, is in the process of recarving its way through the 1980 mudflow. The drainage right at your feet was wiped out, too, when glaciers melted instantly. The contrast between your side of the canyon and the other side, well within the blast zone, couldn't be more stark.

The trail now turns downhill, descending Crescent Ridge, for 1.6 miles to a junction with Toutle Trail #238B, just above the South Fork. It's in this stretch that the trail gets brushy and the tread is poor in places, so take your time to be sure of your footing. Explore to the right of the junction, checking out the mini-gorge the river has cut into the mudflow. Then go back to Toutle Trail #238 and follow its brushy and uneven path through old-growth forest. You'll climb over a small ridge in old-growth forest before arriving at the bridge over Sheep Canyon after 1.5 miles. Sheep Canyon was also gouged out by the 1980 eruption, and for what it's worth, the bridge here is my girlfriend's favorite hiking spot.

Cross that spectacular span, then stay straight at the junction to retrace your steps 3 miles back to your car.

Nearby Activities

If you'd like to learn more about the eruption and its fascinating aftermath, visit the **Mount St. Helens Science and Learning Center** (19000 Spirit Lake Hwy., Toutle, WA 98649). See **mshslc.org** for details.

GPS Information and Directions

N46° 10.028' W122° 15.709'

From Portland on I-5, drive 21 miles north of the Columbia River and take Exit 21/Woodland, Washington. Turn right onto WA 503 (Lewis River Road) and drive 28 miles; then, between Mileposts 35 and 36, turn left onto FR 8100, following a sign for Kalama Recreation Area. Drive 12 miles on Forest Service Road (FR) 8100, then continue straight onto FR 8123 for 2 miles to the Blue Lake Trailhead, at the end of the road.

22 Trapper Creek Wilderness

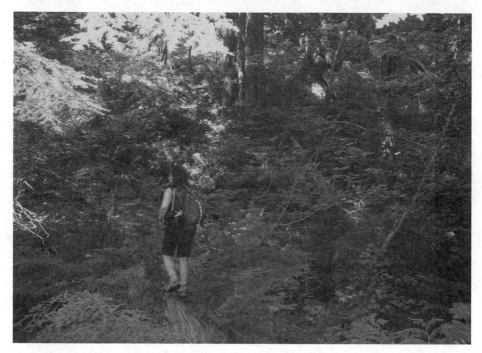

A one-log creek crossing in Trapper Creek Wilderness

In Brief

This is almost a secret hike. Most people have never heard of it, but everybody who goes there loves it. It's quiet and woodsy, with lots of creeks, two waterfalls, great campsites, and—if you want to gain some elevation—a great view from Observation Peak.

Description

I can't explain why so few people have heard of Trapper Creek. It's just over an hour from Portland, it's loaded with trails, and it couldn't be any prettier. If you're a fan of the forest, and especially if you don't mind climbing, this is the place to be. One section of the wilderness was actually set aside in the 1950s as a research area for old-growth Pacific silver firs. And up on the ridge, there are huckleberries—the big, blue, juicy kind—everywhere.

LENGTH 14.5 miles, but options abound	**SEASON** July–October to climb the ridge, May–November for lower elevations
CONFIGURATION Loop	
DIFFICULTY Easy–strenuous	**BEST TIME** September and October
TRAFFIC Moderate on summer weekends, light otherwise	**BACKPACKING OPTIONS** Several nice sites
SCENERY Magnificent forest, two waterfalls, a sweeping mountaintop view	**ACCESS** Northwest Forest Pass required (see page 3)
EXPOSURE A couple of lookouts, otherwise in the woods	**WHEELCHAIR ACCESS** None
	MAPS USFS *Trapper Creek Wilderness*
TRAFFIC Moderate on summer weekends, otherwise light	**FACILITIES** None at trailhead; water everywhere, but it must be treated.
TRAIL SURFACE Packed dirt, rocks	**INFO** Mount Adams Ranger District, 509-395-3400, **www.fs.usda.gov /giffordpinchot**
HIKING TIME 8 hours to do the big loop	
DRIVING DISTANCE 66 miles (1 hour, 30 minutes) from Pioneer Courthouse Square	

The wilderness covers a little more than 6,000 acres, and it's basically one U-shaped watershed, drained by Trapper Creek and its many tributaries. It's heavily forested with firs, hemlocks, cedars, and pines. Wildflowers abound in the spring and early summer, and the animals here include owls, black bears, cougars, and bobcats—though the only sign I've seen of any of those was the sound of an owl and some very fresh, berry-filled bear scat on the trail. You have virtually nothing to fear from a black bear—if you see one, you'll likely see its rump disappearing into the woods.

To explore this area, you have numerous options: casually wander the old-growth forest, climb to a seldom-visited lake, slog up the hill to the big view, or take one of several semi-maintained "adventure trails." Let this challenging 14.5-mile loop serve as an introduction, as it touches on all the other options, or plan for an overnight to break up the work a little.

From the trailhead, start into the woods on Trapper Creek Trail #192, which our loop follows 6 miles to its end. Right off the bat you'll intersect Dry Creek Trail #194, which runs about 4 miles north along Dry Creek. Half a mile out on Trapper Creek Trail, look for a rotting stump in the shape of an hourglass; look also for such forest features as woodpecker holes in snags and new trees growing out of old stumps. Walk 0.9 mile and you'll see Observation Trail #132 on the right; you'll be coming down this one if you do the big loop. For now, continue straight on Trapper Creek Trail—the forest gets even better as you get deeper into the canyon.

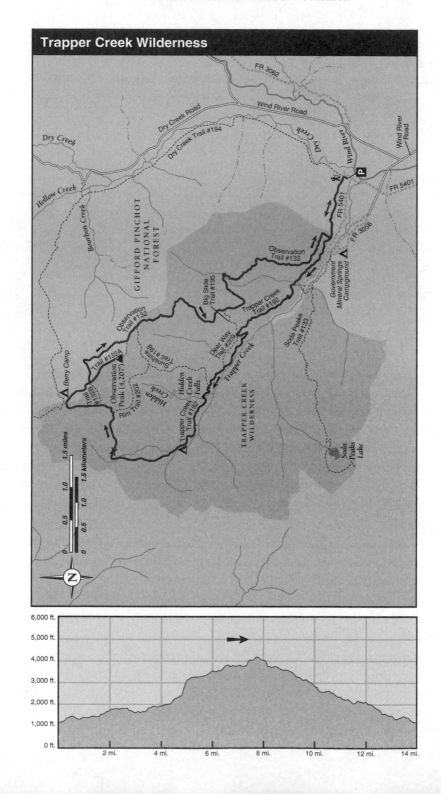

Trapper Creek Wilderness

FR 3062

Wind River Road

Dry Creek Road

Dry Creek Trail #194

Dry Creek

Dry Creek

Wind River

Wind River Road

P

FR 5401

FR 5401

FR 3056

Hollow Creek

Bourbon Creek

GIFFORD PINCHOT NATIONAL FOREST

Observation Trail #132

Government Mineral Springs Campground

Big Slide Trail #195

Trapper Creek Trail #192

Soda Peaks Trail #133

Observation Trail #132

Deer Way Trail #209

Trapper Creek

Berry Camp

Trail #132A

Observation Peak (4,207')

Sunshine Trail # 198

Hidden Creek Falls

TRAPPER CREEK WILDERNESS

Trail #132B

Hidden Creek

Rim Trail #202

Trapper Creek Trail #192

Soda Peaks Lake

1.5 miles

1.5 kilometers

1.0

1.0

0.5

0.5

0

0

N

6,000 ft.

5,000 ft.

4,000 ft.

3,000 ft.

2,000 ft.

1,000 ft.

0 ft.

2 mi.   4 mi.   6 mi.   8 mi.   10 mi.   12 mi.   14 mi.

After another leg-friendly 0.7 mile, you'll cross Lush Creek and encounter Soda Peaks Trail #133, on the left. This leads to the one lake in the wilderness, Soda Peaks Lake; it's a climb of 2,500 feet in about 3 miles, and the trail doesn't loop back to this one. So unless you're looking for another hill to climb—or you want to do some lake-side backpack camping—stay on Trapper Creek Trail #192 to go up and around the end of a ridge, from which you'll get your first good views (or at least sounds) of Trapper Creek on the left.

About a mile later, barely climbing, you'll come to two trails: Big Slide Trail #195 and Deer Way Trail #209. Big Slide, like several other trails in the wilderness, was built and is maintained by the Mazamas, a Portland-based mountaineering club that has adopted this wilderness area. But before you go off on one of their trails, you should know a few things about Mazamas and their trails. For one thing—and I say this as a Mazama—there is an element in that crowd that uses the phrase "get your butt kicked" to mean "have a good time." Some of these trails were designed with that attitude: They're steep scrambles, without such niceties as switchbacks, and they can be tough to follow. And when a log falls across them, rather than cut the log away (as the U.S. Forest Service does), the Mazamas might cut a little notch in the top of it to help you swing your leg over. So these trails are fun—and the Mazamas' signs are really cool—but they aren't what you'd call casual.

Deer Way Trail is basically an easy cutoff that avoids some elevation (plus scenery and campsites) for those in a hurry to get up the hill, so if that's your bag, take it. Otherwise, take Trapper Creek Trail, which dips down, for the first time, to almost touch Trapper Creek. Along the way, it passes Terrace Camp, a lovely spot with room for several tents. The trail continues steeply downhill, passing outrageous Douglas-firs—some of which are on the ground, causing the trail to wind through them—and another campsite, even closer to the creek.

After a total of about 3 miles, the trail seems to disappear at a small side creek. In fact, it continues over a well-worn log, but there's a fun little side trip here, if you're up for it. Pick—and climb and crawl—your way up this creek a couple hundred feet or so, and you'll be rewarded with a view of a tall, hidden waterfall.

Continue 0.4 mile, passing the far end of the Deer Way cutoff, and next you'll cross Sunshine Trail #198 with its cool handmade sign. This Mazamas masterpiece goes straight up about 2,000 feet in less than 2 miles. I've done it and wound up 80 percent lost and 110 percent exhausted; it's a "wonderful" butt-kicking.

Staying on Trapper Creek Trail, you'll have it pretty easy for another 0.5 mile, crossing Hidden Creek and a side trail to view Hidden Creek Falls. A trail on the left, at about 4 miles, leads to Rendezvous Flats, where you can enjoy some creekside loveliness; soon after, you'll pass a campsite at Cliff Creek. Then, if you like, you can start climbing.

You'll put in about 1,700 feet in 2.5 miles, much of it in viewless switchbacks that are better for meditation than for any form of entertainment. There's a mighty nice bridge on the way, and about halfway up is a rocky ledge that makes a fine resting point with a view of a falls off to the left. And this ought to cheer you up: See that ridge over there, the really big one? Observation Peak is 600 feet higher than that.

When the climbing is done—you might notice a rare elevation sign indicating 3,200 feet—you'll be in a dreamland forest. To my mind, there's nothing lovelier than a Northwest forest around 3,000–4,000 feet above sea level. And the crossing (at 3,300 feet) of Trapper Creek, in a berry-filled basin, is about as nice as it gets.

You'll cross one more Mazama trail, Rim Trail #202, before Trail #132B, to the right, cuts off some distance to Observation Trail #132. Turn right here, take another right on Trail #132A in 0.5 mile, and, after just over 0.5 mile of additional climbing, you'll be at Observation Peak. Congratulations: You've now hiked 8 miles and gained a little more than 3,000 feet. Look for Mount St. Helens and its blast zone to the north; from there, around to the right, we have Mount Rainier, the Goat Rocks off on the horizon, and then Mount Adams. See if you can spot, well to the right of that, the meadow atop Dog Mountain—it's rare to see it from "behind"—and across from that the radio towers atop Mount Defiance, the highest point in the Columbia River Gorge. Right of that are Mounts Hood and Jefferson, and closer in are the two Soda Peaks, host to the aforementioned lake. Nice, huh?

Getting down from here is simple: Just go back down Trail #132A, which you came up, and turn right on Observation Trail #132. You can follow this trail 5 pretty boring miles to its end at Trapper Creek Trail #192, a mile up from the parking lot, or you can test your knees going down a Mazama trail. Just turn right on either Sunshine Trail #198 or the much-shorter Big Slide Trail #195, and don't blame me if you have a hard time walking the next day. Seriously, if you want to tackle one of these, go *up* them instead.

Either way you go, you'll come to Trapper Creek Trail #192; your car will be to the left.

Nearby Activities

It's all about springs in this area. When you drive back down Forest Service Road (FR) 5401 on your way out, take a right for Government Mineral Springs and follow the signs to **Iron Mike Well,** for mineral water from an iron pump. Or, when you get back to Carson, go to **Carson Hot Springs Resort,** with its 1901 (now former) hotel and 1923 bathhouse and cabins. You can soak, get a massage, and then get wrapped in hot towels. A new hotel and golf course were in the works as this book was going to press. Call 800-607-3678 or visit **carsonhotspringresort.com** for details.

GPS Information and Directions

N45° 52.891' W121° 58.828'

Take I-84 from Portland, driving 37 miles east of I-205 to Exit 44/Cascade Locks. As soon as you enter town, make your first right to get on Bridge of the Gods, following a sign for Stevenson, Washington. Pay the $1 toll, cross the river, and turn right (east) onto WA 14. Drive 5.9 miles and turn left, following a sign for Carson, Washington—this is Wind River Road. Drive 14.5 miles, then continue straight, leaving Wind River Road and following a sign for Government Mineral Springs. Half a mile later, turn right on FR 5401; the trailhead is 0.4 mile ahead, at the end of the road.

UP THE CLACKAMAS RIVER

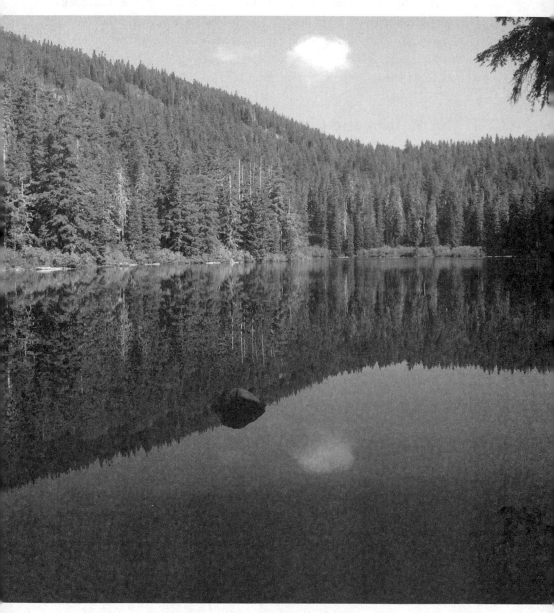

Shellrock Lake, the first of many lakes on the Roaring River trip (Hike 26), offers waterside camping among the trees.

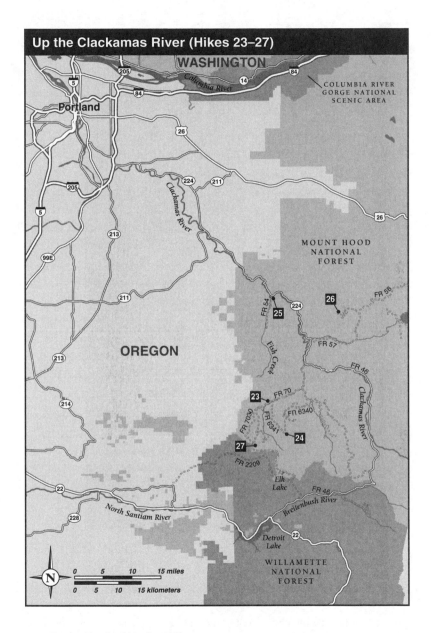

Up the Clackamas River (Hikes 23–27)

23 Bagby Hot Springs

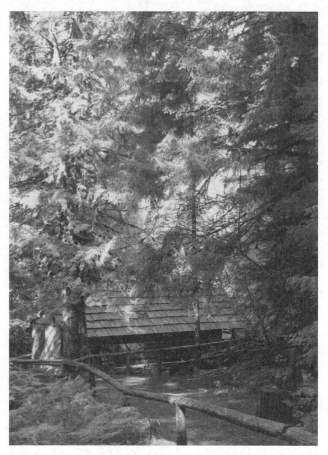

*The rustic bathhouses at Bagby Hot Springs are surrounded
by old-growth majesty and a fine mountain stream.*

In Brief

Unless you're uncomfortable about being among naked people, this is one place
you should absolutely visit; and even if you do dislike the disrobed, just avoid the
bathhouses. The hike isn't much of a challenge, but it passes through sublime ancient-
growth forest. And the springs feature cedar-log tubs, some of them private. It
can get very busy on weekends (though alcohol is now banned at the springs), and
an attendant at the trailhead lot should help reduce car break-ins.

LENGTH 3 miles round-trip to springs, 3.6 miles round-trip to Shower Creek	**BACKPACKING OPTIONS** Several (crowded) sites just past the springs, with many more up in the wilderness
CONFIGURATION Out-and-back	
DIFFICULTY Easy	**ACCESS** No charge just to park and hike; $5 soaking permit can be bought at the trailhead or from the store at Ripplebrook on the way.
SCENERY Old-growth forest, a mountain stream, and wooden tubs of hot water	
EXPOSURE Shady all the way	**WHEELCHAIR ACCESS** None
TRAFFIC Heavy	**MAPS** U.S. Forest Service *Bull of the Woods Wilderness,* U.S. Geological Survey *Bagby Hot Springs*
TRAIL SURFACE Packed dirt and crushed rock with some muddy spots in winter and spring	
HIKING TIME 2 hours (+ time for a soak)	**FACILITIES** Restrooms but no water at the trailhead or the springs; stream water must be treated.
DRIVING DISTANCE 74 miles (1 hour, 35 minutes) from Pioneer Courthouse Square	**INFO** Clackamas River Ranger District, 503-630-6861, **www.fs.usda.gov/mthood**
SEASON March–November; sometimes open in winter, but call ahead for conditions.	**SPECIAL COMMENTS** Don't leave any valuables in your car at this trailhead.
BEST TIME Weekdays April–October	

Description

It seems everybody in the area knows about Bagby, even those who've never been here. Just the word seems to stand for something about life in the Pacific Northwest: soothing, relaxing, a retreat from the hustle and bustle, a journey back to the days of the ancient forest and natural elements.

Well, it's not just that. It can get a little crazy on weekends, and the chances you'll be the only one there on any day are slim. On weekends you might have to wait to get your soak, unless you start early.

From the trailhead parking lot, start up the wide trail and cross the bridge over Nohorn Creek, named for an early pioneer in the area. The hiking is pleasant, the river pools inviting, and the forest inspiring. You might notice some old metal loops tacked high in the trees; those once held telephone wires that connected fire lookouts back in the 1930s. Cross a bridge over Hot Springs Fork Collawash River, and you're almost to the springs.

When you come to the springs area, the first thing you'll notice is the 1913 ranger cabin, which is listed on the National Register of Historic Places but isn't open to the public. It was a central communications station for those fire lookouts and also housed firefighters in season. I should mention that this cabin of 16-inch cedar logs was

Bagby Hot Springs

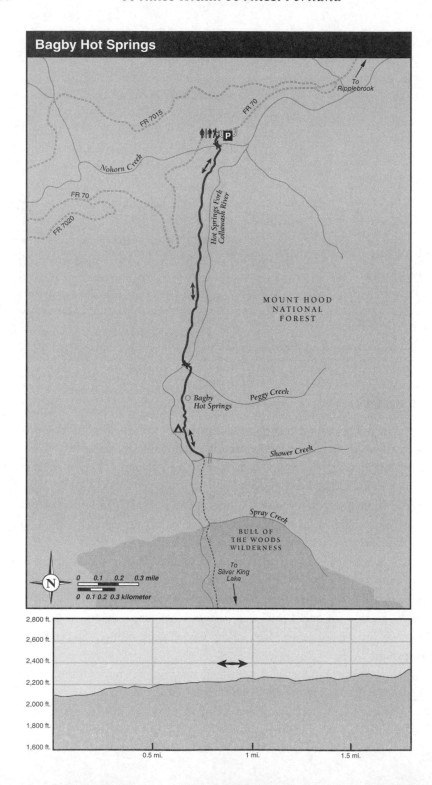

hand-built by one ranger, a certain Phil Putz, who first visited the area after walking 39 miles in one day. Do you think he was happy to arrive at the springs? The path behind the cabin leads to a monumental downed tree; check out the inside, which rotted away long before the giant was felled to keep it from squashing the bathhouses.

The bathhouse on the right has one big tub, with room for five or six adults. The one on the left has an open area with several tubs and five private rooms, each with a two-person log tub. The water comes out of the springs at 136°F and runs through a system of log flumes. To fill a tub, you just open up the valve and let the hot water in, then grab a bucket, fill it with cold water from a nearby tub, and get the temperature where you want it. Typically, a full tub needs four or five buckets of cold water to make it tolerable. As it cools off, just open up the valve and let some more hot water in. It's fantastic. Many bathers don't wear swimsuits, but outside the private rooms you're supposed to. The Forest Service seems to be paying more attention to this recently. If people are waiting, you'll also be asked to limit your soak to 1 hour.

Even if there's nobody around when you get to the springs, consider taking some time to explore farther up the trail before you soak. It's old-growth all the way, up Hot Springs Fork, past Shower Creek and Spray Creek, and eventually into Bull of the Woods Wilderness. You should go at least as far as Shower Creek (0.3 mile past the springs and just 0.1 mile past a camping area on the right) to enjoy the 50-foot falls and a little wooden platform somebody built underneath it so that folks could take a shower.

Beyond that, the trail continues 6 miles and ascends 1,800 feet to reach Silver King Lake, in the heart of the wilderness. Trails fan out from that area to many other great locations.

GPS Information and Directions

N44° 57.440' W122° 9.594'

Take OR 224 from Portland, traveling 44 miles southeast of I-205, through the town of Estacada, to the ranger station at Ripplebrook. Turn right on Forest Service Road (FR) 46, drive 3.6 miles, and make another right, onto FR 63. Drive 3.5 miles and turn right on FR 70. The trailhead is 6 miles ahead, on the left.

24 Bull of the Woods

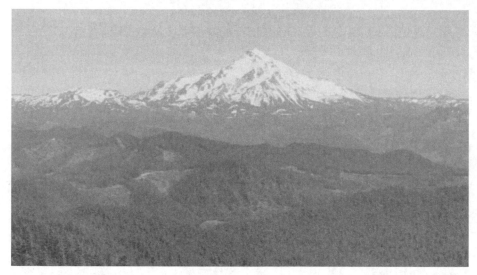

Mount Jefferson from Bull of the Woods lookout

In Brief

This is like two great hikes in one. Choose an easy stroll through old-growth forest past rhododendrons to two beautiful lakes, or a more challenging climb to a fire lookout tower with a panoramic view. Either way it will introduce you to a magnificent wilderness area.

Description

This trail has it all. Come in late June, as soon as the snow has cleared, and enjoy a mind-boggling display of rhododendrons among the old-growth forest on the way to Pansy Lake. (But bring bug repellent!)

Come in late summer and pick huckleberries up on the ridge. Or come in fall, when the ridge is awash in color and the mountains might see their first snow. Just make sure you get here; the long drive is more than worth it.

Bull of the Woods Peak is the second-highest point in the 27,000-acre Bull of the Woods Wilderness, which boasts more than a dozen lakes bigger than an acre,

LENGTH 2.2 miles round-trip to Pansy Lake; 7 miles round-trip to Bull of the Woods

CONFIGURATION Out-and-back, loop

DIFFICULTY Easy to Pansy Lake, strenuous to Bull of the Woods

SCENERY Old-growth forest, a mountain lake, rhododendrons, huckleberries, and a mountaintop panorama

EXPOSURE In the shade to the top of the ridge, then wide open

TRAFFIC Moderate on summer weekends, light otherwise

TRAIL SURFACE Packed dirt with some roots, then a few rocks up top

HIKING TIME 1 hour to Pansy Lake, 4 hours for everything

DRIVING DISTANCE 81 miles (2 hours) from Pioneer Courthouse Square

SEASON Late June–October

BEST TIME August and September

BACKPACKING OPTIONS Sites at Pansy Lake; better ones at other lakes in the wilderness

ACCESS No fees or permits

WHEELCHAIR ACCESS None

MAPS USFS *Bull of the Woods Wilderness,* USGS *Bull of the Woods*

FACILITIES None

INFO Clackamas River Ranger District, 503-630-6861, **www.fs.usda.gov/mthood**

68 miles of hiking trails, and even the world-famous northern spotted owl, which you almost certainly won't see.

From the start, on Pansy Lake Trail #551, you're walking through a beautiful forest on a basically flat trail. In 0.8 mile, you'll cross some nice little creeks, traverse gauntlets of rhododendrons, and ignore an unsigned trail on the right before reaching a signed trail junction. Dickey Lake Trail #549, coming down the hill from your left, is the return portion of the loop—take a right here, following a sign for Pansy Lake.

Just before the lake, you'll pass a sign that says T W I N L A K E S, but ignore it (for now) and continue straight to visit Pansy. A campsite on the right has excellent sitting rocks for picnicking or getting a quick rest and snack before you start up the hill.

Now, return to the trail and take what's now a right turn, following the T W I N L A K E S sign. You'll climb gradually for a while and then start a series of switchbacks. In just less than a mile from the lake, you'll gain 500 feet before you intersect Mother Lode Trail #558, in a saddle between Pansy Mountain and Bull of the Woods. Turn left onto Mother Lode.

While the switchbacks you just did were obviously steep, this trail is what I call "sneaky steep," which means that it doesn't look like much, but you'll feel the elevation gain. You're gaining about 700 feet in 1.1 miles, and since you're now going above 5,000 feet, you may start to feel the relative lack of oxygen. The forest in here is beautiful, though, and should take your mind off the climb. And if you're wondering why the

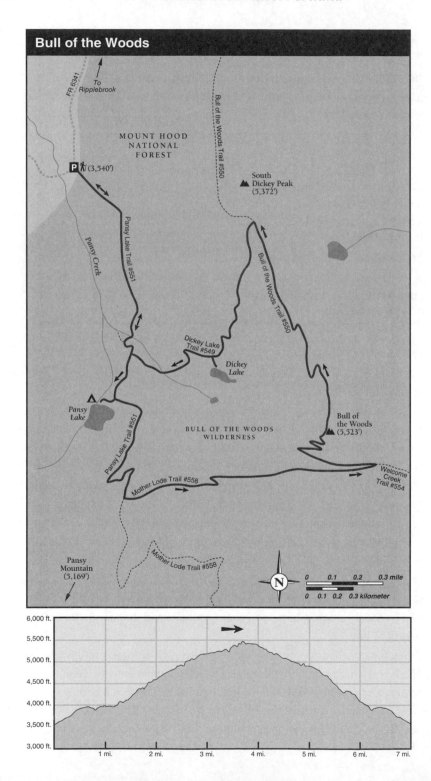

Bull of the Woods

FR 6341

To
Ripplebrook

MOUNT HOOD
NATIONAL
FOREST

Bull of the Woods Trail #550

South
Dickey Peak
(5,372')

P 🚶 (3,540')

Pansy Lake Trail #551

Pansy Creek

Dickey Lake
Trail #549

Dickey
Lake

Bull of the Woods Trail #550

Pansy
Lake

Bull of
the Woods
(5,523')

Pansy Lake Trail #551

BULL OF THE WOODS
WILDERNESS

Mother Lode Trail #558

Welcome
Creek
Trail #554

Pansy
Mountain
(5,169')

Mother Lode Trail #558

N

| 0 | 0.1 | 0.2 | 0.3 mile |
| 0 | 0.1 0.2 | 0.3 kilometer |

moss doesn't grow on the bottom 10 feet of the trunks, it's because that's how high the snow usually gets.

When you gain the top of the ridge and intersect Welcome Creek Trail #554, turn left, and with one more push through some switchbacks you'll pop out at the top of Bull of the Woods, with its old Forest Service fire lookout tower. Walk up onto the deck and have a look around.

You'll see Big Slide Lake below you, but Mount Jefferson, 20 miles away, dominates the view. On a clear day, you can see all the way from the Three Sisters on your right to Mount Rainier on your left. As the crow flies, it's about 175 miles from the Sisters to Rainier. Rest here and feel proud.

To continue the loop, find a trail junction in the trees on the opposite side of the watchtower from Mount Jefferson—this is Bull of the Woods Trail #550. Follow it to your right, along the ridge. You'll see occasional great views and many, many flowers in the next 1.1 miles, at which point you'll intersect Dickey Lake Trail #549. Take Dickey Lake Trail down and to the left, and you'll quickly lose elevation. Just past 0.5 mile, peer through the trees on your left to see Dickey Lake—a lake spied through branches is always a magical sight. Also, look for a trail that leads down to the lake itself; it's just past a meadow on Dickey Lake Trail.

After another 0.5 mile, most of it through a sea of rhododendrons, you'll get back to the trail where this whole thing started, Pansy Lake Trail #551. Turn right here and you'll be back to your car in no time.

Backpacking in the Wilderness

Without getting into too much detail, I'll just say that Bull of the Woods is an awesome place to go backpacking. Get yourself a map and make a couple nights of it. Lake Lenore, about 2 miles east of the lookout, is particularly appealing. The Welcome Lakes burned a few years back and aren't as nice. One great trip, with a reasonable car shuttle, would be to enter here, swing south by Twin Lakes and Silver King Lake, and come out for a soak at Bagby Hot Springs (see previous hike).

GPS Information and Directions

N44° 53.993' W122° 6.977'

Take OR 224 from Portland, traveling 44 miles southeast of I-205, through the town of Estacada, to the ranger station at Ripplebrook. Bear right to take Forest Service Road (FR) 46 and, 3.6 miles later, head right again to access FR 63. After 5.7 miles, turn right on FR 6340, following a sign for Bull of the Woods and Pansy Basin. At a junction 3.5 miles on, continue straight, still on FR 6340. Then, 4.4 miles past that junction (7.9 miles after FR 63), turn right on FR 6341, ignoring a sign to the left for Bull of the Woods Trail. The parking area is 3.6 miles ahead, on the right; the trailhead is across the road, on the left.

25 Clackamas River

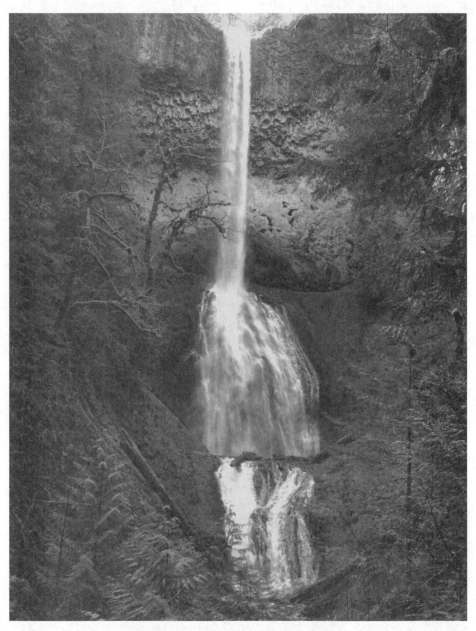

Pup Creek Falls, a highlight of this trail, is about halfway between the two trailheads.

LENGTH 7.8 miles one-way with shuttle, 7.2 miles round-trip to Pup Creek Falls

CONFIGURATION Point-to-point or out-and-back

DIFFICULTY Moderate

SCENERY Old-growth forest, a white-water river, fascinating rock formations, waterfalls

EXPOSURE Shady all the way, with occasional stretches on narrow trail high above the river

TRAFFIC Heavy on nice-weather weekends, light–moderate otherwise

TRAIL SURFACE Packed dirt with roots and rocks; one creek ford if you do the whole thing

HIKING TIME 5 hours for either option

DRIVING DISTANCE 50 miles (1 hour) from Pioneer Courthouse Square

SEASON Year-round; muddy and possibly snowy in winter and spring

BEST TIME May for flowers and much water, October for fall colors

BACKPACKING OPTIONS A few good sites

ACCESS $5 parking fee at Fish Creek (Northwest Forest Pass *not* accepted); no fee at Indian Henry

WHEELCHAIR ACCESS None

MAPS Green Trails *Map 492 (Fish Creek Mountain)*

FACILITIES Restrooms at Fish Creek Trailhead; campgrounds at Fish Creek and Indian Henry; water along the way must be treated.

INFO Clackamas River Ranger District, 503-630-6861, **www.fs.usda.gov/mthood**

SPECIAL COMMENTS Just before press time, two sections of the Clackamas River Trail were closed due to washouts caused by winter storms: 1.8 miles up from the Fish Creek Trailhead and 6 miles down from Indian Henry Campground. The U.S. Forest Service says repairs may take several months to complete, so call ahead or check the website above for the latest info.

In Brief

Convenient, not too tough, and not terribly long, Clackamas River Trail is a great way to stretch your legs and enjoy the scenery among old trees and along a beautiful river. With only one car, do an out-and-back from either trailhead to Pup Creek Falls, but with two do the whole thing with a car shuttle.

Description

As noted above, the Clackamas River Trail was closed at press time in two sections due to winter-storm damage. The route described below assumes the trail is open.

On that rare nice day in early spring—*nice* meaning it's not pouring—when you want to get out and do some hiking, here you'll find ferry slipper orchids and Clackamas lily in bloom. And if it's blazing-hot in summer and you want to visit a cool, shady

Clackamas River

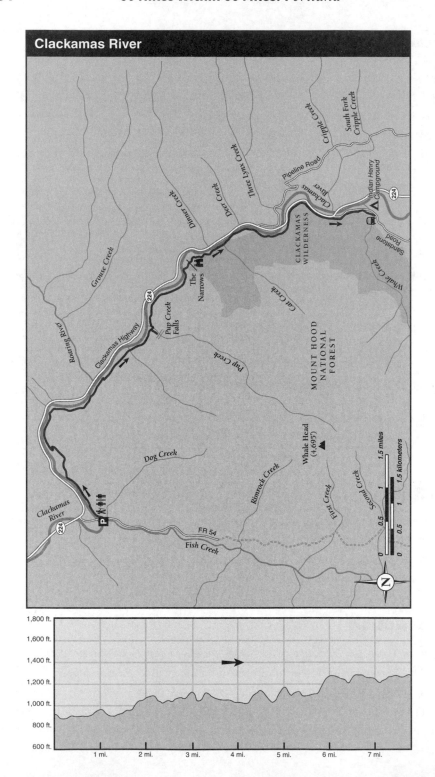

place, or it's autumn and you want to see the fall colors—whatever the time, it's always a nice day to go out and hike the Clackamas River Trail. If you can bring a second car to stash at Indian Henry, it'll be that much better. Otherwise, you can do essentially the same distance and make a fine day of it. (You'll avoid a potentially wet-footed creek crossing if you come in from a single car at Fish Creek.)

From the trailhead, you'll start out in a flat section with the river a short distance to your left. After 0.5 mile you'll come to a river-access point with moss-covered rocks and a sandy beach—perfect for chilling out or perhaps, if you've brought small kids, for turning around. Soon after, you'll come into the first exceptional old-growth forest, featuring 5-foot-thick Douglas-firs and even bigger Western red cedars. In the next mile or so of trail, you'll do a little climbing and occasionally find yourself with some pretty serious drops to and views of the river to your left. Much of this early section burned in 2004, so you can check on how it's recovering.

If you're wondering about a good place to picnic or spend the night, you'll find a campsite 1.5 miles in, but a better one is 2.5 miles up. There's a stupendous Western red cedar right by the water here and plenty of places to sit and gaze at the river. OR 224 is right across the river, by the way, but you'll hardly notice it. Again, if you've brought kids, think about turning around here, because in the next mile you'll go up, down, then up again (a couple hundred feet each time), and occasionally find the river a potentially treacherous 200 feet below you.

After you've hiked a total of 3.5 up-and-down miles and descended a hill to find yourself under power lines, you'll come to a trail on the right, just before Pup Creek. This leads 0.2 mile up the creek to a view of beautiful Pup Creek Falls, with a total drop of some 230 feet. If you didn't stash a car at Indian Henry, turn around here and you'll have a 7.2-mile hike. If you did leave a second car there, keep on trucking.

The ford of Pup Creek, even at low-water times, can be a bit tricky. In spring it would be hard to keep your feet dry, so consider bringing some sandals and hiking poles. Just beyond it, the trail goes under the power lines for a bit, meaning you can get some sunshine and find some flat land to enjoy lunch or a break.

In 0.9 mile a side trail will lead left to another beach, and right after that you'll climb to a view up the Clackamas that includes The Narrows, a spectacular gouge in ancient lava. Down the other side of this hill, a side trail to the left will lead 0.1 mile to The Narrows themselves. Also here, you'll find a nice campsite and enter the new Clackamas Wilderness, created by the Mount Hood Wilderness Act of 2009.

By the way, if you've seen some cables crossing the river in a few spots and wondered what that's about, they were put in by Portland General Electric for cable-car access across the river to maintain their power lines.

In the last 3 miles to Indian Henry Campground, you'll cross several side creeks (the biggest one named Cat Creek), see numerous giant trees, get sprayed by a waterfall, pass two more campsites and a mossy "weeping wall," and go under a cliff and several amazing rock formations—in other words, enjoy a chorus of forest pleasures. I would offer more details, but I've never managed to maintain a GPS connection in here, and besides, let's leave something of mystery in these woods. It's a beautiful and easy stretch of trail that I encourage you to explore.

Nearby Activities

If you haven't had enough riverside fun, stop by **Promontory Park** and its 350-acre **North Fork Reservoir** (40600 SE Highway 224, Estacada, OR 97023). The park has a marina, a campground with showers, and a store where you can get all your fishing supplies and licenses, rent boats, and enjoy an ice cream when you're done fishing. (Small Fry Lake is for kiddie fishing only.) Campsites are $16 per night and can be reserved at 503-622-7229; for more info on the park and marina, call 503-630-5152. You can also visit **portlandgeneral.com** and click "Community & Environment," then "Parks & Campgrounds."

GPS Information and Directions

Fish Creek Trailhead N45° 9.456' W122° 9.051'
Indian Henry Campground N45° 6.529' W122° 4.526'

Take OR 224 from Portland, traveling a total of 33 miles southeast of I-205. Fifteen miles past Estacada, just after crossing two bridges in quick succession, turn right onto Fish Creek Road. Pass Fish Creek Campground, cross another bridge, and park in the parking lot on the right, 0.5 mile up from OR 224 on Forest Service Road 52. The trail starts across the road, on your left. To leave a car at the other end, drive another 7 miles on OR 224 and make a right onto Sandstone Road toward Indian Henry Campground. The trailhead is 0.5 mile up, on the right.

26 Roaring River Wilderness

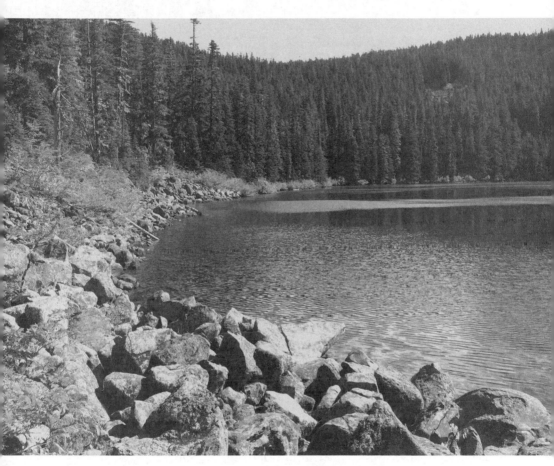

Deep, beautiful Serene Lake offers several nice campsites. The best one is in those trees at the far end.

In Brief

This hike requires an extended drive to a long, up-and-down forested loop. On the upside, it comprises six lakes, a flower-filled meadow, late-summer huckleberries, views of five Cascades volcanoes, and a beautiful forest that you'll probably have largely to yourself. Lovely, shorter options exist, but if you want to do the whole thing, consider backpacking or car-camp at Hideaway Lake, near the trailhead.

LENGTH 1.4 miles round-trip to Shellrock Lake, 5 miles round-trip to the Rock Lakes, 12.6 miles to do the whole thing

CONFIGURATION Out-and-back or balloon

DIFFICULTY Easy to Shellrock, moderate to Rock Lakes, strenuous for the whole loop

SCENERY Peaceful old-growth forest, several lakes, a meadow, a nice viewpoint

EXPOSURE Shady most of the way, with a few open spots

TRAFFIC Light on summer weekends, almost none otherwise

TRAIL SURFACE Packed dirt with roots and rocks

HIKING TIME 1 hour to Shellrock Lake, 3 hours to Rock Lakes, 7 hours for the whole loop

DRIVING DISTANCE 82 miles (2 hours, 10 minutes) from Pioneer Courthouse Square

SEASON July–October

BEST TIME August and September

BACKPACKING OPTIONS Fantastic!

ACCESS No fees or permits

WHEELCHAIR ACCESS None

MAPS Green Trails *Map 492 (Fish Creek Mountain)* and *Map 493 (High Rock)*

FACILITIES Nearby at Hideaway Lake Campground; none at trailhead. Water on trail should be treated.

INFO Clackamas River Ranger District, 503-630-6861, **www.fs.usda.gov/mthood**

Description

It used to be that you could drive to Frazier Turnaround, knocking some 3.6 miles off this hike. And technically, you still can. But I can no longer, in good conscience, send people down this road—I've been cursed for doing so—and besides, hiking in this new way adds another lake and more lovely forest to the experience.

Consider camping at Hideaway Lake before you do this hike; start early in the morning to beat the crowds, and you can go for a swim when you get back in the heat of the afternoon. Although this loop never goes below 4,000 feet or above 5,000 feet, its cumulative elevation gain is more than 2,500 feet!

At the trailhead for Shellrock Lake Trail #700, you may at first wonder why you're here. Hiking through a clearcut for half a mile doesn't exactly scream "wilderness," but there are plenty of flowers, and at least the trail is nearly flat. The reward for your patience is big, beautiful Shellrock Lake, with campsites galore and stocked trout— a fine, easy destination if you have kids or just don't care about putting in the miles.

To keep going, walk along the right side of the lake and climb the hill, following a sign for Frazier Turnaround. It gets rocky in places, and mildly steep, until 1 mile past the lake, where you'll hit Grouse Point Trail #517. Turn right (downhill) here, and in a moment you'll arrive at Frazier Turnaround, the old trailhead.

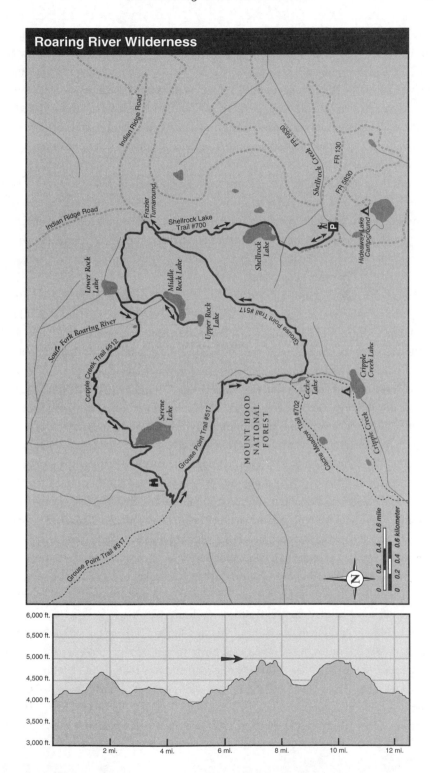

Roaring River Wilderness

Look for Serene Lake Trail #512 going downhill and to the left, and follow it 0.8 mile down to a junction. The loop keeps going here, but you should definitely go left a flat 0.25 mile to Middle Rock Lake, which has a few nice campsites. Turn right when you get to the lake, cross the outlet creek, walk to the far end of the lake, then follow a short trail up the hill to Upper Rock Lake, the smallest of the three—and host to a single, private, dreamy campsite. That trail gets a little brushy and can be tough to follow in early summer. The side trip to Middle and Upper Rock Lakes adds just over a mile to your day.

From the main trail, if you didn't turn left for Middle Rock Lake, go another couple hundred yards and you'll come to a trail leading right, to Lower Rock Lake, which has one inferior campsite. Lower and Middle Rock Lakes are stocked with trout, by the way, so if you're into fishing, get a license and bring your rod. If you've got small kids or you feel done for the day, you're now 3 miles from your car. But for an even nicer lake, and then some, keep going.

You'll put in another mile going downhill, then turn up (steeply at times) for most of a mile to gain the top of a ridge, thick with beargrass. Just over the top of the hill (now 4.3 miles from the trailhead), you'll come to Serene Lake and a signed trail leading left, to a sunny campsite on the shore. Serene Lake is just what its name implies; anglers pull 15-inch trout from its deep, cold, green water, and the same boulders, grassy shallows, downed trees, and thickly vegetated shoreline that hide the fish also make for outstanding scenery for humans. This is the finest lake of the loop. Follow the right-hand shoreline to continue our hike.

If you're camping, you can choose from several excellent spots, one of which in 2013 had an Adirondack chair and table (who put that there?) at the trail junction, one at the far end on a point that sticks out into the lake, and another on the left side. There's also a huge boulder about 100 yards along the shoreline from the trail junction—an awesome spot to jump into the (very cold) lake. A decent trail circles the lake, but you'll have to cross a couple of rockslides to make the full circuit.

Beyond Serene Lake, the trail climbs about 600 feet in less than a mile to the top of a ridge and a junction with Grouse Point Trail #517. Turn left here, climb 200 more feet, and in 0.7 mile you'll reach a clearcut that was put in for helicopters to drop off firefighters. Not a romantic history, but a cliff affords a sublime view back down to Serene Lake and out to Mounts St. Helens, Rainier, Adams, and Hood. The two bare peaks to the right are the Signal Buttes. Also, as you look north toward Hood, you're seeing an area of about 8 miles, as the crow flies, with only one road and two trails to break it up.

The trail now drops 700 feet in a mile, and when you get to the flower-filled Cache Meadow, you'll find an intersection. The right-hand trail leads out to another road; another heads into the meadow, where you can see the lily-filled Cache Lake to the left.

To continue the loop, turn left and go 200 yards to the site of an old shelter. From here, you can cross the seasonal creek on your right and go 0.2 mile to Cripple Creek Lake, yet another mountain beauty with a couple of campsites. They're everywhere!

A minute past the shelter site, turn left to stay on Grouse Point Trail #517 and take it uphill 1 mile (you'll get all of that 700 feet back!) until you come to an abandoned road. Turn right, and in just under a mile you'll be back at the trail leading down to Shellrock Lake and your car. Just keep an eye out, in the clear areas along the road, for a view back to Mount Jefferson. That makes this a six-lake, five-volcano hike!

GPS Information and Directions

N45° 7.627' W121° 58.238'

Take OR 224 from Portland, traveling 44 miles southeast of I-205, through the town of Estacada, to the ranger station at Ripplebrook. Half a mile past the ranger station, turn left onto Forest Service Road (FR) 57. After 7.6 miles, turn left onto FR 58. Drive 3 miles, then turn left onto FR 5830 and follow it 5.7 miles, staying left at one unsigned junction, to the Shellrock Lake Trailhead, on the right just past Hideaway Lake Campground.

27 Whetstone Mountain

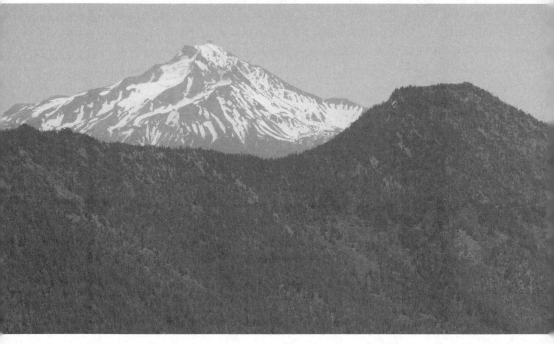

Mount Jefferson and Battle Ax Mountain, viewed from Whetstone Mountain

In Brief

It's a long, tedious drive. And it isn't much of a hike if you're looking for a ton of exercise. But my goodness, what a view you get from Whetstone Mountain! And for what it's worth, you can do an up-close comparison of a clearcut and old-growth forest. This hike is also a gateway into both Opal Creek Wilderness and Bull of the Woods Wilderness.

Description

Whetstone Mountain got its name in pioneer days because of a prevalence in the area of a rock that was useful for sharpening knives. The peak hosted a fire lookout tower for many years, but both it and the useful rock appear to be long gone. What's left, though, is an easy-to-reach viewpoint that rivals anything in the area.

LENGTH 4.8 miles round-trip

CONFIGURATION Out-and-back

DIFFICULTY Moderate

SCENERY Old-growth forest on the way up, a sweeping mountain view up top

EXPOSURE Shady all the way; some mildly sketchy side-hill sections

TRAFFIC Moderate on summer weekends, light otherwise

TRAIL SURFACE Some rock at the very top

HIKING TIME 3 hours

DRIVING DISTANCE 74 miles (2 hours) from Pioneer Courthouse Square

SEASON June–October

BEST TIME June for rhodies, October for fall colors

BACKPACKING OPTIONS Not good on this trail but plentiful in Bull of the Woods Wilderness (see Hike 24, page 128)

ACCESS No fees or permits

WHEELCHAIR ACCESS None

MAPS Green Trails *Map 524 Battle Ax,* USFS *Bull of the Woods Wilderness*

FACILITIES None at trailhead

INFO Clackamas River Ranger District, 503-630-6861, **www.fs.usda.gov/mthood**

SPECIAL COMMENTS Consider doing this hike as part of an overnight trip to the area—it takes almost as long to get here as it does to hike the trail.

You can actually see your destination from the extensive trailhead, which sits in the middle of a lovely clearcut. Whetstone is the forested ridge right in front of you, and a little to the left in the distance you can see flat-topped Battle Ax Mountain (see next hike). Your route to Whetstone is to head toward it, swing to the left, gain that ridge you see, then ascend the other side to the tiny, rocky summit.

When you start out hiking downhill, don't be concerned—you're on the right trail. You'll descend about 0.25 mile, passing rhododendrons (which bloom in late June) and huckleberries (ripe mid-August). This area was cut around 1980 and then replanted, so you have a chance to see how it's recovering. It's when you enter Bull of the Woods Wilderness, about 0.2 mile in, that you'll see the amazing difference between cut and uncut forest. You'll get a bigger-picture view of this later.

Around the time you start uphill, about 0.3 mile in, look for a nice meadow on the right with a spring, then cross a couple of its outlets. Just past 0.5 mile, you'll reach the base of a rockslide with a pond on your left, then go through a few switchbacks— one with a nice view of Mount Hood on the left—as you get up onto the ridge.

At the ridgeline, just over a mile into the hike, you'll intersect Whetstone Mountain Trail #3369. You've been on Whetstone Trail #546, and if you're wondering, you've gone from three digits to four because you've just hiked from Mount Hood National Forest to Willamette National Forest. Turn right on Whetstone Mountain

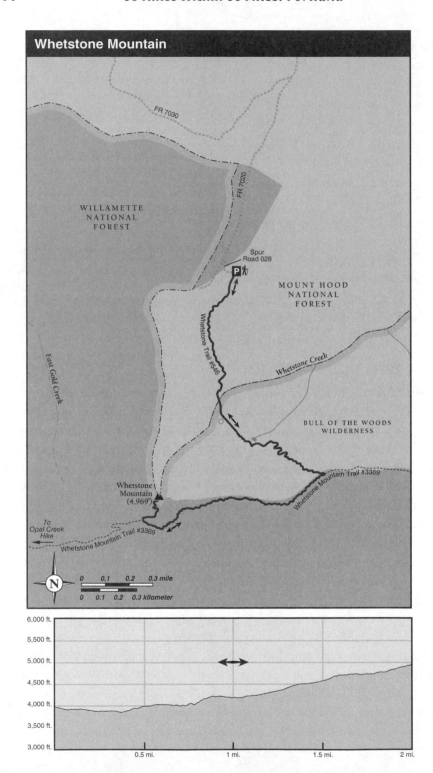

Trail #3369 and start a slow ascent along the north side of the ridge, with occasional views down and to the left into Opal Creek Wilderness. In a couple of places you'll be walking on a side-hill section of trail with a fairly steep drop to the left, but the good news is you'll also be, in August, walking through Huckleberry Heaven.

When you've gone about a mile since the turn, you'll reach another right turn, this time up the short, steep trail to the rocky summit; going left here would drop you 3.5 miles to an intersection early in the Opal Creek hike (Hike 30, page 158). Gaining Whetstone's summit requires a few steps on rocky terrain, but nothing challenging. Besides, when you get there, the summit is so small, and so high relative to its surroundings, you may feel like you're airborne.

Catch your breath, then let's do the visual tour. The easy way to start is to find Mount Hood to the northeast. Left of that is Mount Adams, and left of that is Mount Rainier. To the right of Hood, and seemingly at your feet, a ridge heads east toward unseen Silver King Lake, in the heart of Bull of the Woods (Hike 24) and at the top of the Bagby Hot Springs hike (Hike 23). The right side of that ridge is the drainage for Battle Ax Creek, which joins Opal Creek at Jawbone Flats, almost directly beneath you.

In the distance to the east is knob-topped Olallie Butte, and right of that is Mount Jefferson, 25 miles away but seemingly right behind Battle Ax, which is 5 miles away. Still moving right, look for crumbly Three-Fingered Jack; the next pointy one to the right is Mount Washington, followed by tiny-looking Coffin Mountain and then the Three Sisters and Broken Top, and way out there is Diamond Peak, just north of Crater Lake. Near as I can figure, the straight-line distance from Diamond to Rainier is about 225 miles.

Quite a view, eh? Worth the drive? Thought so. If you're looking for some back-packing options, you won't find anything good on this trail, but Bull of the Woods is filled with lakes and trails and campsites—just turn left at the intersection on the ridge, instead of right as you did to get here. But if you're thinking of a car shuttle to Opal Creek, consider this: You could hike from this trailhead to that one in about 6 miles, but the drive on Forest Service Road (FR) 46 is more than 60 miles!

GPS Information and Directions

N44° 52.522' W122° 12.157'

From Portland on OR 224, drive 44 miles southeast of I-205, through the town of Estacada, to the ranger station at Ripplebrook. Turn right onto FR 46 and then, 3.6 miles later, right again onto FR 63. After 3.5 miles on FR 63, turn right onto FR 70 and drive 9.6 miles—stay right at an unmarked junction around 8 miles—before turning left onto FR 7030. Drive 5.7 miles on FR 7030, turn right onto FR 7020, and then drive 0.6 mile to Spur Road 028, on the left. The trailhead is at the end of that road, 0.1 mile ahead.

UP THE SANTIAM RIVER

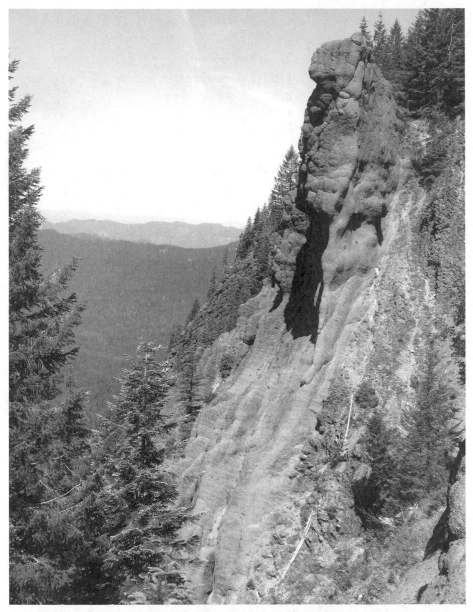

Rock formations just below Battle Ax Mountain (see Hike 28)

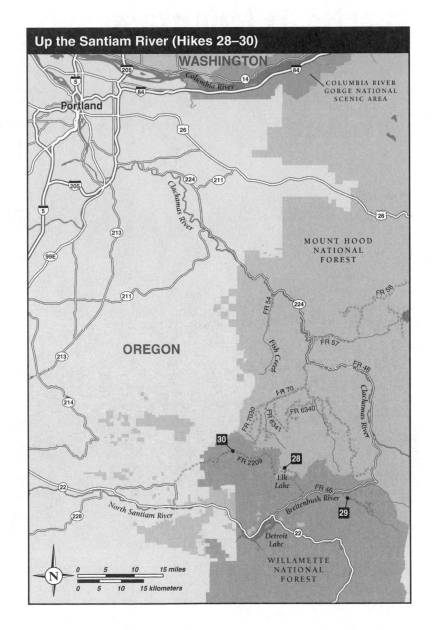

Up the Santiam River (Hikes 28–30)

28 Battle Ax Mountain

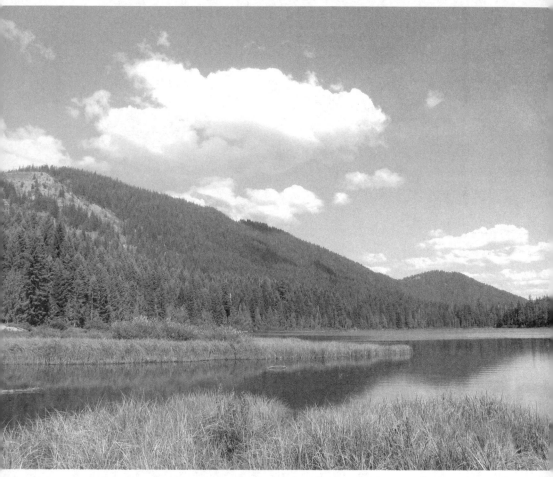

It's a rough road to Elk Lake, but the camping is free and the hiking tremendous.

In Brief

It's a long drive on a bumpy road. And parts of the hike up are rather dull. So why hike Battle Ax? Three reasons: one of the greatest views among all the hikes in this whole book, few fellow hikers, and easy access to a fantastic, lake-filled wilderness area.

LENGTH 5.1 miles from the trailhead, 6.5 miles from the campground	**BEST TIME** August and September
CONFIGURATION Loop	**BACKPACKING OPTIONS** Plenty in the vicinity, though limited on this trail; see end of profile for details.
DIFFICULTY Strenuous	**ACCESS** No fees or permits
SCENERY Forest, rock formations, mountain vistas	**WHEELCHAIR ACCESS** None
EXPOSURE Lots of time in the open; some rocky slopes and side hills	**MAPS** U.S. Geological Survey *Bull of the Woods Wilderness*
TRAFFIC Light	**FACILITIES** Restrooms (but no drinkable water) at nearby Elk Lake Campground
TRAIL SURFACE Rocky in places	
HIKING TIME 4 hours	**INFO** Detroit Ranger District, 503-854-3366, www.fs.usda.gov/willamette
DRIVING DISTANCE 102 miles (2 hours) from Pioneer Courthouse Square	**SPECIAL COMMENTS** The road to this trailhead is pretty bumpy; check ahead for current conditions.
SEASON June–October	

Description

OK, let's start with the road, because there's a chance that when you mentioned Battle Ax Mountain or Elk Lake to friends, they told you some horror story about having their teeth rattled out of their heads while driving up there. First, the road has been worked on quite a bit in the last few years, and second, I got my 1992 Nissan Sentra up there with no problem. Sure, I was going 5 miles an hour at times, but I made it just fine. Just drive around the bigger potholes and rocks, and you'll be all right. And while you're up there, consider spending the night at the campground, which costs only $10 but has a reputation for a little weekend rowdiness.

Now, the hike. If you drive to the trailhead, you'll knock 1.4 miles off your walk, and I'll describe it as if you did that. (If you're parked at the campground, just walk back up to the fork and go left to reach the trailhead.) It isn't too exciting at first, winding up Bagby Trail #544 through thick forest. The initial 0.6 mile gains 500 feet to reach a pair of small ponds, and 0.2 mile past them it flattens out to start a 1-mile traverse along the northeast side of Battle Ax. So, at this point, you're actually walking away from the peak, which will be visible over your left shoulder.

Halfway across this traverse, you'll enter an impressive rockslide where, if you give a shout, you'll notice that the sound really bounces around. The far end of this slide offers a great view back to Battle Ax; and don't worry, you're not going up that side of it. You'll next cross a series of brushy, spring-fed forks of Battle Creek, with views north into the heart of Bull of the Woods Wilderness.

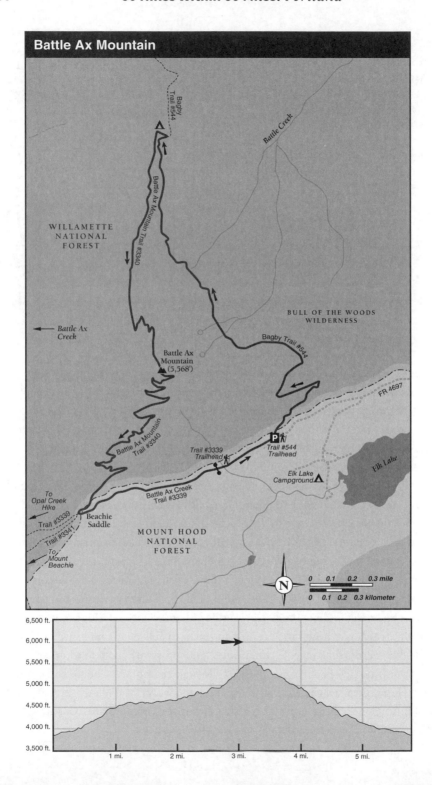

Battle Ax Mountain

Bagby Trail #544

Battle Creek

Battle Ax Mountain Trail #3340

WILLAMETTE NATIONAL FOREST

Battle Ax Creek

Battle Ax Mountain (5,568')

BULL OF THE WOODS WILDERNESS

Bagby Trail #544

FR 4697

Battle Ax Mountain Trail #3340

Trail #3339 Trailhead

Trail #544 Trailhead

Elk Lake Campground

Elk Lake

To Opal Creek Hike

Trail #3339

Trail #3341

Beachie Saddle

Battle Ax Creek Trail #3339

MOUNT HOOD NATIONAL FOREST

To Mount Beachie

N

0   0.1   0.2   0.3 mile

0   0.1   0.2   0.3 kilometer

6,500 ft.

6,000 ft.

5,500 ft.

5,000 ft.

4,500 ft.

4,000 ft.

3,500 ft.

1 mi.   2 mi.   3 mi.   4 mi.   5 mi.

When you're 1.8 miles from the trailhead, the trail intersects Battle Ax Mountain Trail #3340, heading up and to the left. You'll also see, on the right, one of the more pitiful campsites of your life. It's a nice place for a rest or snack before you start climbing, but if you're looking to camp overnight, check the backpacking options below.

While you're resting and snacking, perhaps you'd like to know where Battle Ax got its name. One theory is pretty simple: From some views, it's shaped like an ax. Another theory is that an old woodsman named it for a brand of chewing tobacco that was popular in the 1890s; apparently he chewed a lot of it while exploring the area. I say we go with that one.

To get up Battle Ax, take the trail from this junction, and soon you'll be climbing and in the sun, as the forest thins out and you approach 5,000 feet in elevation. Another rockslide offers a view southeast to Mount Jefferson, as does a rocky bowl 0.3 mile up. After 0.5 mile of climbing, you'll cross over the ridge, and then your view will be west, down Battle Ax Creek—not to be confused with Battle Creek (on the other side)—and into the Opal Creek Wilderness.

Now you'll switchback up 0.6 mile, gaining a final 600 feet to put you at the north end of the broad, flat summit. Look for remnants of the old fire lookout, and a 1947 benchmark from the U.S. Coast and Geodetic Survey, which hasn't been an independent agency since 1970.

A big rock at the southern end of the peak offers a great view back down to Elk Lake, 1,800 feet below. Otherwise, you can see from Mount Hood to the Three Sisters. Try to spot the distinctive Coffin Mountain and Whetstone Mountain (see previous hike), both of which are on the far side of Opal Creek Wilderness (Hike 30, page 158).

To go down, we'll aim for Beachie Saddle, between Elk Lake and Battle Ax Creek. Take the trail that heads to the right (when looking at the lake) from near the southern end of the summit, and descend a series of rocky, dusty, sun-drenched switchbacks. (This is why you came up the other way!) Some of this trail is also mildly exposed on steep, rocky sidehills—nothing life-threatening, but a fall would ruin your day.

A little less than a mile downhill, you'll pass some neat rock formations. Check out Mount Beachie, across the way. It looks like somebody took a saw to the summit, cut out a rectangular chunk, and planted a tree in it. You can go up there later, if you want.

A mile and a half below the summit, you'll come to Beachie Saddle and an old road that is now Battle Ax Creek Trail #3339, to your right; this leads 4 miles down to Jawbone Flats in the middle of Opal Creek Wilderness, passing lots of old railroad and mining relics along the way. So the walk from Elk Lake to Jawbone Flats on the trail is about 5.5 miles; the drive is 46 miles. (I think these facts are fascinating.) Above you is Mount Beachie, with a well-shot-up sign marking the start of that 1.5-mile, 800-foot climb.

To get to your car, head left and down the gravel road, which is at times a trail and at times something less than that. You'll pass the trailhead for Battle Ax Creek Trail #3339—imagine driving there!—0.2 mile before our original trailhead, which is 0.7 mile from the campground and the lake you now deserve to jump into.

Backpacking Options

Since you're at the corner of two wilderness areas, why not use this simple hike as a way into the backcountry? Options abound—as do a dozen lakes at least an acre in size—in Bull of the Woods. From the pitiful campsite at the junction above, it's about 3 miles (descending 800 feet!) to Twin Lakes, which are right in the middle of the wilderness. Get a map and go for it; with a long car shuttle, you could even end the hike at Bagby Hot Springs! So many choices . . .

GPS Information and Directions

N44° 49.513' W122° 7.500'

Take I-5 South from Portland, driving 45 miles to Exit 253/Detroit Lake. Drive east 49 miles on OR 22 to the town of Detroit, then turn left onto Forest Service Road (FR) 46, following signs for Breitenbush Hot Springs. After 4.4 miles, turn left on FR 4696—note that from here on, many intersections have no signs. Drive 0.8 mile on FR 4696 and turn left on FR 4697, following it 2.2 miles to a T-intersection, where you'll turn right. Drive 1.8 miles and make a left. This is where the road gets rough(er). Follow it 2.1 miles to another left, then 0.3 mile to a fork just above the campground: Here, you can bear right—on an even bumpier road—and drive 0.4 mile to reach the trailhead, on the right, or you can turn left and drive 0.3 mile to park in the campground.

29 Breitenbush Hot Springs Area

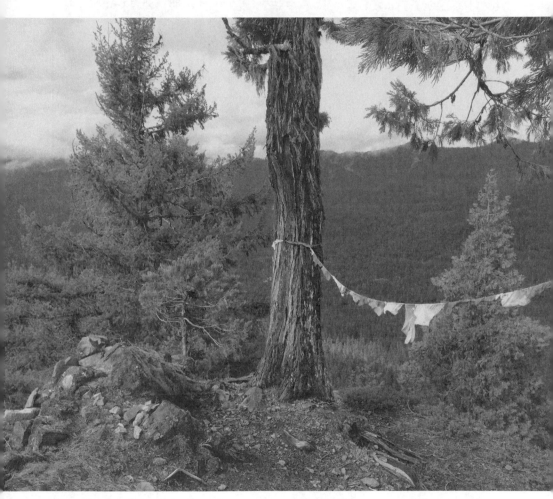

Tibetan prayer flags fly at Devils Lookout, the best vista point on Devils Ridge Trail.

In Brief

With its combination of old-growth majesty and New Age spirituality, the area around Breitenbush Hot Springs is one of the most serene and inspiring places in Oregon. The trails are plentiful and (mostly) easy, the surroundings are sublime, and the water is hot.

LENGTH 1–8 miles round-trip	**BACKPACKING OPTIONS** A few options along the South Fork Breitenbush
CONFIGURATION Out-and-back or point-to-point with shuttle	**ACCESS** Northwest Forest Pass (see page 3) to park on FR 4685, day-use fee to park at hot springs (see Nearby Activities)
DIFFICULTY Easy–strenuous	
SCENERY Ancient forest, river, a narrow gorge, a mountain viewpoint	**WHEELCHAIR ACCESS** None
EXPOSURE Shady all the way, except some rocky areas on the hilltops	**MAPS** USGS *Breitenbush Hot Springs;* free maps at resort office
TRAFFIC Moderate–light	**FACILITIES** None at trailhead; full services at hot springs
TRAIL SURFACE Packed dirt, a few roots	
HIKING TIME 30 minutes–5 hours	**INFO** Breitenbush Hot Springs Resort, 503-854-3320, **breitenbush.com;** Detroit Ranger District, 503-854-3366, **www.fs.usda.gov/willamette**
DRIVING DISTANCE 103 miles (2 hours) from Pioneer Courthouse Square	
SEASON April–November	**SPECIAL COMMENTS** Even if all you plan to do is hike, you need to check in at the resort; there's now a welcome desk at the parking lot.
BEST TIME September and October, for fall colors and fewer crowds	

Description

Like a refuge of tranquility amid a sea of logging operations, the area along the South Fork Breitenbush River is often described with words like *peaceful, magical,* and *special.* The resort is itself a draw—with its pools, tubs, well-being programs, massage, and other healing arts—but easy, pleasant walks through the forest and along the river beckon.

Starting at the Resort Lot

One option is simply to register for a day pass at the hot-springs resort (see Nearby Activities) and start your hike at the Spotted Owl Trailhead, across from the parking lot. After 1.1 miles on that trail, you'll come to a junction with Cliff Trail. Turn right on Cliff Trail and climb a fairly steep 0.5 mile, including some semiexposed sections along a cliff, to an intersection with Devils Ridge Trail, which climbs steeply to Devils Lookout and Devils Peak. (If you'd rather stay on Spotted Owl Trail instead of turning on Cliff Trail, you'll come to Emerald Forest Trail in 0.5 mile at a junction that we'll describe below.) The hot springs also has a hiking map, so you can just ignore my directions and take an unplanned spiritual walkabout, if you prefer. Call ahead for day use and get in a soak afterward.

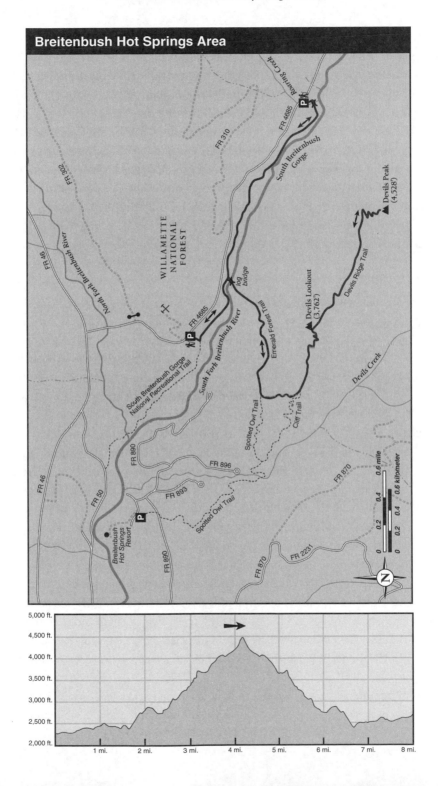

Breitenbush Hot Springs Area

Breitenbush Gorge

For the shortest hike in the area, walk about a mile round-trip to see Breitenbush Gorge, a 100-yard-long, 40-foot-deep chasm that the river rips through. From the upper trailhead on Forest Service Road (FR) 4685, start downhill and, after a couple of minutes, turn right at a sign for Breitenbush Gorge. Cross Roaring Creek on a log bridge and look for a nice river viewpoint on the left just afterward. After 0.3 mile, you'll pass through an open area where lots of trees were blown down by a storm on Thanksgiving Day in 1999.

To find the gorge from this area—the junction is strangely unsigned—walk a couple more minutes and look for two parallel logs pointing downhill between a big cedar and a root ball with ferns and hemlock saplings. The "trail" drops 100 feet or so to a viewpoint; here, the gorge has several big logs lying across it. A little trail heading left and under some logs leads to a view of the upper part of the gorge.

Emerald Forest and Devils Ridge

The most recommended hike starts at the lower parking area on FR 4685. From here, walk 0.1 mile downhill and turn left onto South Breitenbush Gorge National Recreation Trail. You will hear only the river at this point, so for views you'll have to "settle" for the big Douglas-firs, hemlocks, and Western red cedars towering over you and the cloverlike oxalis and early-summer wildflowers. Rhododendrons bloom here in June.

After 0.7 mile, you'll come to a descending trail on the right, signed E M E R A L D F O R E S T. (If you opt to continue straight and bypass the Emerald Forest Trail, it's a 1-mile flat hike to the gorge.) Take the Emerald Forest Trail 0.1 mile downhill to the South Fork Breitenbush River, which hikers used to cross on an official bridge. The same 1999 storm rolled this one-log bridge over on its side, officially closing it; you can still see it to the left. But subsequent storms blew several more trees down over the river, and someone added a helpful handrail to one of these logs. Cross it, and on the other side climb 0.5 mile on Emerald Forest Trail through as pretty a forest as you'll ever see.

When you've gone 0.8 mile past the bridge, your path intersects Devils Ridge Trail. Along the way, you may notice a sign referring to the Neotropical Migratory Bird Conservation Program, which was a program of small grants that improved habitats for birds in Central and South America; many of those birds come here for the summer. Make a right, toward Spotted Owl Trail, if you want to return to the hot springs. But if you're looking for some serious exercise and a spectacular view, turn left onto Devils Ridge Trail, which soon becomes quite steep in its 0.3-mile climb to a junction with Cliff Trail.

From this intersection, you can turn right and loop back, again toward Spotted Owl Trail and the resort, passing a viewpoint atop steep cliffs about 0.2 mile from here. Or you can turn left and keep doing the horribly steep thing. You'll pass a decent viewpoint after climbing 200 feet in 0.2 mile, then Devils Lookout after climbing 700 feet in 0.5 mile—dang! Whenever I've been to this place, I've found Tibetan prayer flags. Beyond Devils Lookout, Devils Peak is 1 mile away and 800 feet up, but you actually *lose* some elevation on the way, and it gets crazy steep, but you do get a pretty view of Mount Jefferson. It's worth it, if you're feeling energetic.

Like I said, you have a lot of hiking options here, but all of them are beautiful, and all of them are close to the hot springs.

Nearby Activities

Breitenbush Hot Springs Resort & Conference Center is open (except for occasional closures of up to a week) daily, 9 a.m.–6 p.m., to day-use visitors, but it often fills. Advance reservations are required and give you access to the pools, steam room, and daily well-being programs for a sliding-scale fee (that is, one based on your ability to pay) of $13–$26. Lunch and dinner, both vegetarian, are $11 each. Overnight rates, depending on the season, include meals and range from $56 for a dorm room to $124 for a cabin with a bathroom. You can also camp here in the summer. For more information, call 503-854-3320 or visit **breitenbush.com.**

GPS Information and Directions

Breitenbush Hot Springs Resort **N44° 46.896' W121° 58.527'**
Lower Trailhead (FR 4685) **N44° 46.508' W121° 57.214'**
Upper Trailhead (Gorge) **N44° 45.972' W121° 55.666'**

Take I-5 from Portland, driving 35 miles south of I-205 to Exit 253/Stayton–Detroit Lake. Turn left (east) on OR 22 and follow it 49 miles to Detroit. Turn left onto FR 46.

For the hot springs, from Detroit drive 9 miles on FR 46 and turn right onto a one-lane bridge just past Cleator Bend Campground. Over the next 1.2 miles, keep left at three junctions to reach the resort parking lot.

For the trailheads on FR 4685, drive 2.5 miles past the right you made off of FR 46, turn right onto FR 4685, and drive 0.6 mile to the trailhead, on the right. The trailhead nearest the gorge is another 1.5 miles up the road, on the right.

30 Opal Creek Wilderness

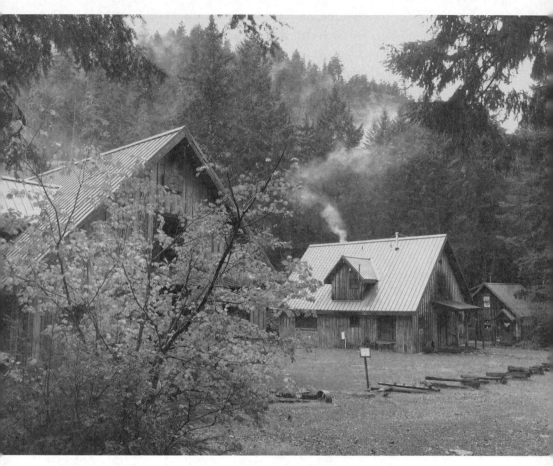

Some of the cabins in Jawbone Flats can be rented for the night; others host programs of the Opal Creek Ancient Forest Center.

In Brief

Opal Creek's history stretches from ancient times to a modern-day legislative show-down, but its value can hardly be measured. It's an almost completely preserved sample of what the Northwest used to be, a place that hasn't been logged and where the water runs clear. The largest such low-elevation area in the state, it doesn't even require that you work hard to see most of it.

LENGTH 7 miles round-trip to Opal Pool, 10 miles round-trip to Cedar Flats, 13 miles to see it all

CONFIGURATION Out-and-back

DIFFICULTY Easy–moderate

SCENERY Uncut forest, clear-water pools, historic mining structures

EXPOSURE Shady

TRAFFIC Heavy on summer weekends, moderate otherwise

TRAIL SURFACE Packed road for 3.1 miles; otherwise dirt, roots, rocks

HIKING TIME 4 hours to Opal Pool, 5.5 hours to Cedar Flats, 6 hours to see it all

DRIVING DISTANCE 92 miles (2 hours) from Pioneer Courthouse Square

SEASON April–November

BEST TIME July–September for weather, October for fall colors

BACKPACKING OPTIONS Plentiful

ACCESS Northwest Forest Pass required (see page 3) and can be purchased at trailhead

WHEELCHAIR ACCESS None

MAPS U.S. Forest Service *Opal Creek Wilderness*

FACILITIES Outhouses at trailhead; composting toilet in meadow at Jawbone Flats

INFO Opal Creek Ancient Forest Center, 503-892-2782, **opalcreek.org**

Description

For thousands of years, the Santiam Indians maintained their summer camp at the confluence of what we now call Opal and Battle Ax Creeks. Other tribes would come here to trade such items as fish from the Pacific Ocean and obsidian from east of the Cascades. In the 1850s, pioneers arrived and started mining for silver and gold. Not much of either was found, but there were enough other minerals to keep mining alive here until the early 1980s. A mining town was built at the confluence in the 1920s, and it came to be known as Jawbone Flats; the story has it that while the men were out mining, the women were back there "jawboning." A sawmill was also built nearby, but it burned in the 1940s. In 1992, the mining company donated 4,000 acres of land to a nonprofit group now known as the Opal Creek Ancient Forest Center, asking that it be preserved. Meanwhile, the U.S. Forest Service announced plans to log 15,000 acres of the Little North Santiam Valley.

This is when Opal Creek became famous; a massive effort was launched to save it from the saw. National TV crews visited, a book was written, and the fight went all the way to the U.S. Congress, where in 1998 the 35,000-acre Opal Creek Wilderness and Scenic Recreation Area was finally established. Today the Opal Creek Ancient Forest Center operates educational programs at Jawbone Flats, and a sprawling system of mostly easy trails brings visitors into the magical land of what used to be.

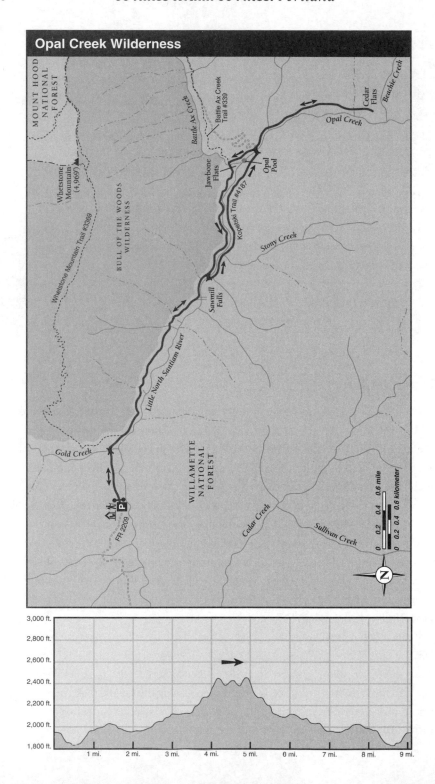

Opal Creek Wilderness

MOUNT HOOD NATIONAL FOREST

Whetstone Mountain (4,969')

Whetstone Mountain Trail #3369

BULL OF THE WOODS WILDERNESS

Battle Ax Creek

Battle Ax Creek Trail #339

Cedar Flats

Beachie Creek

Opal Creek

Jawbone Flats

Opal Pool

Kopetski Trail #4187

Stony Creek

Sawmill Falls

Little North Santiam River

Gold Creek

WILLAMETTE NATIONAL FOREST

Cedar Creek

Sullivan Creek

FR 2209

0.6 mile
0.4
0.2
0
0.6 kilometer
0.4
0.2
0

From the gate, start by walking slightly downhill on an old road. Most of the big trees are still ahead, but a Douglas-fir on the right is thought to be between 700 and 1,000 years old; a side trail leads to it at about 0.2 mile. Soon after, another old road leads down to the right, to two mine shafts on either side of the Little North Santiam River. At 0.3 mile, a high bridge crosses Gold Creek; 0.1 mile past that, you'll see Whetstone Mountain Trail #3369 on the left. This 3.5-mile trail climbs 3,000 feet to a superb view from atop Whetstone Mountain, but if you want to see that, it's much easier to do the Whetstone Mountain hike instead (see Hike 27, page 142). About 0.2 mile past that trailhead, you'll cross a series of "half-bridges"; keep an eye out for another old mining shaft on the left just past them.

The most impressive forest along the road occurs between 1 and 1.5 miles out, where you'll find 6-foot-thick Douglas-firs. At a wide spot in the road 1.5 miles out, look for a trail to the right that leads 100 yards to a rocky viewpoint. At 1.9 miles, you'll see a tiny creek on the left, flowing between exposed cedar tree roots. In fact, if it has rained recently, there will be water coming down all over the place.

At 2 miles, you come to a trail on the right leading into an area filled with old mining equipment and the burned-out remains of the sawmill's steel and masonry boiler. Behind the one building still standing, a trail leads 100 feet to a falls, known as either Sawmill Falls or Cascadia de los Niños ("Waterfall of the Children"), depending on whom you ask.

Just past the sawmill site, you'll come to a junction. From here, head straight ahead on the road to reach a river-access point, on the right 0.2 mile farther on; Jawbone Flats is 1.2 miles past that. Here, you'll find several cabins from the 1920s and 1930s (some can be rented overnight) and two built since a fire in 1999. They were all constructed largely of wood cut and milled right on the site. To reach the local highlight, Opal Pool, from here, take the road straight through the camp, following signs to make a right-hand turn and pass a collection of old vehicles that includes, oddly, a U.S. Navy fire truck. The pool is 0.1 mile past the cars.

Back at the first fork in the road, I recommend taking the right turn, across a bridge and then left, onto Kopetski Trail #4187. (Then–U.S. Congressman Mike Kopetski sponsored the Opal Creek Forest Preserve Act of 1994.) Along this trail, several side trails lead left to the Little North Santiam; you'll also pass several campsites on both sides of the trail; the best of them are on the left, down by the river. The trail will also be muddy and swamped if it's rained recently.

Continue 1.4 miles to a sign directing you to the sublime Opal Pool, on the left. In summer you may see people jumping off the rocks into the amazingly clear, cold water. You're now looking at Opal Creek itself, probably the clearest water you'll ever see, and the best bet in Oregon for a stream you can drink from. I have ingested several

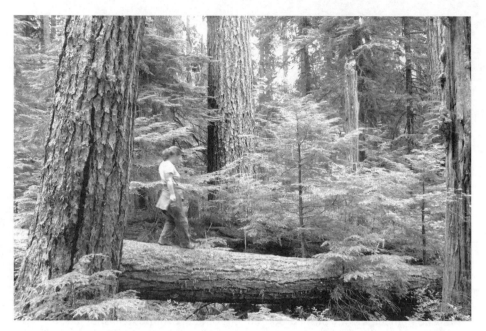

A hiker crosses Beachie Creek on a giant log. You'll encounter a lot of these crossings past Cedar Flats—they're a fun way to explore the forest.

gallons of Opal Creek and never gotten sick; take that for what it's worth and make your own decisions.

Just past the pool, the trail swings left to cross a bridge between the pool and a mini-gorge where the water is either babbling or raging, depending on the time of year. On the other side, climb briefly to a junction with Battle Ax Creek Trail #3339, coming up from Jawbone Flats. Go left to head back toward your car, or go right, sticking with the Kopetski Trail to head for Cedar Flats. This is a new trail section, built in 2013 because a bridge just up Opal Creek was wiped out. It passes one place with mild exposure, then crosses Flume Creek between two waterfalls; this latter bit is sketchy if the water is high.

A mile up from the junction—a total of 5 miles from the gate—the trail more or less ends at Cedar Flats, where Beachie Creek flows into Opal Creek from the left and three 1,000-year-old cedars frame the trail. You'll also find good camping in this area.

I say "more or less ends" because the trail beyond there is not maintained, but it is possible, even recommended, to go off exploring. One way to go is to look for a big log over Beachie Creek and then just go with it. Sometimes there's a trail; sometimes there are logs to walk on; sometimes there are logs to climb over. If a trail dead-ends near a log, hop up on it, walk a ways, and look around; you just might find some more trail. I can't give any specifics—not that I'm unwilling; I just can't explain it—but there is at least one more waterfall and one more pool like Opal Pool up there. Some folks just wander up the creek itself, which can be OK at low-water times; you might even find Poster Falls, made famous by a poster during the save-the-forest campaign.

There are long-term plans to relocate the trail and build a new 4-mile section up to Opal Lake. There are also plans to connect Opal Creek Trail with Little North Santiam Trail, which currently ends several miles down the Little North Santiam River. None of that work had begun when this book was written, but one day you may be able to hike from the Elkhorn Recreation Area (back on Little North Santiam Road) to Opal Lake, 17 miles one-way.

And Opal Creek has still more to offer. Battle Ax Creek Trail #3339 goes 4 miles and 1,800 feet up to a junction near Elk Lake and the Battle Ax Mountain hike (Hike 28, page 148), passing old mining equipment and railroad sections along the way. From the start of Opal Creek Trail, near the bridge, another trail leads up Stony Creek to a hidden waterfall. There's even a trail that branches off Whetstone Mountain Trail, heading up Gold Creek; beyond Whetstone Mountain, you can hike 14 miles through Bull of the Woods Wilderness to Bagby Hot Springs (Hike 23, page 124).

Basically, this is hiker heaven. Get some friends together, rent a cabin in Jawbone Flats for a few days or pitch a tent in the woods, and go for it.

Nearby Activities

A mile back on OR 22, you may have noticed **The Gingerbread House** (503-859-2247). It's on your left as you head home, at the junction of OR 22 and OR 226 in Mehama. Stop in for some fresh, warm gingerbread with ice cream after your hike, and your day will be complete.

GPS Information and Directions

N44° 51.591' W122° 15.864'

Take I-5 from Portland, driving 35 miles south of I-205 to Exit 253/Stayton–Detroit Lake. Turn left (east) onto OR 22 and follow it 22 miles, then turn left onto North Fork Road, following a sign for Little North Santiam Recreation Area. In just over 15 miles, the pavement ends and the road becomes Forest Service Road (FR) 2209. Keep left on FR 2209 at a junction; the trailhead is at the end of the road, 5.6 miles after you leave the pavement.

AROUND
MOUNT HOOD

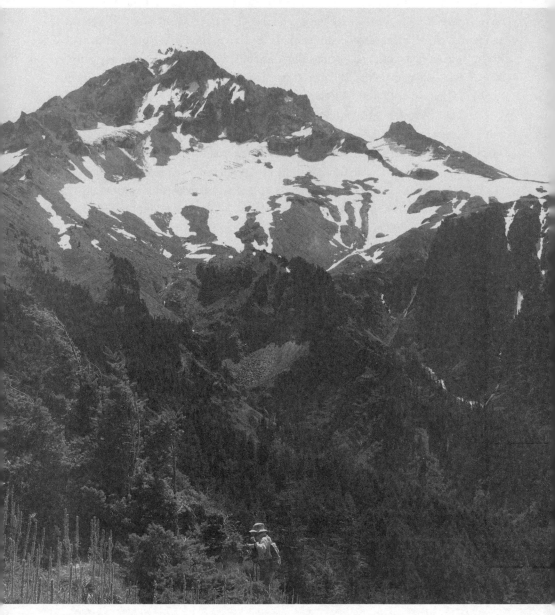

Dwarfed by Mount Hood, a happy hiker picks huckleberries on the way to McNeil Point (Hike 36).

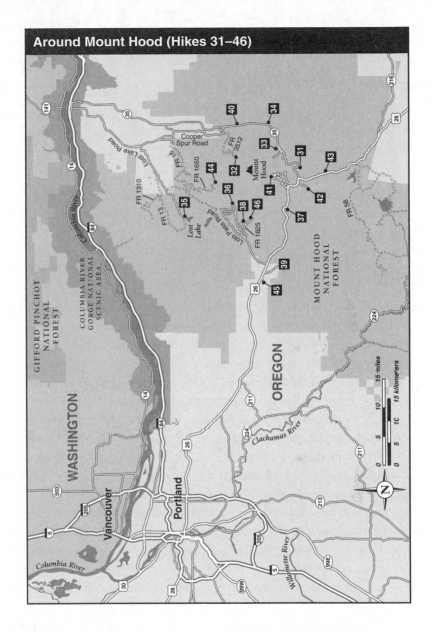

Around Mount Hood (Hikes 31–46)

31 Barlow Pass

In Brief

There's a great view of Mount Hood at the top, along with a one-way car-shuttle option that ends at Timberline Lodge, but this convenient, not-too-tough hike is all about the forest, traversing some of the finest high-elevation old-growth around and ending at an Oregon landmark.

Description

There are more-spectacular hikes in the Mount Hood area, but none offers the combination of solitude and old-growth beauty that this one does. It's also perfect for a picnic or just a dose of sunshine, in a high-altitude meadow with Mount Hood towering above. You can do the one-way option with a shuttle, possibly combining this hike with the Twin Lakes trip (Hike 43, page 223), and wind up at Timberline Lodge.

From the trailhead, walk across Forest Service Road (FR) 3531 and into the woods on Pacific Crest Trail (PCT) #2000. Stop to admire the relief map of the PCT in Oregon and contemplate some of the distances. People who hike the whole PCT in five or six months average about 20 miles a day—and when they get to Oregon, it's often more like 30. You'll get in 4–5 miles today—a distance most PCT long-haul hikers fly through, with dreams of showers and food up at the lodge.

At the sign, take the leftmost fork of the trails before you, walking north on the PCT toward Mount Hood. You'll take a few steps across historic Barlow Road and, after 0.1 mile, carefully cross OR 35. The trail continues in a small draw on the far side.

The first part of the trail isn't too exciting; in fact, after 0.5 mile you'll traverse a fairly recent clearcut. But right after that you enter a glorious stand of mostly noble fir, with its long, straight, branchless trunks. In early summer the ground will be blanketed with wildflowers. In late summer you'll see several species of huckleberries, and in fall, red-and-orange vine maple. If you're quiet, especially early in the day, you'll hear birds and possibly see deer or elk. It's just a pleasant place to be, and the trail's altitude gain—less than 400 feet per mile—is entirely manageable.

If you're wondering about those blue diamonds up on the trees early in the hike, they mark winter trails for cross-country skiers and snowshoers. Their height should give you a sense of how much snow falls in these parts. The white diamonds mark the PCT all the way from Mexico to Canada.

LENGTH Up to 10 miles round-trip, 5 miles one-way with shuttle	**BEST TIME** August and September
CONFIGURATION Out-and-back or point-to-point	**BACKPACKING OPTIONS** One good creekside site along the way
DIFFICULTY Moderate	**ACCESS** Northwest Forest Pass required (see page 3)
SCENERY Forest, meadows, views of Mount Hood, two river canyons	**WHEELCHAIR ACCESS** None
EXPOSURE Forest on the way up, open on top	**MAPS** Green Trails *Map #462 (Mount Hood)*, U.S. Forest Service *Mount Hood Wilderness*
TRAFFIC Light	**FACILITIES** None; water along trail must be treated.
TRAIL SURFACE Packed dirt with some roots	**INFO** Hood River Ranger District, 541-352-6002, **www.fs.usda.gov/mthood;** Pacific Crest Trail Association, **pcta.org**
HIKING TIME 3.5 hours one-way	
DRIVING DISTANCE 62 miles (1 hour, 30 minutes) from Pioneer Courthouse Square	**SPECIAL COMMENTS** Consider doing this hike as a one-way, 5-mile trek with a second car parked at Timberline Lodge.
SEASON July–October	

At the 2-mile mark, you'll enter a more diverse forest that includes firs and hemlocks, then cross a creek beside a small campsite at 2.7 miles. A little more than 3 miles into the hike, you'll reach an overlook of Salmon River Canyon and the headwaters of the Salmon River. The Salmon is the only river in the lower 48 states classified as a Wild and Scenic River from its headwaters to its mouth. The river flows from a glacier above Timberline Ski Area, snaking its way down to the Sandy River along US 26. Two hikes along the lower Salmon—Salmon River Trail and Wildwood Recreation Site—are described elsewhere in this book (see Hikes 39 and 45, pages 204 and 234, respectively).

Just past here, the forest will start to open up; in July and August, you'll see meadows filled with wildflowers, especially the spectacular beargrass, which looks like a giant cotton swab. In a few minutes, your trail intersects Timberline Trail #600 in just such a meadow, with Mount Hood rising above you. Relax here if you like, then turn around; or continue 0.3 mile left on Timberline Trail to reach a spectacular lookout with views of the White River Canyon, hundreds of feet deep.

If you've opted to park a car up at Timberline, keep going up Timberline Trail (which, at this point, is also the PCT) toward the mountain. It's 1.25 miles to the lodge—700 feet up—so it's not *too* much more work. However, most of the climbing is along the first part of the trail, which is also, at points, as sandy as a beach. So it can get arduous. And if cold weather is in the forecast, it's a sure thing up here, so bring a coat. There's nothing to stop the wind this high on the mountain.

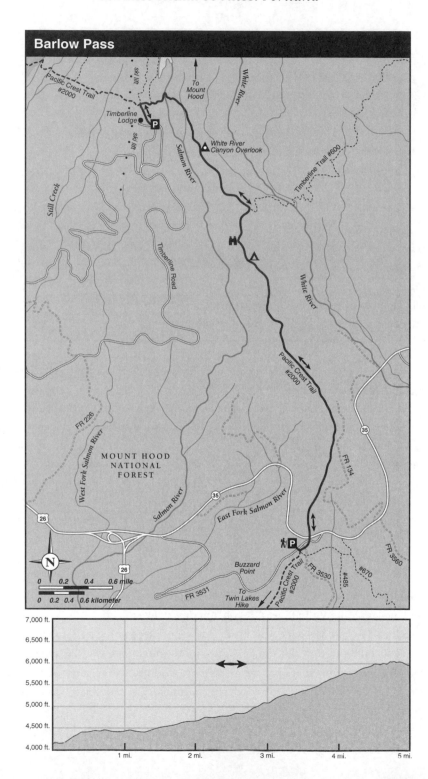

Barlow Pass

Pacific Crest Trail #2000

ski lift

To Mount Hood

White River

Timberline Lodge

P

ski lift

White River Canyon Overlook

Salmon River

Timberline Trail #600

Still Creek

Timberline Road

White River

Pacific Crest Trail #2000

35

FR 226

West Fork Salmon River

MOUNT HOOD NATIONAL FOREST

FR 134

Salmon River

26

35

East Fork Salmon River

FR 3560

N

FR 3530

FR 670

#485

P

0   0.2   0.4   0.6 mile

0   0.2   0.4   0.6 kilometer

26

Buzzard Point

To Twin Lakes Hike

Pacific Crest Trail #2000

FR 3531

7,000 ft.

6,500 ft.

6,000 ft.

5,500 ft.

5,000 ft.

4,500 ft.

4,000 ft.

1 mi.   2 mi.   3 mi.   4 mi.   5 mi.

You first go along the edge of the White River Canyon and then through meadows and across the tiny Salmon River; this crossing has no bridge but is manageable. Look for views south to Mount Jefferson, some 45 miles away, and a sign on the PCT with mileages to Canada and Mexico. You'll also encounter Mountaineer Trail, which loops up to Silcox Hut, then back down to Timberline Trail west of the lodge, in a section that's part of Hike 42, Trillium Lake (see page 219). When you get close to the lodge, trails will go every which way, so just aim for the hot chocolate and finish the hike with style.

It's possible to hike just the upper part of this walk from Timberline Lodge—an especially good idea if you have kids with you. This shorter option is an easy, scenic alternative with very little elevation gain; if you go to the White River Canyon overlook, it's about 1 mile round-trip.

And if you're wondering about those PCT thru-hikers, the main "herd" of them typically passes through here in late August or early September—look for (usually) young, thin, filthy people with small backpacks. It's fun to do something nice for them and practice some "trail magic" by offering them chips or candy bars, or taking out their garbage. And if you get to see what they do to the breakfast buffet at the lodge, you'll really have a story to tell.

Nearby Activities

If you've got some clearance on your vehicle, you can drive **Barlow Road** for miles, eventually making your way to The Dalles—though the road improves dramatically a long way before The Dalles. The drive is fun for the historical value and a few campsites along the way.

Though it's crowded, spend some time exploring **Timberline Lodge.** Watch the film *The Builders of Timberline* to hear the story of how artists and artisans came together during the Depression to create this masterwork. Then learn the details of their accomplishment, especially those of the Head House and its massive central stone tower. More info: 503-272-3311, **timberlinelodge.com.**

GPS Information and Directions

Barlow Pass Trailhead **N45° 16.957' W121° 41.116'**
Timberline Lodge **N45° 19.841' W121° 42.551'**

Take US 26 from Portland, driving 51 miles east of I-205, then turn left (north) on OR 35, following signs for Hood River. Drive 2.5 miles on OR 35, make a right onto FR 3531, and follow signs for Barlow Pass and the Pacific Crest Trail. The trailhead is 0.2 mile ahead, on FR 3531.

32 Cooper Spur

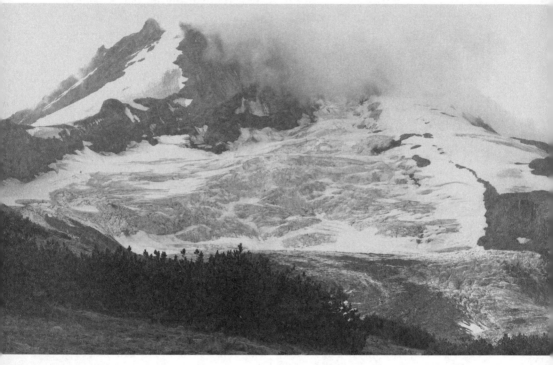

Even when the weather doesn't quite cooperate, the scenery at Cooper Spur is tremendous. This is a view from just beyond the shelter.

In Brief

Though it's not the toughest trail in this book, it is the highest—right up into the realm of the mountain climber. But while you'll be in the world of rock and snow, you won't wear yourself out getting here—well, not completely. You'll also get to see the oldest buildings on Mount Hood and the results of a massive landslide and a recent forest fire.

Description

If you want to get way, way up there, this is your hike. In the days before Timberline Lodge and the road to it were built, Cooper Spur was the standard climbing route to Mount Hood's 11,239-foot summit, and people still climb it that way today.

LENGTH 7.5 miles	**BACKPACKING OPTIONS** One site at Cooper Spur Shelter, but access to water is tough from here.
CONFIGURATION Balloon	
DIFFICULTY Strenuous	**ACCESS** Northwest Forest Pass (see page 3); $5/vehicle/day without pass
SCENERY Old-growth forest, glaciers, wide panoramas, the upper reaches of Mount Hood	**WHEELCHAIR ACCESS** None
EXPOSURE Mostly out in the open, with plenty of wind	**MAPS** Green Trails *Map 462 (Mount Hood)*, U.S. Forest Service *Mount Hood Wilderness*, U.S. Geological Survey *Mount Hood North*
TRAFFIC Moderate on summer weekends, light otherwise	**FACILITIES** Outhouse and water at trailhead
TRAIL SURFACE Packed dirt, sand, rocks	**INFO** Hood River Ranger District, 541-352-6002, **www.fs.usda.gov/mthood**
HIKING TIME 4.5 hours	**SPECIAL COMMENTS** No matter the forecast, bring warm clothing—weather at this altitude can change quickly. Also, Cloud Cap Road (FR 3512) was closed all of 2013 for removal of hazardous trees, so check ahead to make sure it's open for the 2014 season.
DRIVING DISTANCE 88 miles (2 hours, 15 minutes) from Pioneer Courthouse Square	
SEASON July–October	
BEST TIME August and September	

The whole area, in fact, is historically significant. Just up a hill from the trailhead, at the end of the road, is Cloud Cap Inn. Built in 1889 by two prominent Portland families as a recreation destination, it's the oldest building on Mount Hood. The hotel venture never took off, however, and by World War II the property was given to the U.S. Forest Service. In 1956 the Crag Rats, a Hood River–based climbing and rescue organization, took it over, and they maintain it to this day. Although officially the public isn't allowed in, if you're nice to the folks there, they might let you pop in for a bit. The Forest Service also offers public tours on occasion.

In 2008 a forest fire swept through this area, and dramatic measures were taken to save the buildings, including wrapping them in a protective material. As you start the hike, you'll get to see how the forest is recovering, and hopefully you'll feel grateful to the folks who saved the area's historic legacy.

More history later—now, for the hike. The trail starts at the far end of the campground. Take Timberline Trail #600 up and to the left and enter a rare snow-zone, old-growth forest, where mountain hemlock and Pacific silver firs get bigger than you'd think possible in an area that usually has 10 feet of snow by the end of December. Walk 1.2 miles to reach a junction after winding through the rocks and sand;

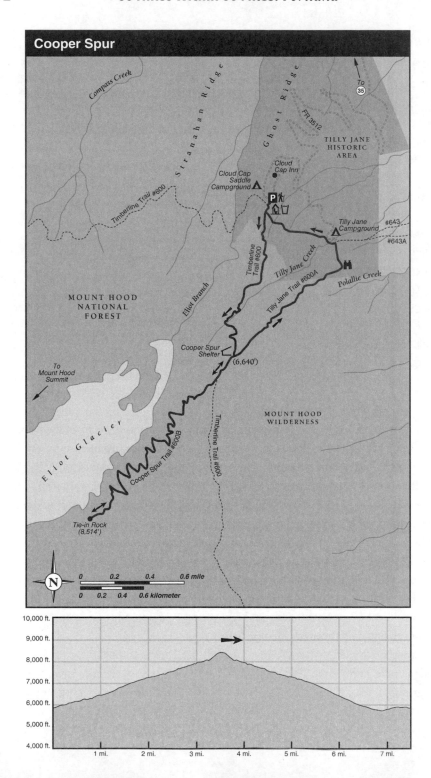

Cooper Spur

Compass Creek

Stranahan Ridge

Ghost Ridge

To 35

FR 3512

TILLY JANE HISTORIC AREA

Timberline Trail #600

Cloud Cap Saddle Campground

Cloud Cap Inn

P

Tilly Jane Campground

#643

#643A

Timberline Trail #600

Tilly Jane Creek

Tilly Jane Trail #600A

Polallie Creek

Eliot Branch

MOUNT HOOD NATIONAL FOREST

Cooper Spur Shelter

(6,640')

To Mount Hood Summit

MOUNT HOOD WILDERNESS

Eliot Glacier

Cooper Spur Trail #600B

Timberline Trail #600

Tie-in Rock (8,514')

N

| 0 | 0.2 | 0.4 | 0.6 mile |
| 0 | 0.2 | 0.4 | 0.6 kilometer |

10,000 ft.
9,000 ft.
8,000 ft.
7,000 ft.
6,000 ft.
5,000 ft.
4,000 ft.

1 mi.   2 mi.   3 mi.   4 mi.   5 mi.   6 mi.   7 mi.

following a sign for Cooper Spur Trail #600B, turn right and uphill—and get used to the climbing.

Just a hundred yards up, back among the twisted whitebark pines on your right, sits the Cooper Spur Shelter, at the end of a small side trail. This thing has been standing for some 70 years; imagine what weather it's been through! You can pitch a tent here or even sleep in the shelter, but for our purposes, have a snack and keep climbing. The trail will switchback through the sand and rocks, and Eliot Glacier will gradually come into view to the right. You'll hear it pop and rumble as it carves the side of the mountain, and if you're lucky, especially on late-summer afternoons, you'll see big boulders tumbling down its face.

After 2 miles of tough climbing, gaining 1,900 feet, you'll come to the top of the ridge, where you should look for a rock with some impressive carvings. JULY 17, 1910 is engraved in the stone here, commemorating a Japanese climbing party's ascent. Since you've climbed all the altitude at this point, you might as well go another 0.2 mile along the ridgetop—just be aware that this ridge is thin, rocky, and usually windswept.

Just before the snow line, you'll come to a plaque attached to the side of what's known as Tie-in Rock, so named because it's here that climbers tie themselves to one another to venture out onto the glacier. Heed my warning, though: Do *not,* under any circumstances—short of having ropes and crampons and relevant experience—go out onto the glacier. Be satisfied with having reached the top of your local hiking world, and relax among the sheltering rocks to take in the view.

From left to right, with Mount Hood behind you, you can see Eliot Glacier and, way off in the distance, the bare face of Table Mountain in the Columbia River Gorge, Mount St. Helens, Mount Rainier, Mount Adams, Elk Meadows, and Gnarl Ridge at your feet. Lookout Mountain is on a ridge to the east; there's a building below you on a Mount Hood ridge, which is the top of a ski lift at Mount Hood Meadows Ski Area.

Now look up at Mount Hood. The Cooper Spur climbing route begins on the snow-field right in front of you and proceeds up through the rocks, tending slightly to your left. (As climbers like to say, it's not as steep as it looks.) Look for a prominent rock called The Chimney, just below the summit, and Pulpit Rock more to your right. The Crag Rats say that whenever somebody falls on the Cooper Spur climbing route, they generally wind up within about 200 feet of the same falling spot at the top of Eliot Glacier.

When you've descended to the junction where you originally turned right, continue straight, leaving Timberline Trail #600 for Tilly Jane Trail #600A. Hike 0.6 mile and you'll come to an overlook of a large, bare bowl on your right. That's what was left behind by the Polallie Slide, a massive debris flow and flood in December 1980 that wiped out parts of OR 35.

A short distance on, you'll find yourself at some old buildings. This is part of the 1,400-acre Tilly Jane Historic Area, which is immensely popular with cross-country skiers and snowshoers, who come up a 2.7-mile trail from near Cooper Spur Ski Area and spend the night here. (In fact, during winter you can rent the **Tilly Jane A-Frame,** which is managed by the Oregon Nordic Club, at **reserveamerica.com.**) And if you're wondering about that name, Tilly Jane was the nickname of the matriarch of the Ladd family, one of the builders of Cloud Cap Inn—and the former owners of what's now the Ladd's Addition neighborhood in Portland.

In this area you'll also find a campground, an amphitheater that's been there since at least the 1950s, and a 1938 guard station, managed by the Oregon Nordic Club and available for rent in the winter. A sign at the parking lot tells more about the local history.

To get back to your car, just put Mount Hood on your left and follow Tilly Jane Trail #600A for 0.5 mile back to the trailhead. You'll find the trail over by the amphitheater, heading across the creek.

Nearby Activities

When you get back to OR 35, go north (left) and indulge yourself at some of the berry and fruit stands in the Hood River Valley. Some let you pick your own. See **hoodriver fruitloop.com** for details.

GPS Information and Directions

N45° 24.141' W121° 39.297'

Take US 26 from Portland, driving 51 miles east of I-205; turn left (north) on OR 35, following signs for Hood River. Continue 17 miles on OR 35, then turn left at a sign for Cooper Spur Ski Area. Drive 2.4 miles, turn left, and follow another sign for Cooper Spur Ski Area. In 1.4 miles, continue straight, leaving the pavement. Go 8.3 winding miles on Cloud Cap Road (Forest Service Road 3512) to a T-junction, and turn right. The trailhead is 0.5 mile ahead on the right, in Cloud Cap Saddle Campground.

33 Elk Meadows

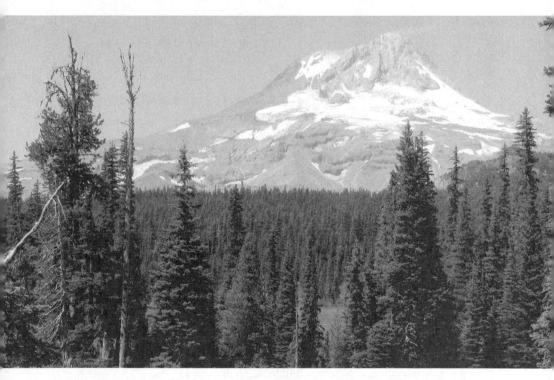

You'll enjoy this view of Hood—and be knee-deep in wildflowers—if you make it to Elk Meadows.

In Brief

One of the most spectacular sights in the Mount Hood area, sprawling and flower-filled Elk Meadows is relatively easy to reach. And beyond it lies Gnarl Ridge, with its awesome close-up view of the mountain.

Note: This makes an excellent snowshoe or ski trip, but you'll have to start at the Clark Creek Sno-Park on OR 35. The Green Trails map shows winter trails.

Description

If I were to tell you there's a place where you can skip through meadows and over creeks, picking berries all the way, and wind up in a flower-filled wonderland with

LENGTH 2 miles to Newton Creek, 5.5 miles to Elk Meadows, 12 miles to see it all

CONFIGURATION Out-and-back with optional loop

DIFFICULTY Moderate to Elk Meadows, strenuous to Gnarl Ridge

SCENERY Meadows, mountain streams, extreme close-ups of Mount Hood, a fire-recovery area

EXPOSURE In and out of the trees, with two bridgeless creek crossings

TRAFFIC Moderate on summer weekends, light otherwise

TRAIL SURFACE Dirt, some roots and rocky areas

HIKING TIME 3.5 hours to Elk Meadows, 6 hours for the whole loop

DRIVING DISTANCE 69 miles (1 hour, 30 minutes) from Pioneer Courthouse Square

SEASON July–October

BEST TIME August and September

BACKPACKING OPTIONS Several good ones

ACCESS No fees or permits

WHEELCHAIR ACCESS None

MAPS Green Trails *Map 462 (Mount Hood),* USFS *Mount Hood Wilderness*

FACILITIES Outhouse at trailhead; water on trail must be treated.

INFO Hood River Ranger District, 541-352-6002, **www.fs.usda.gov/mthood**

a snow-covered peak above it, and if you wanted, you could climb up through more meadows to a rocky point with a huge view of everything around, right up where the water blasts out from under the glaciers . . . you'd be interested in that, right?

That's this hike. And if all you're doing is going to Elk Meadows, there's only one moderate hill between you and your destination. In fact, you and the kids could walk a flat mile, see two mountain streams, and have a ball. And you could do the whole thing in an easy day or spend the night on an easy introductory backpack.

From the trailhead, follow Sahalie Falls Trail #667C through moss-draped forest, pocket meadows with wildflowers, and huckleberries that ripen in late August. You may notice that some of these meadows aren't entirely natural (they're filled with stumps); that's because they're actually Nordic ski runs, part of Mt. Hood Meadows Ski Resort.

Pass Umbrella Falls Trail #667 on the left, and now you're officially on Elk Meadows Trail #645. After hiking 0.5 mile, you'll cross Clark Creek on a bridge, which skiers and snowshoers can attest is a lot more interesting with about 2 feet of snow on it. There's also a campsite at this crossing, but better ones await.

Keep going straight—ignore the trails leading left—and after another 0.6 mile you'll cross Newton Creek—on logs, one hopes. If you're here early in the season and the logs aren't in place yet, this crossing (and a later one) might be tricky. Check **portlandhikers.org** for the latest conditions.

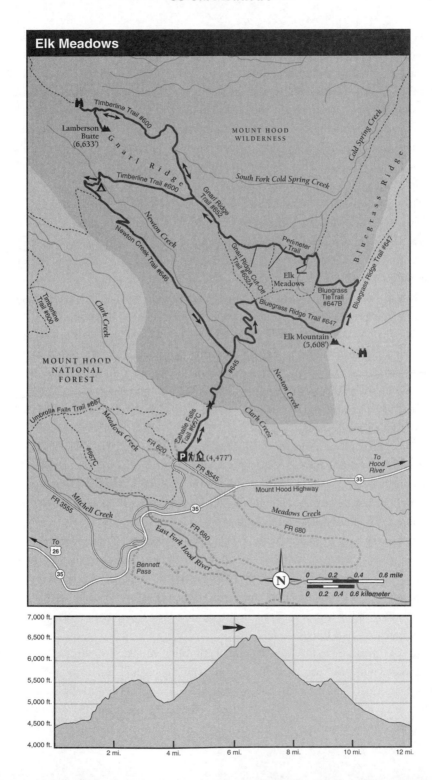

Elk Meadows

While we're here, a few words about the names of these creeks: They both flow from Newton Clark Glacier. What many people don't realize is that Newton Clark was just one guy, a teacher and surveyor who moved from South Dakota to Hood River Valley in 1877 and lived until 1918. He also has a county in South Dakota named for him.

Safely across Newton Creek, you're at the hill. Hike 0.8 mile to gain almost 700 feet in a series of long switchbacks; consider this the price of admission to Elk Meadows. Just over the top, you'll come to a four-way intersection—for Elk Meadows, go straight and you'll be there in just a few minutes; for a side trip to Elk Mountain, turn right, into an area that burned in 2006.

The trail to Elk Mountain isn't spectacular in and of itself, but it's quiet and woodsy, and it leads to a nice view east across OR 35 and to Mount Jefferson to the south. To get to the lookout, climb 0.6 mile on Bluegrass Ridge Trail #647, then stay straight at a junction with Elk Mountain Vista Trail #647C; the lookout is 0.3 mile ahead. When you come back, take Bluegrass Ridge Trail, now right, and follow it 0.5 mile along the ridgetop—through the heart of the burned area—before turning left, at a large stone cairn, and plunging 0.4 mile down Bluegrass Tie Trail #647B to Elk Meadows.

Elk Meadows is almost unbelievable. It's basically a circular area of meadows about half a mile in diameter, with islands of trees throughout and streams crisscrossing it. For the good of the flowers and grass, resist the temptation to go meadow-stomping, but by all means find a log or rock on the perimeter and take a load off. To complete a loop around the meadows, or to explore the other loop on this hike, follow the trail to the right.

When you come to a sign for Polallie Campground 0.1 mile later, stay left on Perimeter Trail #645A, and 0.1 mile later you'll come to another trail leading left. Take it and continue straight, out into the middle of the meadows, where a stone shelter hosts backpackers most summer nights (additional tent sites are behind the shelter in the woods). It's a lovely place for a picnic.

On the way back from the shelter, take a left on Perimeter Trail and start climbing along the side of the meadow, passing a couple more campsites along the way. In about 0.5 mile, you'll come to a junction with Gnarl Ridge Cut-Off Trail #652A. To return to your car, turn left here, finish the loop around the meadows, and then turn right at the junction with Elk Meadows Trail. But to climb a little toward Mount Hood, stay straight here on Gnarl Ridge Trail.

After a little more than a mile of gradual climbing, you'll join Gnarl Ridge Trail #652 and, 0.3 mile past that, reach Timberline Trail #600. Here you have another choice to make: Turn left to start back toward the car, or turn right to climb another 900 feet in 1.5 miles to the top of Gnarl Ridge. That trail leads through more meadows and an ever-thinner forest, with views of Mount Adams to your right and Lookout

Mountain (see next hike) behind you. You can also clearly see the whole of Bluegrass Ridge, the scene of that 2006 fire.

The gravelly viewpoint of Gnarl Ridge offers one of the finer vistas around. The glaciers of Mount Hood loom above you, with the headwater of Newton Creek bursting out from under them, and across the way you can make out a ski-lift building on the resort. Mount Jefferson and the Three Sisters are out beyond that. A short trail leads up to Lamberson Butte (6,633 feet), the official summit of the ridge.

Keep wandering up Timberline Trail—it's out in the open for quite a while now and leads just a couple miles over to Cooper Spur (see previous hike)—or head back down to the junction and turn right. A gradual descent will bring you back to another crossing of Newton Creek, where again (one hopes) logs will help you across. On the far side, pass another fine campsite next to a spring creek, climb about 0.3 mile, and then turn left at the ridgetop onto Newton Creek Trail #646. Two miles down that heavily huckleberried trail, your path intersects the trail you started all this wandering on: Elk Meadows #645. Turn right to hike less than a mile back to the trailhead.

I know all this is a lot of numbers and letters and junctions—just bring this book and the Green Trails map with you, and enjoy the ride.

Nearby Activities

For a little piece of Oregon history, pay your respects at the **Pioneer Woman's Grave,** off OR 35 on Forest Service Road (FR) 3531, just east of its intersection with US 26 (GPS: **N45° 16.928' W121° 42.004'**). Workers building the old Mount Hood Loop Highway found the woman buried beneath a crude marker; her remains have since been moved twice, and to this day people lay crosses or flowers on the pile of rocks marking her grave.

GPS Information and Directions

N45° 19.399' W121° 38.125'

Take US 26 from Portland, driving 51 miles east of I-205. Turn left (north) on OR 35, following signs for Hood River. Drive 7 miles and turn left onto FR 3545, at the second entrance for Mount Hood Meadows Ski Resort (the one for the Nordic Center). The trailhead is 0.5 mile ahead, on the right.

34 Lookout Mountain

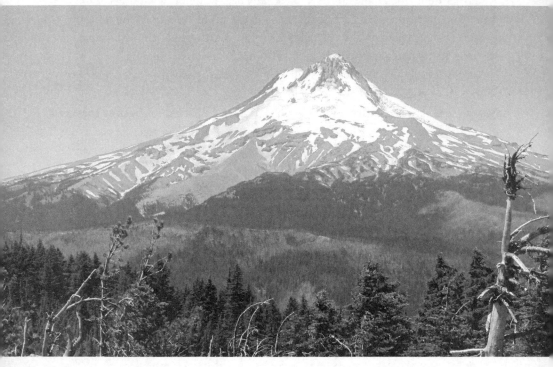

You won't find many better views of Mount Hood than the one from Lookout Mountain. You can see the Columbia River, too.

In Brief

One of the easternmost points in this book, Lookout Mountain is also one of the widest and most wonderful viewpoints, stretching from south of the Three Sisters all the way to Mount Rainier and including desert, lakes, and the Columbia River.

Description

First, for the "studly" out-and-back route, which is a whole lot more work but comes with a lot of benefits: From the trailhead on OR 35, the first couple of miles are relentlessly uphill. On Gumjuwac Trail #460, you'll gain 1,400 feet in 1.8 miles to a nice view of Mount Hood, then catch a little break over the last 0.5 mile to Gumjuwac Saddle. All this is in the forest—think of it as your price of admission.

LENGTH 3 miles for the loop (starting from High Prairie), 9.6 for the out-and-back (starting at OR 35)

CONFIGURATION Loop or out-and-back

DIFFICULTY Easy on the loop, strenuous on the out-and-back

SCENERY Meadows, forest, and one of the great vistas in Oregon

EXPOSURE Shady, exposed rock at the top

TRAFFIC Moderate on weekends, light otherwise

TRAIL SURFACE Packed dirt, rock

HIKING TIME 1 hour for the loop, 5 hours for the out-and-back

DRIVING DISTANCE 60 miles (1 hour, 30 minutes) from Pioneer Courthouse Square

SEASON July–October

BEST TIME August and September

BACKPACKING OPTIONS Not great; some sites around Senecal Spring

ACCESS Northwest Forest Pass (see page 3) required at High Prairie Trailhead

WHEELCHAIR ACCESS None

MAPS Green Trails *Map 462 (Mount Hood)*, USGS *Badger Lake*

FACILITIES Outhouse at High Prairie Trailhead; 1 spring on the way up from Gumjuwac Trailhead and another near the summit

INFO Barlow Ranger District, 541-467-2291, **www.fs.usda.gov/mthood**

At Gumjuwac Saddle, on Forest Service Road (FR) 3550, you'll encounter several trails. Gumjuwac Trail crosses the road and drops to the other side of the ridge, into Badger Creek Wilderness. Coming in from the right is Gunsight Butte Trail #685, popular with mountain bikers because it's 4.5 miles along the ridge with very little elevation change. In case you're thinking of driving FR 3550 to this point, you'd better have some clearance. But if you insist, turn right at the BADGER LAKE sign mentioned in the directions to High Prairie, then bounce about 3 miles to the saddle.

And in case you're wondering about the name *Gumjuwac,* it comes from a sheepherder named Jack. Apparently, Jack liked gum shoes, hence "Gum Shoe Jack." Somehow that morphed into "Gumjuwac" over the years.

To keep going to Lookout Mountain, simply walk across FR 3550 and start walking to your left, on Divide Trail #458. You'll encounter a lovely spring 0.9 mile up; on this stretch you'll also have a view of Lookout Mountain straight ahead (the summit is actually to the right and appears lower than the one on the left). And you'll see why this trail is called Divide Trail. Technically, it splits two watersheds—Hood River from The Dalles—but it also exhibits the amazing contrast between east and west. Coming up Gumjuwac Trail, it's all shady, with a view of glacier-covered Mount Hood, but on this side you'll encounter meadows, flowers, and views of the desert. As you climb with Mount Hood on your left, look for views over your right shoulder to Badger Lake.

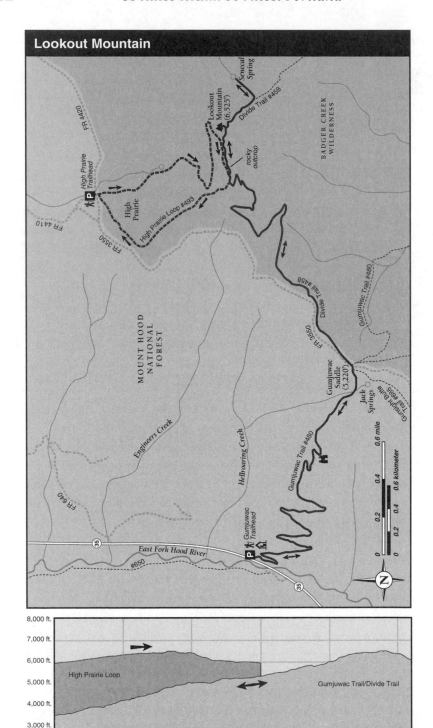

Lookout Mountain

Watch for wildlife, too: I once saw two falcons chasing each other around here, and another time I scared up an owl in the woods.

After the spring, the trail gets a little steeper. Keep climbing, and just below a summit of sorts, continue straight and uphill where High Prairie Loop #493 cuts down to the left. This will put you on a rocky outcrop with an amazing view; many people stop here, but it's not the top of Lookout Mountain. To get there, put Mount Hood behind you and keep going, staying on Divide Trail. You'll walk along a rocky ridge looking down into the Badger Creek drainage; keep right where an old road goes left, then climb a short way to a trail leading left, to the wide-open summit and the foundation of an old fire lookout. For a description of the view, see below.

There's one more spring up here that's worth visiting. To reach Senecal Spring—named for a U.S. Forest Service ranger from the turn of the 20th century—take Divide Trail 0.2 mile past the summit and turn left on a trail that's barely visible and whose sign is often lying on the ground. The (very cold) spring is 0.25 mile below Divide Trail.

The Shorter Loop

Now, if you're more into driving up long hills than walking up them, here's High Prairie Loop. Lookout Mountain has many trails, some of which aren't marked on maps. So take our map with you and remember that just about all these trails go to the same two places: Lookout Mountain and the trailhead.

From the parking area on FR 4410, walk straight across 4410 and up the wide path—so well worn it's practically paved—into the meadows. The fields of daisies and lupines might make you want to stop there, but keep going. And try to resist the temptation to wander into the meadows. The trail you see immediately on your right, labeled for horses, is High Prairie Loop #493, which heads back to the trailhead. Ignore it for now.

Follow the wide trail ahead 0.7 mile until, in an area of reddish rock, it splits into three. The faint path through the trees on the right is a cutoff to the return portion of Loop Trail—ignore it. The path straight ahead and up the hill is a cutoff to Divide Trail—ignore that, too. If you stay on the wide trail, you'll loop around to the left to a point with a fine view east of the Cascades, out into the Oregon High Desert. The road then loops back around to the right and intersects Divide Trail #458. Turn left on Divide Trail, climb a bit, and follow a narrow trail to the left to reach the summit. Like Gumjuwac Trail, this approach is listed on our elevation profile.

The Summit

The view from Lookout Mountain's 6,500-foot summit is one that you just can't get from the western side of the Cascades, or for that matter from most points in the

Cascades. From left to right, on a clear day, you can see Diamond Peak, the Three Sisters, and Mounts Jefferson, Hood (absolutely huge, just 7 miles across the way), St. Helens, Rainier, and Adams. From Diamond Peak to Mount Rainier, as the crow flies, it's about 225 miles. You can also see, if you look closely, a stretch of the Columbia River to the northeast.

If you came up from Gumjuwac, you might as well see some new country on the way back by completing High Prairie Loop: When you're on Lookout Mountain, walk toward Mount Hood on Divide Trail, retracing your steps from the trip up. At 0.3 mile, take the signed Loop Trail to your right and follow it as it crosses the face of Lookout Mountain and dives into the woods. Walk 0.7 mile, then turn right at a sign and walk back through the meadows to rejoin the wide, packed trail that leads to the right and back to Divide Trail.

GPS Information and Directions

High Prairie Trailhead **N45° 21.124' W121° 31.866'**
Gumjuwac Trailhead **N45° 20.396' W121° 34.197'**

Take US 26 from Portland, driving 51 miles east of I-205. Turn left (north) on OR 35, following signs for Hood River. For the longer hike, on Gumjuwac Trail, drive 11 miles on OR 35 and park along the shoulder on the right, just after the road crosses the East Fork Hood River.

For the shorter loop, at High Prairie, drive 2.5 miles farther on OR 35 and turn right onto FR 44. Drive 3.7 miles and turn right, following a sign for High Prairie, onto gravel FR 4410. Over the next 4.6 miles—during which the road occasionally rides like a washboard—take the larger, more uphill road at all the junctions. At a sign for Badger Lake, on the right, follow FR 4410 around to the left; the parking area is 100 yards ahead.

35 Lost Lake

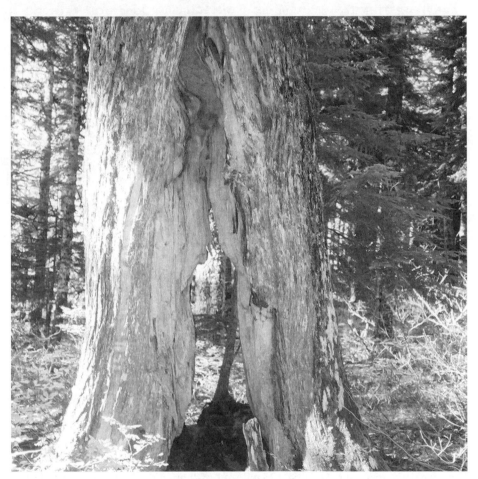

A hollowed-out snag on Lost Lake Trail

In Brief

The rustic resort at Lost Lake is a great place to spend a night or two, with boats for rent, picnic tables with grills, a campground, and a beautiful lake stocked with trout. It's also a lovely walk around the natural 240-acre lake, including an interpretive, barrier-free, old-growth trail and one of the most photographed views of Mount Hood—all this, plus two optional longer hikes, one of them to a fine lookout point.

LENGTH 3.3 miles around the lake, 4 miles round-trip to Lost Lake Butte, 16 miles round-trip to Buck Peak	**DRIVING DISTANCE** 88 miles (1 hour, 45 minutes) from Pioneer Courthouse Square
CONFIGURATION Loop plus 2 out-and-back options	**SEASON** June–October; call the resort to make sure the road is snow-free before June.
DIFFICULTY Easy around the lake, moderate to Lost Lake Butte, strenuous to Buck Peak	**BEST TIME** August and September
SCENERY Lake, beaches, views of Mount Hood, huge trees	**BACKPACKING OPTIONS** Sites along the Pacific Crest Trail on the way to Buck Peak
EXPOSURE Shady except for at the lake and atop the butte	**ACCESS** $7/vehicle day-use fee
TRAFFIC Heavy on summer days, very heavy on weekends	**WHEELCHAIR ACCESS** 2 miles of lakeside trails, including old-growth boardwalk
TRAIL SURFACE Packed dirt and boardwalk	**MAPS** Available free at Lost Lake General Store
HIKING TIME 1.5 hours around the lake; add 2 hours to Lost Lake Butte and 6 hours for Buck Peak.	**FACILITIES** Full-service camping resort
	INFO Lost Lake Resort, 541-386-6366, **lostlakeresort.org**

Description

Whether you're looking for a pleasant family campout or a good day of hiking, Lost Lake has what you need; that's why there are often so many people there. But as is always the case, their number decreases in direct proportion to how far you walk.

Around the Lake

For the 3.3-mile trail around the lake, start in front of the general store. Walk to the boat dock and turn right. The first 0.25 mile of Lost Lake Trail #620, which parallels the road, is dotted with lakeside picnic tables. Soon you'll come to a platform with a view of Mount Hood that will look quite familiar if you've ever seen a calendar with Hood in it. Come back here at the end of the day for the best photographic light.

Beyond the platform, the trail leaves the road and you start to feel like you're actually out in the woods. In late summer, your progress will be slowed by plump, ripe huckleberries; you can pick a handful or two, then choose a little beach off the trail, sit on a log, and peacefully enjoy your snack. Keep an eye out for signs identifying tree species.

After just less than a mile, you'll come to a marshy area where the trail becomes a boardwalk. At 1.6 miles there's a rockslide with excellent swimming. After you've

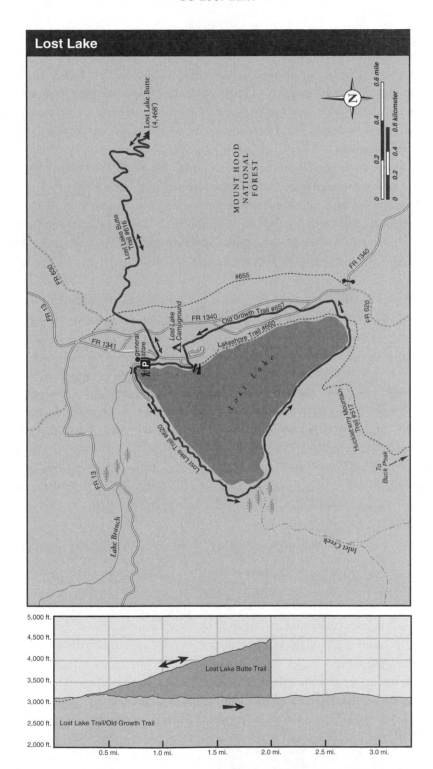

hiked another mile, you'll see Huckleberry Mountain Trail #617 leading right 2.5 miles to an intersection with the Pacific Crest Trail (PCT). More on that in a bit.

Just past Huckleberry Mountain Trail, veer right and away from Lakeshore Trail #660, then stay left as you approach a group of buildings. This will put you on a road; Old Growth Trail #657 begins 100 yards ahead on a boardwalk and immediately passes between two of the largest cedars you're ever likely to see—both in the neighborhood of 12 feet in diameter.

This 1-mile trail is great for kids because it's not too long and includes educational signs explaining the roles that nurse logs, the forest canopy, the weather, and pileated woodpeckers and other animals play in a forest's life. Some of these trees are hundreds of years old and more than 200 feet tall. When the boardwalk runs out, continue another 0.3 mile, follow Lakeshore Express Trail through the campground and down to the lake, and turn right to get back to your car.

To Lost Lake Butte

To climb Lost Lake Butte for a view of, as the resort's hiking map puts it, "pretty near everything worth seeing," start in the general store's parking area. Walk back up the road and, at the turnoff for the main exit, look for a sign and a trail heading into the woods. You'll come to an unsigned trail intersection; turn right and uphill here. A hundred yards later, you'll cross another road—aim for a sign that reads L O S T L A K E B U T T E T R A I L H E A D. It can get confusing here, but when in doubt, keep going uphill. It's a steady climb of 1,300 feet in 2 miles to the former site of an old fire lookout.

Mount Hood, of course, is the dominant view to the south, but you can also see as far north as Mount Rainier (but not Mount Baker, as the resort map and website claim). Then just come back down the way you went up and get yourself a cool drink or some ice cream at the store as a reward for all your effort. (Constant access to refreshments is one of the great things about Lost Lake.)

Note: A one-day fishing license, required for visitors ages 14 and up, costs $16.

To Buck Peak

This one's a bit of a slog, but it offers some amazing forest, a little introduction to the PCT, and a nice lookout at the end. Across Lost Lake from the general store, start up the Huckleberry Mountain Trail . . . which goes nowhere near anything called Huckleberry Mountain.

The trail is steep for the first mile, gaining 700 feet, and passes some undesirable campsites along the way. A flatter mile leads to the PCT junction, where you turn right. Very soon you'll pass a much better site at Salvation Spring, which for years had a handwritten (and misspelled) sign reading S A L V A T O I N S P R I N G.

Now the trail climbs gently for a mile through towering forest to a saddle between Preachers Peak and Devils Pulpit. A Forest Service ranger named the former for his dad, a local minister with a bum foot who rode a horse to the summit, and the latter got its name because somebody remarked that if a preacher is here, the devil can't be far away.

Passing between those peaks, the PCT offers views of Lost Lake and Mount Adams to the east as it loses elevation for 0.5 mile to a rock pile on the left. Here, you can scramble up for a rare view west into Bull Run watershed, the uncut, off-limits drainage that supplies Portland with its water. From this rocky point, you can just make out Bull Run Lake off to the left.

At a total of 6.8 miles since the trailhead (about 2.5 miles since you got on the PCT), you'll round a ridge where the view north takes in a large bowl with two peaks at the far end—the one on the right is our destination, Buck Peak. Work your way around the bowl, and 1 mile north from the viewing point, an unsigned, brushy trail heads up to the right; this is your 0.5-mile-long summit trail.

The view from 4,751-foot Buck Peak takes in Mounts Hood, Adams, Jefferson, and Defiance (the forested one with the radio towers), as well as Lost Lake and the upper parts of the Hood River Valley. Along the summit to the left are the rusty remains of an old lookout tower, in a small meadow that makes a fine picnic site.

Nearby Activities

The **Apple Valley Country Store** (2363 Tucker Rd., Hood River, OR 97031) is one of my favorite places in the world. They use local fruits to create walls of jams, jellies, syrups, and preserves; a freezer stuffed with pies; a dozen mustards and other sauces; and various baking mixes. Annual events include summer country barbecues and fall weekends when pear dumplings are served. (Trust me—you want a pear dumpling!) Find out more at 541-386-1971 or **applevaleystore.com.**

GPS Information and Directions

N45° 29.789' W121° 49.141'

Take I-84 from Portland, driving 55 miles east of I-205 to Exit 62/West Hood River. Make a right at the end of the off-ramp, then immediately turn right again, onto Country Club Road, following signs for several wineries. At the end of Country Club Road, 3 miles on, turn left at a stop sign onto Barrett Drive. Continue 1.3 miles and turn right on Tucker Road, the second stop sign you'll come to on Barrett Drive. Go 2 miles up Tucker and turn right on Dee Highway, where a sign reads PARKDALE. Drive 6.5 miles on Dee Highway, then turn right again onto Forest Service Road (FR) 13, following signs for Lost Lake. The resort is 14 miles ahead, at the end of FR 1341—just keep following the signs for Lost Lake.

36 McNeil Point

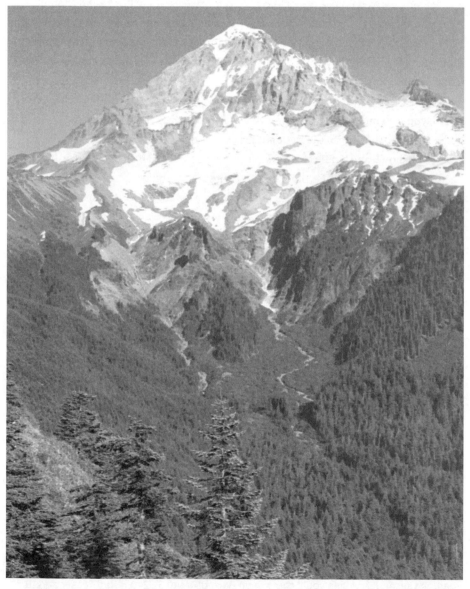

Mount Hood and Sandy Glacier from Bald Mountain. This view is barely a mile from the Top Spur Trailhead.

LENGTH 12 miles round-trip	**SEASON** July–October
CONFIGURATION Out-and-back	**BEST TIME** August and September
DIFFICULTY Easy to Bald Mountain view-point, strenuous to McNeil Point	**BACKPACKING OPTIONS** Excellent
	ACCESS Northwest Forest Pass required (see page 3)
SCENERY Old-growth forest, meadows, rugged mountainside	**WHEELCHAIR ACCESS** None
EXPOSURE Shady, with a few stretches on rock and snow	**MAPS** USFS *Mount Hood Wilderness*
TRAFFIC Heavy on summer weekends, light otherwise	**FACILITIES** None at trailhead; water on trail must be treated.
TRAIL SURFACE Packed dirt with roots, a few small stream crossings, some rocks and snow	**INFO** Zigzag Ranger District, 503-622-3191, **www.fs.usda.gov/mthood**
	SPECIAL COMMENTS No matter what the weather is like when you start, bring warm clothing if you're going to McNeil Point—it's above the tree line, and weather changes quickly up here.
HIKING TIME 5.5 hours	
DRIVING DISTANCE 58 miles (1 hour, 30 minutes) from Pioneer Courthouse Square	

In Brief

You don't have to do this whole trail to make it worthwhile—it opens with a great view, passes through a cathedral forest to wildflower meadows and alpine ponds, then gets up close and personal with Mount Hood. But if you do go all the way up, you can see the trickle that is the source of the Sandy River and hear glaciers pop and rumble.

Description

This is a honey of a hike! Start out on Top Spur Trail #785, which climbs gradually for 0.5 mile to a veritable highway interchange of trails. First you'll reach the Pacific Crest Trail (PCT); turn right on that. Hike 100 feet to a four-way junction with Timberline Trail #600. From here, the PCT, on the right, leads down 2.2 miles to Ramona Falls Trail (see Hike 38, page 199).

To simply head for McNeil Point, follow Timberline Trail #600 uphill and to the left. But it's well worth it to see the magnificent view from the open side (not actually the top) of Bald Mountain, a mere 0.4 mile the other way on Timberline Trail. Head out there—that's the middle path at the four-way junction—to take in the sweeping view of Mount Hood and the Muddy Fork Sandy River. Then keep going, toward Mount Hood, and look for a faint cutoff trail that goes over the ridge to your left, just

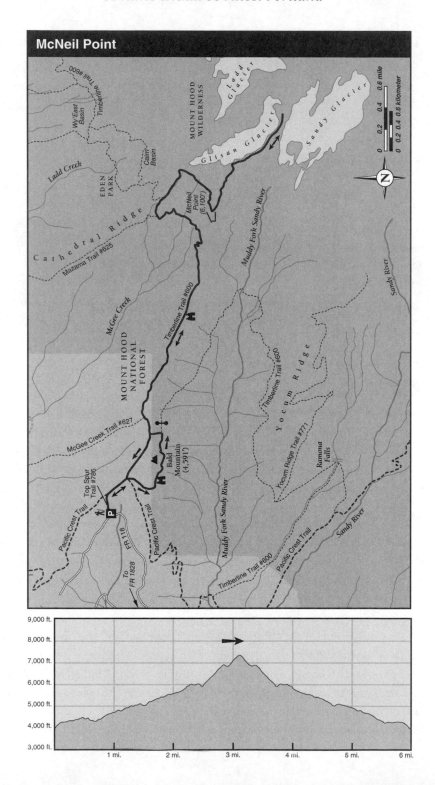

before the trail heads back into the woods; if you come to a gate on the trail, you just missed it. The cutoff extends about 100 yards over the ridge and back to Timberline Trail—turn right for McNeil Point.

This stretch of Timberline Trail lies in a true cathedral forest—the tall, straight trees, mostly hemlocks, have no branches on their lower portions, creating a forest scene that's both open and lofty. Adding to the pleasure are the many huckleberry bushes that make up the ground cover; their juicy morsels are typically ripe in late August. You'll hardly notice that you've started climbing in earnest.

On Timberline Trail, at the first big view of Mount Hood you come to (you'll have gone 2.3 miles), look for the large, unnamed waterfall across the valley on Hood's flank. At 3.5 miles, you'll cross a fork of McGee Creek and, if it's around August, arrive in the land of wildflowers. Lupines, daisies, pasqueflowers, lilies, and butterflies will welcome you to the high country. Just a bit farther are a couple of ponds, which make ideal places to stop for lunch and also host some fine campsites. You can skip and frolic in this area and call it a day, or you can keep going to even higher country.

At 3.9 miles, soon after Mazama Trail #625 has come in from the left, you'll see the old McNeil Point Trail, now closed for revegetation. Timberline Trail next passes through one more patch of forest—look for the Mount Adams view on the far side—and then intersects the new trail to the point, heading up and to the right.

If you just want more meadows without more climbing, stay on the main trail as it swings left, negotiate a stream crossing that can be mildly dangerous in high water, and connect with the outer reaches of the Vista Ridge trip (see Hike 44, page 228) for Cairn Basin and Eden Park. If you're set on McNeil Point, turn right and climb the braided trail that seems to wander a bit. It all goes to the same place, so just stick to the ridge.

About 0.5 mile up, the trail crosses a rockslide and, in most years, a snowfield. Be careful on both these terrains: They aren't steep, but remember that even big rocks move and that even packed snow is slippery. The trail keeps ascending the ridge face, crossing occasional small patches of snow. At a Y-junction, head right for the official McNeil Point, or go left to stay higher.

One mile from the turnoff at the creek, you'll reach the 1930s-era stone shelter at McNeil Point. From here the view is stupendous: Mount Hood soaring above you, the valley of the Muddy Fork Sandy River stretching out below you, the other Cascade volcanoes beyond. As you look at Mount Hood, the sprawling glacier on your right is Sandy Glacier, and the trickle coming out the bottom of it is the beginning of the Muddy Fork Sandy, which flows into the Columbia River down at Troutdale. See if you can also spot Lost Lake to the north and Bald Peak, which you just visited, looking like a green gash on the side of a hill. Evidence of the 2011 Dollar Fire on Mount Hood is clearly visible to your right.

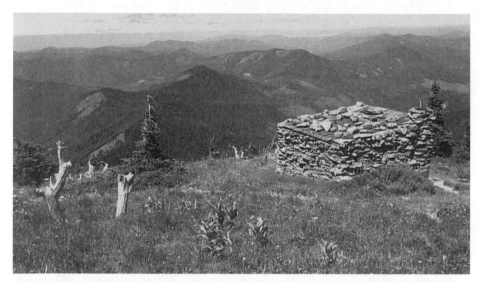

Built in the 1930s, the stone shelter at McNeil Point is a terrific lunch spot.

Also, as you look at Mount Hood, you'll notice more trail above you, heading into the Really High Country. It's not on any maps, but if you follow it you'll (1) soon run out of breath as you approach 7,000 feet in elevation with virtually no switchbacks, and (2) find yourself on a narrow, rocky ridge between Glisan (on your left) and Sandy (on your right) Glaciers.

I sat up here one day listening to the glaciers pop and moan as they slid slowly but relentlessly down the face of the mountain. You might even see massive boulders tumbling down the slope; you can certainly pick out their trails on the snow. At all costs, be careful up there, and most definitely resist the temptation to hop onto the snow.

You may hear or see reports of another, more direct trail between McNeil Point and Timberline Trail, connecting with the latter at a point west of the ponds. The word from many hikers, including this one, is to avoid that trail. It's steep, rocky, difficult, and unnecessary. The one described here is easier and more scenic.

GPS Information and Directions

N45° 24.467' W121° 47.149'

Take US 26 from Portland, driving 36 miles east of I-205 to Zigzag, and turn left onto Lolo Pass Road at the Zigzag Store. Go 10.6 miles to Lolo Pass and make a right onto paved Forest Service Road (FR) 1828, which is the first right at the pass. Go 3.1 miles and turn left onto gravel FR 118, following a sign for Top Spur. The trailhead is 1.5 miles ahead, on the right.

37 Mirror Lake

PHOTO: Clackamas County Tourism & Cultural Affairs

Mount Hood reflected in Mirror Lake

In Brief

You can go a short way on this hike and join the weekend throngs at a lovely little lake with a great view of Mount Hood. Or you can put in a little more effort and leave most of the crowds behind to claim an even better view at the top of, believe it or not, Tom, Dick, and Harry Mountain.

LENGTH 2.8 miles round-trip to the lake, 7 miles round-trip to the top of the ridge

CONFIGURATION Out-and-back

DIFFICULTY Easy to the lake, strenuous to the ridge

SCENERY Rhododendrons; deep forest; a small, placid lake; a big view

EXPOSURE Shady on the way up, open at the lake, wide-open atop the ridge

TRAFFIC Heavy all summer, insane on weekends

TRAIL SURFACE Packed dirt, rocks

HIKING TIME 2 hours to the lake, 4 hours to the ridgetop

DRIVING DISTANCE 52 miles (1 hour, 15 minutes) from Pioneer Courthouse Square

SEASON Late June–October

BEST TIME August and September

BACKPACKING OPTIONS A few sites at the lake

ACCESS Northwest Forest Pass required (see page 3)

WHEELCHAIR ACCESS None

MAPS Green Trails *Map 461 (Government Camp),* USFS *Mount Hood Wilderness,* USGS *Government Camp*

FACILITIES Portable restroom at trailhead

INFO Zigzag Ranger District, 503-622-3191, **www.fs.usda.gov/mthood**

SPECIAL COMMENTS Though this trail is very popular as a snowshoe destination, parking at the trailhead between November 1 and April 30 is prohibited, and your car will be towed. Even in the summer, parking outside the signs marking the lot will get you towed.

Description

When you come around the corner on US 26 and see 75 cars parked on the side of the road, know that it's not a fair: It's the Mirror Lake Trailhead. The interest in this trail is well justified, so think about starting early or going on a weekday to have a decent chance for some quiet time.

The lower portions of Mirror Lake Trail #664 have rhododendrons that bloom pink in late June, and the upper portions are cool and shady, keeping you from warming up too much as you head up the hill. But it isn't even much of a hill, gaining less than 700 feet in 1.4 well-graded miles. Just below the lake, you'll come to the outlet creek and a trail junction. You can go either way to loop 0.4 mile around the lake, but if you're headed up the ridge, bear right.

The lake itself is a beauty. The beaches are on the right side, the (unimpressive) campsites are on the left, and the view of Mount Hood you're looking for is at the far end, on the boardwalk in a marshy area.

To get to the top of Tom, Dick, and Harry Mountain, walk to the far right side of the lake (as you face it when you arrive), and follow a trail that goes right and steadily climbs the face of the ridge. Your destination is actually right above you, but you have

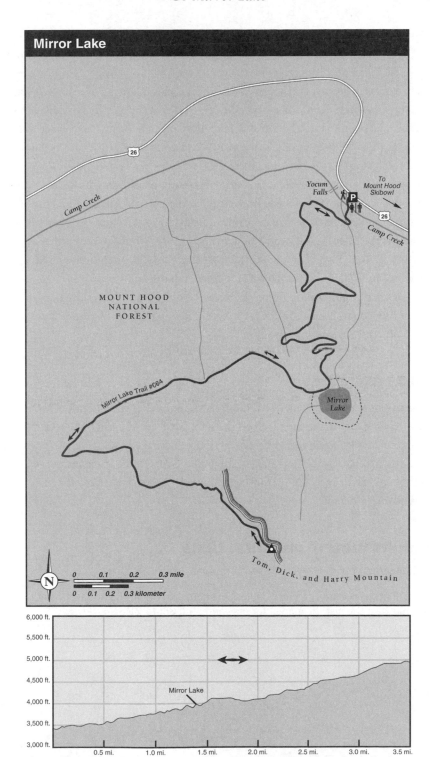

to walk almost 2 miles to get there. As for the mountain's name, it indicates the three peaks on the ridge—not, as some would suggest, the fact that every Tom, Dick, and Harry hikes this trail.

The trail is really just two lengthy switchbacks, each almost a mile long. It's time to turn left when you get to some very odd, large piles of rocks, which no one has ever been able to explain to me. The forest opens a little more here and, as you approach the summit, the trail gets a smidgen steeper. When you reach a rocky area (neither steep nor dangerous), you're almost there.

The view from atop this ridge is really something, considering how close you still are to your car. For starters, look at how pitifully small Mirror Lake is—and how far down it is. It never ceases to amaze me how quickly you gain elevation when hiking. Right across the highway is Mount Hood, in all its glory. Mount Adams is actually blocked by it. To the left is Mount St. Helens. What looks like a shoulder on St. Helens is in fact Mount Rainier, some 100 miles to the north of you.

In case you're still feeling energetic, resist the temptation to explore the other two peaks on this ridge—Tom and Dick, as it were. They're off-limits because they're home to protected peregrine falcons.

Nearby Activities

The easternmost peak of Tom, Dick, and Harry Mountain is the summit of **Mt. Hood Skibowl,** which, in the summer, is like a constant carnival. You can bungee-jump, ride the alpine slide, play mini-golf, drive go-carts, take a trip in a helicopter, or ride the chairlift to the top of the hill and hike or mountain-bike down. The entrance is 1 mile east of the Mirror Lake Trailhead on US 26. Call 503-222-B O W L (2695) or see **skibowl.com** for details.

GPS Information and Directions

N45° 18.410' W121° 47.534'

Take US 26 from Portland, driving 45 miles east of I-205. Park at the trailhead, on the right. It's 0.5 mile past the historic marker for the Laurel Hill Chute, also on the right.

38 Ramona Falls

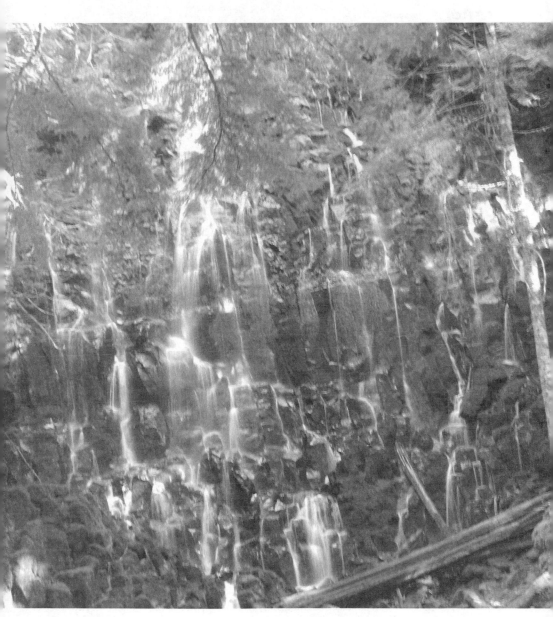

Ramona Falls—lovely to visit, really hard to photograph!

LENGTH 7.1 miles to the falls, 15.4 miles up Yocum Ridge	**BACKPACKING OPTIONS** Campsites very near the falls and up on Yocum Ridge
CONFIGURATION Balloon	**ACCESS** Northwest Forest Pass required (see page 3)
DIFFICULTY Easy	
SCENERY A pleasant stream, a historic cabin, a one-of-a-kind waterfall, and maybe a trip to the high country	**WHEELCHAIR ACCESS** None
	MAPS Green Trails *Map 461 (Government Camp)*, USFS *Mount Hood Wilderness*, USGS *Bull Run Lake*
EXPOSURE In the woods all the way, with occasional open spots	
	FACILITIES None at trailhead; campground with water and toilets less than a mile away
TRAFFIC Heavy use, especially on summer weekends	
TRAIL SURFACE Packed dirt	**INFO** Zigzag Ranger District, 503-622-3191, www.fs.usda.gov/mthood
HIKING TIME 4 hours to the falls, 9 hours to Yocum Ridge	**SPECIAL COMMENTS** A hiking bridge over the Sandy River is in place only from mid-May to mid-October, so call ahead or check online. Also, many hikers have had their cars broken into at this trailhead—leave valuables at home, and consider leaving the door unlocked so they won't take out your window.
DRIVING DISTANCE 53 miles (1 hour, 10 minutes) from Pioneer Courthouse Square	
SEASON May–October	
BEST TIME July–September	

In Brief

This trail is immensely popular, and no wonder: It's a fairly easy hike to a uniquely beautiful falls, with plenty of room for a picnic when you get there. There's even a side trip that takes you up onto a shoulder of Mount Hood.

Description

This hike starts on a trail that looks like a highway; that's because it's basically flat and thousands of people make the trek to Ramona Falls every year. Walk 0.2 mile and cross Sandy River Trail #770, a connector from Riley Horse Camp. Continue on Ramona Falls Trail #797, pausing to admire a very large, cracked boulder near the junction.

A short walk rewards you with a nice view of Mount Hood up the main stem of the Sandy River. You'll also see the results of a massive flood that occurred in November 2007. The deep cut you see here didn't exist before that flood, and the trail has been moved in a few places to replace sections that are probably now down in the Columbia River. In fact, at one point about a mile up, you can see the trail reappearing on the far edge of a big bend in the gorge. Gives you some perspective, huh?

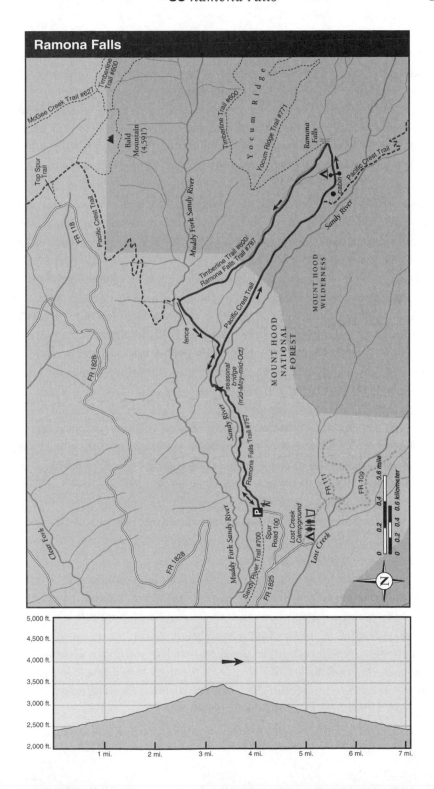

At 1.2 miles, you'll reach the Sandy River crossing. The bridge here is in place from mid-May to mid-October; you'll generally find signs at the trailhead alerting you to its status, but call ahead if you're in doubt. In the fall, the river can often be crossed without the bridge—if there hasn't been much rain.

After crossing the river, follow the ribbons across the new debris flow, eventually putting in 0.25 mile to reach the junction with the Pacific Crest Trail (PCT), which here makes its way around the west side of Mount Hood. This is also where your loop starts, so for now turn right (south) onto the PCT and continue your gradual climb over moss-covered ground and under some very large rhododendrons. A mile past the junction, you'll reach the top of a bluff from which the Sandy River, below you to the right, is more audible. Keep an eye out for eroded cliffs across the way, which offer a cross-section of Mount Hood's volcanic deposits. Those deposits are much older than the ones you just left.

When you're 1.5 miles past the junction (and 3 miles from your car), the PCT dips to the right and toward the river; follow it for a little scenic side trip. At the bottom of a short descent, you'll reach a pretty sad campsite near the Sandy's shore. The PCT crosses the Sandy here and starts a long climb toward Timberline Lodge; it's worth walking out to the crossing to stand on the 2007 debris and catch some cool views up the canyon toward Hood and some big-time waterfalls. Follow pink ribbons if you get confused.

Back at the far end of the campsite, look for log steps leading up the hill to a 1935 ranger station, built to keep hikers out of the protected Bull Run watershed. The rangers are long gone, but hikers can spend the night here. The leaky cabin is lousy with mice and has been boarded up for years, but there are some tent sites nearby, along with a nice view of Sandy River Canyon, about 100 yards uphill.

Follow the PCT back up the hill to Ramona Falls Trail, turn right, and in 0.2 mile you'll come to a horse gate that protects the entrance to the falls area. From here, you can descend to the left to find campsites; camping is not allowed at the falls itself. Pass through the gate and enter the falls area.

Ramona Falls is a perfect example of how a tiny stream can make one heck of a waterfall. These falls are best compared to one of those pyramids of Champagne glasses: As the water cascades over broken columns of basalt, it spreads across a 120-foot-wide expanse, the force of the water sending a cool, misty spray into the open air. No wonder so many people come here with kids and dogs and picnic supplies! Just beware of the gray jays that haunt the area—they'll take food right out of your hands if you're not careful. The falls are also famous for being tough to photograph, owing to their size and the lighting.

There's a nice story, by the way, behind the naming of Ramona Falls. In 1933, a U.S. Forest Service employee came across the falls while scouting the area for a trail; at the time, he was courting his future wife and named the falls after a popular romantic song of the time called "Ramona."

Continue over the bridge to reach a junction at the far end. To head back to your car, go straight. Or, if you're looking for an adventure, make a right onto Timberline Trail #600, the 42-mile wonder trail around Mount Hood. You can follow this trail 5 or so miles around the headwater of the Sandy River's Muddy Fork to wind up on the flanks of Bald Mountain (also part of the McNeil Point hike; see page 190). That trail, though, has suffered over the years from mudslides and washouts, despite crews working to keep it open. It can be really sketchy, especially the river crossings and washouts, so call the ranger district ahead of time to check on conditions before heading this way.

What you can still do is put in just over 0.5 mile on Timberline Trail and then head right, up Yocum Ridge Trail #771, an occasionally steep affair that gains 2,100 feet in 4.1 miles. The reward for that effort is an amazing bit of alpine splendor, far enough from any trailhead that it receives relatively few visitors—certainly compared with other hikes in this book, like Vista Ridge or McNeil Point. Campsites are found on the ridge, and chances are you won't see more than one other party up there.

To complete the much simpler loop back to the parking lot from Ramona Falls, follow the trail straight ahead and down Ramona Creek, perhaps singing a romantic tune as you go. It's a gentle 1.6-mile descent, featuring several log-bridge crossings of the creek, with views of fantastic rock walls on the right. See if you can spot a little section of "underground" creek as well.

Rejoin the PCT when it comes in from the right; continuing straight ahead on Ramona Falls Trail #797, go through a fence 0.1 mile later, and then turn left and walk 0.5 mile back to where your loop started. Backtrack across the Sandy River to your car, which is 2 miles down from where you hit the PCT.

GPS Information and Directions

N45° 23.220' W121° 49.905'

Take US 26 from Portland, driving 36 miles east of I-205 to Zigzag. Turn left (north) onto Lolo Pass Road, which is 0.6 mile past Milepost 41. Go 4.2 miles and make a right onto Forest Service Road (FR) 1825, which is 0.1 mile past a sign for Mount Hood National Forest and is marked CAMPGROUNDS AND TRAILHEADS. Stay right at 0.7 mile, cross a bridge, and continue another 1.7 miles to turn left onto Spur Road 100, which leads 0.5 mile to the trailhead. (This intersection is occasionally without signs, so trust your odometer.) Going right at this last fork would take you 0.3 mile to Lost Creek Campground, which has water and restrooms.

39 Salmon River

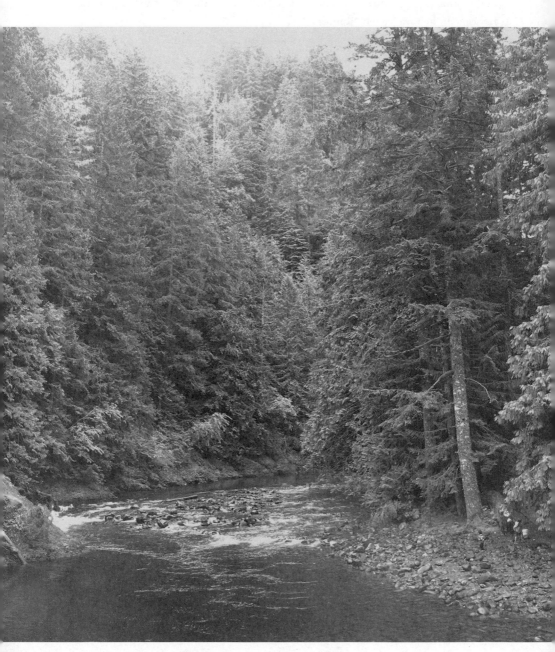

There's plenty of peace along the Salmon River.

LENGTH Lower section, 5.2 miles round-trip; upper section, 6.6 miles round-trip	DRIVING DISTANCE 50 miles (1 hour, 15 minutes) from Pioneer Courthouse Square
CONFIGURATION Out-and-back	SEASON Year-round; gets snow in winter
DIFFICULTY Easy all the way to the campsites in the upper section, moderate–strenuous beyond that	BEST TIME October, for the colors and salmon
SCENERY Old-growth forest, spawning salmon in the spring and fall, a canyon view at the top	BACKPACKING OPTIONS Nice sites in the upper section
	ACCESS Northwest Forest Pass required (see page 3)
EXPOSURE Shady all the way to the top, where there are exposed rocks	WHEELCHAIR ACCESS None
	MAPS USFS *Salmon-Huckleberry Wilderness*
TRAFFIC Heavy all summer long	
TRAIL SURFACE Packed dirt, with rocks and roots	FACILITIES None at trailheads; water and restrooms at Green Canyon Campground
HIKING TIME 2 hours for the lower section, 3.5 hours for the upper section	INFO Zigzag Ranger District, 503-622-3191, www.fs.usda.gov/mthood

In Brief

The Salmon River, which starts on the slopes of Timberline Ski Area, is the only river in the lower 48 states that is classified as a Wild and Scenic River from its headwater to its mouth. (To see its headwater and ford it where you can skip across, do the Barlow Pass or Timberline Lodge trip; see pages 166 and 213, respectively.) The trail along the Salmon can be thought of as having three sections. The upper and lower sections, described here, are extremely easy to get to, and in the fall they host—wait for it—spawning salmon. The uppermost section, accessed by a different road near Trillium Lake, is less interesting than these and tougher to find; its only advantage is that hardly anybody hikes it. For hardier hikers, I've also included an optional side trip to Devils Peak.

Description

Lower Section (EASY)

This is Old Salmon River Trail #742A. From the roadside parking area (the first one you came to while driving in), you'll start out downhill through a beautiful forest of Douglas-firs and Western red cedars. You'll be close to the river after 0.1 mile and

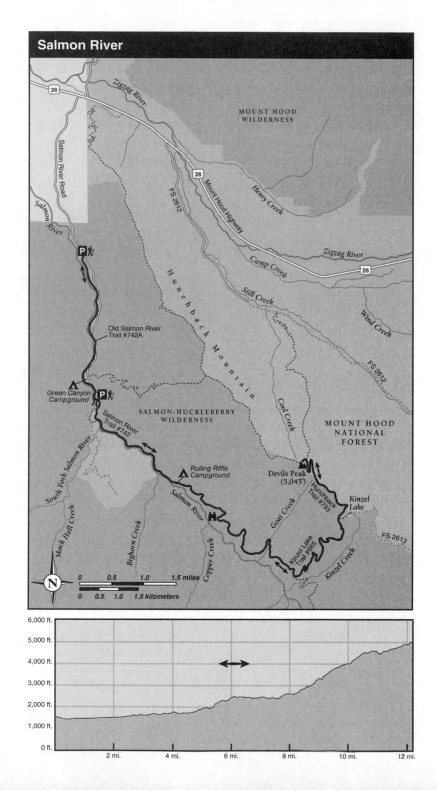

follow it most of the rest of the way. After two little footbridges over side creeks, you'll come to the first of several trails leading down to the river. You'll pass two more small bridges and, after 0.4 mile, come to a campsite where a log sticks out over the river. It's perfectly sturdy, but be sure of your balance before you go out on it.

The best thing about this trail, other than its convenience and the river itself, is the nature of the old-growth forest. Look for "nurse logs"—fallen trees that are now the home of new trees. Just past the campsite with the suspended log, you'll climb a set of steps, at the top of which is an absolutely massive Western red cedar. You can't miss it— it's right next to the trail and about 10 feet thick at its base. At about the 1-mile mark, look for a hollowed-out cedar stump with a new tree growing from it; just past it is the biggest Douglas-fir (about 8 feet in diameter) on this stretch of the trail.

At about the 1.5-mile mark, you'll come to the first of two sections where the trail briefly joins the road. Take the second trail back into the woods; the first trail is used by anglers and dead-ends at the river. Continue 50 yards and look for three large trees—two firs and a cedar—that are almost bonded together. Just past here, where a downed tree lies along the bank, I came across several spawning salmon on a late-September hike. They were in the shallows just a few feet from shore. The fish will actually go several miles farther upstream; if you hike the upper section of this trail in the fall, you'll get more chances to see them.

There are two more highlights to this trail. One is a cedar tree so large that a hollowed-out area in its base is big enough to be called a cave. The other is a nurse log, cut into three pieces for trail-construction purposes, which is now host to no fewer than eight saplings.

When you've hiked a little more than 2 miles, you'll come to Green Canyon Campground, which has an outhouse and water. Then, after a second section on the roadside, you'll briefly drop back into the woods before emerging at the upper trail-head, where the road crosses the river.

Upper Section (EASY–MODERATE)

Now for Salmon River Trail #742. From the trailhead at the bridge, walk upstream through a forest replete with massive Douglas-firs. Just less than 0.5 mile up, you'll pass a deep pool, where anglers often gather. A short distance past this, when you get another view of the river from about 40 feet above it, look (in September and October) for dark shapes swirling about in the pools. Those are salmon: The black-gray ones are chinook, and the less-often-seen gold ones are coho. Consider that they have spent their lives in the ocean and have swum some 75 miles up the Columbia River, about 41 miles up the Sandy, then about 20 miles up the Salmon.

At the 2-mile mark, a series of campsites on the right offers yet more chances to get close to the river and look for fish. Just past that, a trail leads right, to a nice little falls and deep pool—both formed by a huge log that fell across the river. Beyond the falls trail, you'll embark on just about your only climb of the day, picking up nearly 600 feet in 1.3 miles as you climb toward an overlook of Salmon River Canyon. After you pop out into the open, make sure you go as far as the rock outcrop for the best view. Just be very careful around here, and don't try any of the trails heading down toward the river—you might descend farther and faster than you ever intended.

Devils Peak Option (STRENUOUS)

That scenic view is your recommended turnaround, as you're now 3.3 miles from the upper trailhead, but the trail actually goes another 10.8 miles upstream to the road near Trillium Lake. If you're feeling truly industrious, or perhaps you camped back along the river and you have more time, consider putting in the big climb to the lookout tower at Devils Peak. Just continue 2.3 miles up Salmon River Trail #742, then turn left to climb Kinzel Lake Trail #665, following it 2.3 miles (and 1,600 feet) up to Hunchback Trail #793, which leads 1.6 miles (and another 700 feet) up to the 5,045-foot lookout. So if you started at the bridge, you're looking at 9.8 miles one-way with a climb of 3,400 feet. Good luck with that. You have other options for getting up there, but this one would be good as part of an overnight trip.

Nearby Activities

Start your day with breakfast at the **ZigZag Inn,** 0.1 mile east of Salmon River Road (70162 US 26, Welches, OR 97055; 503-622-4779). They do good things with French toast here.

GPS Information and Directions

N45° 18.646' W121° 56.615'

Take US 26 from Portland, driving 36 miles east of I-205. Turn right on Salmon River Road, which is 0.1 mile before Lolo Pass Road, on the left. Continue 2.7 miles straight down this road to reach the lower trailhead, just beyond the sign for Mount Hood National Forest, or drive 4.9 miles to the upper trailhead, at a bridge over the river.

40 Tamanawas Falls

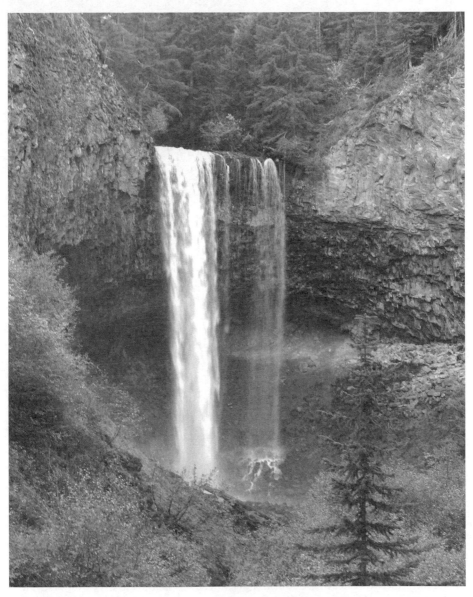

The prize at the end of the trail. You can even slip behind the falls.

LENGTH 3.4 miles	**SEASON** June–November
CONFIGURATION Out-and-back	**BEST TIME** July–September
DIFFICULTY Easy	**BACKPACKING OPTIONS** None
SCENERY Two mountain streams, a plunging waterfall	**ACCESS** Northwest Forest Pass required (see page 3)
EXPOSURE Shady all the way, then open at the end	**WHEELCHAIR ACCESS** None
TRAFFIC Heavy on summer weekends, moderate otherwise	**MAPS** Green Trails *Map 462 (Mount Hood),* USFS *Mount Hood Wilderness,* USGS *Dog River*
TRAIL SURFACE Packed dirt and rocks	**FACILITIES** None at trailhead; water and restrooms 0.5 mile south on OR 35, at Sherwood Campground
HIKING TIME 2.5 hours	
DRIVING DISTANCE 75 miles (1 hour, 40 minutes) from Pioneer Courthouse Square	**INFO** Hood River Ranger District, 541-352-6002, **www.fs.usda.gov/mthood**

In Brief

This is a classic falls in a dramatic setting at the end of an easy, beautiful hike that's perfectly suited for a family outing. *Tamanawas* (pronounced ta-**MAH**-na-was) is a Chinook word for a friendly guardian spirit, and it's an appropriate name for this easy, pleasant hike.

Description

So many people like this trail that even a flood in 2000, which wiped out two trail bridges, didn't keep folks away. Officially, the trail was closed that entire summer, but Oregonians displayed their typical respect for the government by hiking the "closed" trail in such numbers that the U.S. Forest Service acquiesced and made the new, hiker-created trail the official one. The Forest Service hasn't rebuilt the bridges, so the trail you hike today is what the locals came up with in 2000.

From the trailhead, walk to your right and cross the East Fork Hood River on a one-log bridge with handrails. Note the milky color of the river; that's glacial silt. At the far end of the bridge, join East Fork Trail #650 and follow it to the right, where it parallels the road for 0.5 mile. Ignore the mileage on that sign, by the way—you're 1.6 miles from the falls, not 2.

At 0.7 mile, you'll leave East Fork Trail and cross Cold Spring Creek on Tamana-was Falls Trail #650A. Now enjoy a lovely stretch right along the creek, passing numerous cascades, creekside picnic areas, and forest features, and in 0.7 mile come

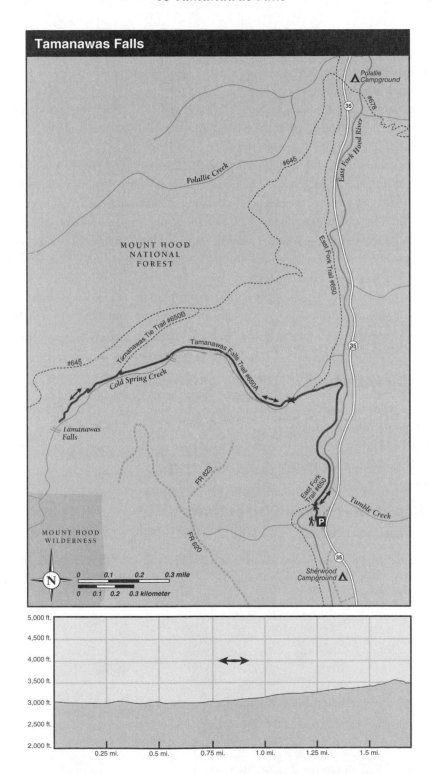

Tamanawas Falls

to a rockslide area where Tamanawas Tie Trail #650B splits off to the right. The original Tamanawas Falls Trail crossed the creek on a bridge, but that was one of the bridges wiped out in 2000. The new route goes slightly left to cross a rockslide where hikers made their way in 2000.

This larger rockslide has been here for a long time; it is, in fact, the reason the trail crossed the creek in the first place. The path winds through the boulders, and from the far side it's about 0.2 mile to the falls.

What makes this falls so special is that even in late summer there's plenty of water coming over it, and it's rimmed by basalt walls, many of which are pink because pieces have so recently fallen into the chasm. For this reason, take care if you want to go nearer (or even behind) the falls, as you'll be walking on wet rocks with no official trail and with cliffs above you—cliffs that provide ample evidence that rocks could come crashing down at any time. These are just little reminders from Mother Nature that we are, after all, just visitors in her world.

One other feature to note: A few of the trees around the falls are western larches, which you wouldn't know unless you're here in late October and they've turned their brilliant shade of gold. Assuming it isn't raining *too* hard, it's a lovely time to visit.

Nearby Activities

Drive 7.5 miles north of the trailhead on OR 35, then turn left to visit the **Hutson Museum** (4697 Baseline Rd., Parkdale, OR 97041), which features local history, Indian artifacts, and memorabilia of the early settlers. Open April–October; for more info, call 541-352-6806 or see **tinyurl.com/hutsonmuseum.**

GPS Information and Directions

N45° 23.831' W121° 34.305'

Take US 26 from Portland, driving 51 miles east of I-205. Turn north (left) on OR 35, following signs for Hood River. Drive 15 miles on OR 35; 0.2 mile past Sherwood Campground, park at the trailhead, on the left.

41 Timberline Lodge

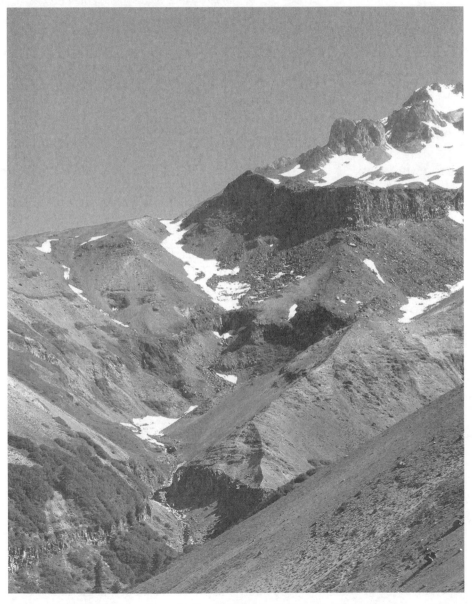

A view of Zigzag Canyon from the Pacific Crest Trail. To get to Paradise Park, you have to pass through this!

LENGTH 13 miles round-trip to Paradise Park, 4.8 miles round-trip to Zigzag Canyon overlook, 2.2 miles round-trip to Silcox Hut, 1 mile round-trip to White River Canyon	**DRIVING DISTANCE** 64 miles (1 hour, 30 minutes) from Pioneer Courthouse Square
	SEASON July–October
	BEST TIME August and September
CONFIGURATION Paradise Park, balloon; Zigzag and White River Canyons, out-and-backs; Silcox Hut, out-and-back or loop	**BACKPACKING OPTIONS** Good sites in Paradise Park
	ACCESS No fees or permits
	WHEELCHAIR ACCESS A few patches of road around the lodge
DIFFICULTY Easy–strenuous depending on the hike	**MAPS** Green Trails *Map 462 (Mount Hood),* USFS *Mount Hood Wilderness*
SCENERY Flower-filled meadows, deep canyons, overhead glaciers	**FACILITIES** Full services at Timberline Lodge
EXPOSURE Both shady and open	
TRAFFIC Heavy all summer long	**INFO** Zigzag Ranger District, 503-622-3191, **www.fs.usda.gov/mthood**
TRAIL SURFACE Dirt, rock, pavement, sand	**SPECIAL COMMENTS** No matter what the weather looks like, bring warm clothing for this hike.
HIKING TIME 30 minutes–7 hours	

In Brief

If you spend just one day in Oregon, you should spend it at Timberline Lodge. If you go on only one hike, you should go to Paradise Park in August or early September. But fear not—if you aren't up to a 13-mile loop, options abound at this spectacular mountain palace.

Description

Timberline Lodge is the greatest human-made thing in Oregon. It was built in 1937 by the Works Progress Administration and dedicated by President Franklin D. Roosevelt the same day that he dedicated Bonneville Dam. But as astounding as the interior is, it's the setting of the place that requires one to spend time here. Only a few peaks in Oregon rise above it, and with few trees around, the views are amazing, especially views to the summit of Mount Hood—the highest point in the state— 3 miles away, and to Mount Jefferson, 45 miles to the south. In August, wildflowers bloom everywhere.

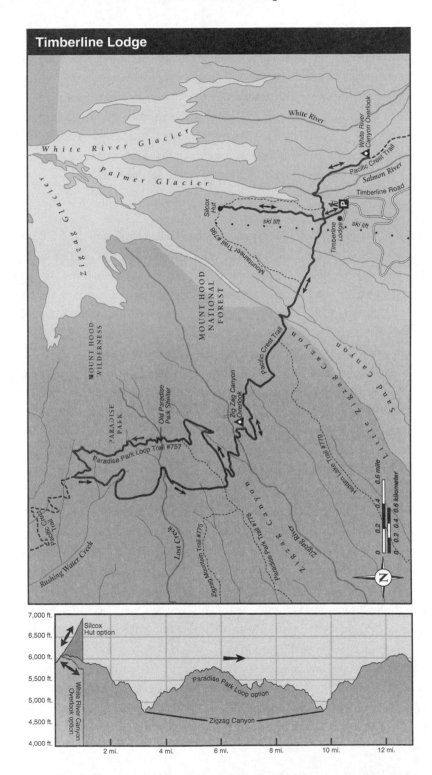

Timberline Lodge

White River Canyon Overlook (1 MILE)

Let's start with the shortest hike. Follow a sign to the right of the lodge, pointing you to the Pacific Crest Trail (PCT). You'll walk uphill a couple hundred yards, perhaps wondering why you're suddenly breathing heavily: It's because you're now at 6,000 feet elevation. At the PCT, turn right (that would be toward Mexico) and walk 0.5 mile to the overlook; note that you'll have to skip over a couple of small creeks along the way.

If you'd like to do a one-way hike with a car shuttle, this trail connects in another 0.5 mile with the top of the Barlow Pass trip (see Hike 31, page 166).

Silcox Hut (2.2 MILES)

For our next-toughest destination, go straight ahead when you get to the PCT junction and follow the road uphill 1.1 miles to Silcox Hut. There seem to be a lot of small trails, but you can see the hut at the top of the chairlift, so just head for it. The last part of the hike is on a dirt road. Timberline Lodge rents this hut out to groups of 12 or more during the winter. For about $100 per person, they take you to the hut, cook your dinner, then come back in the morning to cook your breakfast. And in the summer, you can ride the Magic Mile chairlift up here, then walk down.

To loop back to the lodge, go back the way you came or take the service road under the chairlift. For a slightly longer loop, take Mountaineer Trail #798, which goes right (as you look down) from the top of the lift. It drops to the PCT 1 mile west of the lodge, in forest broken up by flowered meadows. Turn left and walk 0.8 mile to the lodge.

Zigzag Canyon Overlook (4.8 MILES)

But enough with the preliminaries: Let's head for Zigzag Canyon and Paradise Park. From the lodge, follow the PCT to your left; it will cross under two chairlifts and start descending slowly as it enters the woods. Hike 0.8 mile, ignoring Mountaineer Trail, which leads up to Silcox Hut. Continue 1.4 miles, ignoring Trail #779 to the left, leading to Hidden Lake (it's a nice lake, but it's 3 miles below you). Just keep on truckin' through meadows and forests, past flowers and little springs. The best of these are around 2 miles out from the trailhead: great vertical bands of grass and color, the farthest one with a cool view of Mt. Hood Skibowl and Tom, Dick, and Harry Mountain, described in the Mirror Lake profile (see Hike 37, page 195).

At 2.4 miles, you'll find yourself standing agog at the edge of a massive gash in the hillside, with Mount Hood rising to your right. This is Zigzag Canyon. If you've had enough at this point, head back and you'll have done a 4.8-mile out-and-back trip. But for the real prize of this part of the mountain, keep going.

Paradise Park (13 MILES)

Looking at a map or elevation profile, you may have noticed that Paradise Park is actually below Timberline Lodge, making it sound pretty easy. But what you need to know, standing at Zigzag Overlook, is that in the next 3 miles, while crossing Zigzag Canyon and climbing up to Paradise Park, you'll descend 600 feet and then climb 900 feet. Just believe that it's worth it, and press on.

You'll have to hop across the Zigzag River—look for the waterfall just upstream—and, 0.7 mile up the other side, take the first right, onto Paradise Park Loop Trail #757. Then, yes, keep climbing toward Paradise Park—that's if you want to climb up to the best attractions. You can also stay on the PCT/Timberline Trail #600 for 2.1 miles to the lower end of our loop, and you'll save yourself several hundred feet of climbing but still see some great waterfalls.

As you head up Paradise Park Loop Trail, things start to get really spectacular. The number and variety of flowers in this area—lupines, daisies, lilies, and bushy-looking pasqueflowers—and, of course, the plump sweetness of huckleberries in late summer make it a prime destination. Another big flower highlight is the beargrass show in July. Hike 1 mile to reach Paradise Park Trail #778 coming in from the left; you can take it 0.6 mile down to the PCT and shorten your walk by 3.8 miles. But those 3.8 miles are fairly flat and very beautiful, so keep going.

Staying on Paradise Park Loop Trail, in 0.25 mile you'll cross Lost Creek, spy an amazing campsite on a ledge above it, and 100 yards later come to the site of the old Paradise Park Shelter, one of several built in the 1930s for people hiking the Timberline Trail.

The trail turns right just before the shelter foundation and starts a long, wonderfully flat traverse through Paradise Park: heather, flowers, creeks, Mount Rainier, Mount St. Helens, a big cliff above you called Mississippi Head, the Zigzag Glacier above that . . . not bad at all for a flat walk. After 1.2 miles of this, you'll descend into the forest again, where your trail intersects the PCT and Timberline Trail; this area provides great views down Sandy River Canyon and across it to Slide Mountain, a literal cross-section of Mount Hood.

Turn left here and start back toward the lodge. After an easy 0.5 mile, you'll come to Rushing Water Creek and its wonderful canyon, where you'll pass just under its waterfall; below you are an amazing slot canyon and a view down into Sandy River Canyon. Hike another 0.5 mile, slowly descending now, to return to Lost Creek. Look for a trail that leads uphill just after the crossing; it first passes a little double waterfall, then a magical, hidden cove with yet another waterfall. They're everywhere! It's not hard to find campsites in this area, either.

Another 0.7 mile brings you to the lower end of Paradise Park Trail #778, where a horse corral and its smell will encourage you to keep moving. The descent is steeper now, and in 0.4 mile you'll have returned to the junction where your loop started, Paradise Park Loop Trail #757. Follow the PCT back down into the canyon, and, well, hate to tell you, but from here—with 9.5 miles under your belt—you've got 3.5 miles to go, gaining 1,200 feet, and you've seen it all before.

But hey, it was worth it, right? Besides, you've got Timberline Lodge to enjoy now. The hot chocolate and coffee drinks are sublime, the food's not bad (or cheap), you can watch an interesting film about its construction, and its main lobby is about as nice a place to recover from a hike as you could ask for. And you deserve it.

Nearby Activities

Though it's crowded, spend some time exploring **Timberline Lodge.** Watch the film *The Builders of Timberline* to hear the story of how artists and artisans came together during the Depression to create this masterwork. Then learn the details of their accomplishment, especially those of the Head House and its massive central stone tower. More info: 503-272-3311, **timberlinelodge.com.**

GPS Information and Directions

N45° 19.841' W121° 42.551'

Take US 26 from Portland, driving 48 miles east of I-205. Turn left onto the well-marked Timberline Road, 2 miles past Government Camp. Follow Timberline Road 6 winding miles to the parking lot.

42 Trillium Lake

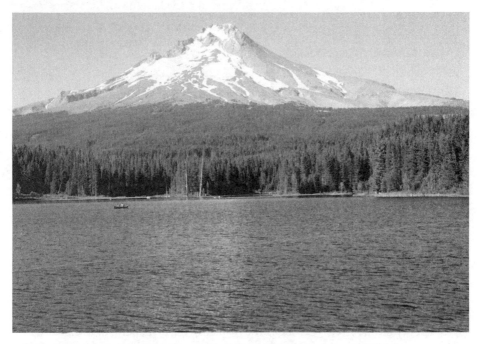

If you can get here when it isn't crowded, few places are more peaceful than Trillium Lake, which offers camping, boating, fishing, and hiking.

In Brief

A prime place to take the kids or to stretch your legs after driving up from Portland, Trillium Lake is a tiny body of water with a friendly scene and an impressive and popular view of Mount Hood. In addition to some short, easy hikes, you'll have opportunities to fish, boat, or picnic—or just lie around, catch some rays, and watch the ducks.

Description

Most outdoorsy Portlanders know Trillium Lake as a cross-country-skiing area, famed for the terror felt by many beginners on the long hill one drives down from US 26. But in the summer the lake is a beautiful, peaceful place to get a little taste of what the

LENGTH 2 miles	**SEASON** June–October
CONFIGURATION Loop	**BEST TIME** August and September
DIFFICULTY Easy	**BACKPACKING OPTIONS** Not great
SCENERY Marshes, lake, birds, forest	**ACCESS** Northwest Forest Pass (see page 3); $5/vehicle/day without pass
EXPOSURE Shady, except when crossing the dam	**WHEELCHAIR ACCESS** The trail was built to be barrier-free, with boardwalk and finely compacted rock.
TRAFFIC Heavy all summer long, moderate when school is in session	**MAPS** Green Trails *Map 462 (Mount Hood)*, USFS *Mount Hood Wilderness*
TRAIL SURFACE Packed dirt, boardwalk, pavement	**FACILITIES** Restrooms in day-use area near the dam; water at campground
HIKING TIME 1.5 hours	
DRIVING DISTANCE 61 miles (1 hour, 20 minutes) from Pioneer Courthouse Square	**INFO** Zigzag Ranger District, 503-622-3191, **www.fs.usda.gov/mthood**

Mount Hood area has to offer. And if you've got kids along, they can swim, fish, and paddle in the lake all day.

To hike around it, start at the day-use area, just before the road crosses the dam at the lake's southern end. Stop here and take the picture of Mount Hood that so many other people have taken. In case you're wondering, that square area of snow high up on the mountain is Palmer Glacier, the scene of summer-long skiing and snowboarding at Timberline Ski Area. Walk along the road atop the dam, perhaps ask how the fishing is, and, at the far end of the dam, follow Trillium Lake Trail #761 to the right, into the woods.

On the first part of the trail, you won't be right by the lake because the shore on that side is marshy and covered with tall grass. So you'll have to enjoy the forest. At 0.6 mile, a short boardwalk heads right, providing a glimpse of the shoreline. At 0.8 mile, a campsite on the right affords access to a relatively private lakeshore spot. Beyond this point, the trail becomes a boardwalk that traverses a marshy area thick with vegetation. It will seem like you're swimming through the wildflowers late in the summer.

As you round the northern end of the lake, you'll pass from marsh to meadow, with a view of a corner of the lake that's covered with lily pads. Then, coming back to the more crowded eastern shore, you'll find numerous beaches for the kids to romp on or for you to sun yourself on. At 1.8 miles—just 0.2 mile from where you started, going the other way—there's a boat ramp and another parking lot. Just beyond that is a dock you can walk out onto (it has rails, so you don't have to worry about the kids). I was out there late one summer, with the sun setting and a few pink-hued clouds hanging

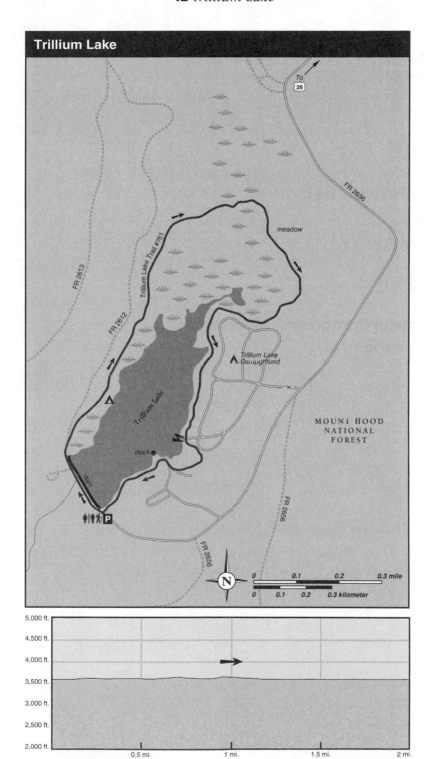

around Mount Hood across the way, and some grown-ups on the dock were talking about the stock market and housing prices. Some people just don't get it.

When you drive out, go past the lake for a piece of Oregon history. Head across the dam and drive 1 mile on the unpaved road, turn right and go 0.5 mile, and then make another right and park immediately on the right, near a white picket fence. That's a pioneer-era graveyard. Across the road is Summit Prairie, where Barlow Road travelers rested the day before tackling the infamous Laurel Hill.

Nearby Activities

You have to stop at some point at the **Huckleberry Inn** in Government Camp (503-272-3325, **huckleberry-inn.com** for directions and a map). They've got huckleberry pies, pancakes, milkshakes, and ice cream, and they serve pretty good cheeseburgers, too. I love this place.

GPS Information and Directions

N45° 15.992' W121° 44.483'

Take US 26 from Portland, driving 49 miles east of I-205. Turn right at a sign for Trillium Lake. At the bottom of the hill, proceed straight ahead for the day-use areas. The hiking trail, as described here, starts in the second day-use area you come to.

43 Twin Lakes

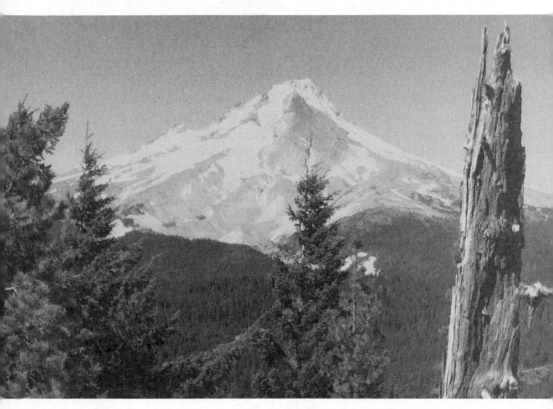

Palmateer Point is sort of a hassle to get to, but it affords this great view of Mount Hood.

In Brief

Whether you're a dayhiker or an overnighter, you won't find much of a challenge here: The total elevation gain averages less than 200 feet per mile, making this an easy-to-reach, easy-to-hike introduction to the Pacific Crest Trail (PCT) and the world of mountain lakes.

Description

For long-distance hikers on the PCT, the Twin Lakes are a diversion used mainly for water or camping—and even then they're often ignored. Long-distance hikers passing

LENGTH 4 miles to Lower Twin Lake, 8.5 miles to both lakes and Palmateer Point

CONFIGURATION Out-and-back or balloon

DIFFICULTY Moderate

SCENERY Two mountain lakes, old-growth forest, nice view of Mount Hood

EXPOSURE Shady all the way, except at the viewpoint

TRAFFIC Heavy on summer weekends, light otherwise

TRAIL SURFACE Packed dirt, with rocks and roots

HIKING TIME 2 hours to Lower Twin Lake, 6 hours to see it all

DRIVING DISTANCE 58 miles (1 hour, 20 minutes) from Pioneer Courthouse Square

SEASON June–October

BEST TIME August and September

BACKPACKING OPTIONS Sites at both lakes

ACCESS Northwest Forest Pass required (see page 3)

WHEELCHAIR ACCESS None

MAPS Green Trails *Map 462 (Mount Hood)*, USFS *Mount Hood Wilderness*

FACILITIES Restrooms at trailhead; water at nearby Frog Lake Campground

INFO Hood River Ranger District, 541-352-6002, **www.fs.usda.gov/mthood**

SPECIAL COMMENTS This hike is also a very popular snowshoeing and Nordic-skiing trip.

through these parts are just a few miles from both a US highway and Timberline Lodge, so there's not much here for them.

In fact, this trail was originally part of the Oregon Skyline Trail, and later the PCT, but the PCT was moved up the hill when the lakes started becoming overused.

What's here now are two lovely lakes and a nice viewpoint, all within easy reach. You can simply hike in to a lakeside campsite with only 4 round-trip miles of hiking and in half a day see all the sights this area has to offer. Another suggestion, before we get started: Consider combining this with the hike from Barlow Pass to Timberline Lodge (see Hike 31, page 166); by adding a car shuttle, you've got a one-way hike of just under 10 miles that winds up high on the slopes of Mount Hood.

One more thing: I did this hike once in mid-August in the midst of a monarch butterfly migration. If you find yourself at the center of this, it's astonishing—hundreds of butterflies fluttering around you, seemingly oblivious to your presence. The migration is fascinating because the butterflies are born in California, fly to Oregon, lay eggs, and die; the ones born in Oregon then fly to Washington, lay eggs, and die; and those monarchs fly to Canada, lay eggs, and die. Some of the ones born in Canada then return to California, often flying 100 miles in a day. Unreal.

At the parking lot at Frog Lake Sno-Park, head for the west end of the lot and walk into the woods near a hiker sign. You'll see a picnic table and garbage can here,

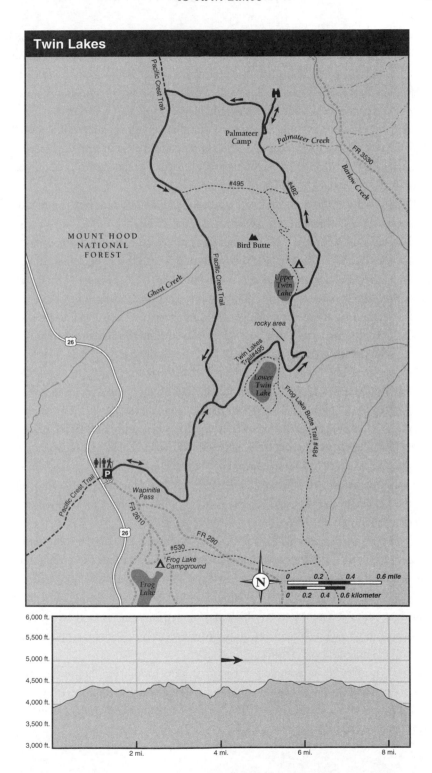

Twin Lakes

Pacific Crest Trail

Palmateer Camp

Palmateer Creek

FR 3530

Barlow Creek

#495

#482

MOUNT HOOD
NATIONAL
FOREST

Bird Butte

Ghost Creek

Pacific Crest Trail

Upper
Twin
Lake

rocky area

Twin Lakes
Trail #495

Lower
Twin
Lake

Frog Lake Butte Trail #484

26

Wapinitia
Pass

Pacific Crest Trail

FR 2610

26

FR 290

#530
Frog Lake
Campground

Frog
Lake

N

| 0 | 0.2 | 0.4 | 0.6 mile |

| 0 | 0.2 | 0.4 | 0.6 kilometer |

6,000 ft.

5,500 ft.

5,000 ft.

4,500 ft.

4,000 ft.

3,500 ft.

3,000 ft.

2 mi.   4 mi.   6 mi.   8 mi.

along with two outhouses nearby. Go 100 feet and turn right to take the PCT; you'll notice some evidence of the annual snowfall here, such as the height of the sign on your right, and that of the blue-diamond marker on a nice hemlock on the trail. That's all related to winter sports; this trail is wildly popular with the ski and snowshoe crowds for its easy access and excellent grade.

You'll appreciate that grade as you head uphill on a highway of a trail, wide enough for two people to walk shoulder-to-shoulder, and of such a mellow steepness (gaining 500 feet in 1.5 miles) that you'll hardly notice it—especially if the abundant huckleberries are ripe.

When you reach the beginning of Twin Lakes Trail #495, turn right on it and you'll soon descend a hill and spy Lower Twin Lake through the trees on your right. You'll also see a social trail or two plunging down the hillside to the shore, but don't use them—you'll add to erosion, and the main trail goes to the same place. After a total of 2 miles (including a short stretch past the lake, up a drainage), you'll arrive at a junction with Frog Lake Butte Trail #484 at the northeast shore of the lake. You'll find camping enough for a village here, and practically nothing alive on the ground, but there's also a trail that goes all the way around the lake, leading to other campsites along the way.

To head for Upper Twin Lake and the rest of the hike, stay on Twin Lakes Trail #495. You'll round a bend, climb briefly, and, in 0.7 mile, come to a rocky area with a view (on the left) looking back down to Lower Twin in its steep-sided, forested bowl. Hike another 0.25 mile to reach Upper Twin and its own round-the-lake trail. Staying on Twin Lakes Trail, you'll go along the east side of the lake, passing a big campsite from which a small trail heads into the woods on the right—to a toilet, believe it or not. Not an outhouse, mind you, just a toilet. Bizarre, and quite uncomfortable-looking.

Upper Twin, by the way, gets less use, but that might be because it's smaller, much more shallow, and not well suited to swimming.

A half-mile north of the Camp Toilet, you'll come to a trail on the right marked PALMATEER VIEW. Great name, huh? Sounds like a pirate or something, but alas, it's the name of a sheepherder from pioneer days. This trail is a shortcut to Palmateer Trail #482, which you'll reach in a few minutes—turn left here and you'll descend to the headwater of Palmateer Creek (which may be dry for your visit), then climb briefly to a large meadow called Palmateer Camp. From here, a moderately steep trail on the right leads 0.3 mile to the viewpoint.

This view gives you a rare perspective on Mount Hood, from the southeast, and the local stretch of the PCT. Climbing behind the ridge on your left, the PCT drops off its end to Barlow Pass, then climbs to Timberline Lodge, the gray roof of which is visible from your viewpoint.

You're also looking straight across (to the north) at Barlow Butte, where meadows unfold on the side facing you. The drainage between you and the butte is that of Barlow Creek, traced by the historic Barlow Road, which was an overland portion of the Oregon Trail used by people who didn't want to risk their lives on the Columbia River. You can still drive this road all the way to The Dalles if your car has some clearance; access it just off OR 35, at the trailhead to the Barlow Pass trip.

Descending from the viewpoint, turn right on Palmateer Trail #482 at Palmateer Camp, and in 0.7 mile you'll be back at the PCT. You're 1.2 miles south of Barlow Pass now, but to return to the car, turn left. You'll pass the upper end of Twin Lakes Trail #495 in 0.3 mile, climb slightly for just less than a mile, then cruise the last 2 miles on the PCT, heading for your car. Pick some more huckleberries, while you're at it.

Nice and easy, huh?

GPS Information and Directions

N45° 13.757' W121° 41.982'

Take US 26 from Portland, driving 55 miles east of I-205 to reach Frog Lake Sno-Park. The trailhead is in the left-hand corner as you enter, and the parking spots to the left of it will be in the shade all day.

44 Vista Ridge

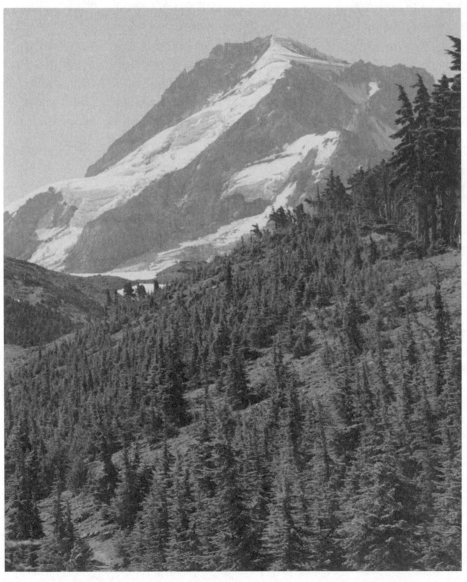

Wy'East Basin, at the top of Vista Ridge Trail. This photo was taken before the Dollar Lake Fire of 2011.

LENGTH Options of 4.4–11 miles	**DRIVING DISTANCE** 77 miles (2 hours, 10 minutes) from Pioneer Courthouse Square
CONFIGURATION Balloon	
DIFFICULTY Moderate, with one tricky river crossing	**SEASON** July–October
SCENERY Mountain streams, rocks, glaciers, meadows, flowers, and the results of a recent forest fire	**BEST TIME** August and September
	BACKPACKING OPTIONS Plentiful
	ACCESS No fees or permits
EXPOSURE In a burned forest for a couple of miles, then in and out of healthy forest and meadows	**WHEELCHAIR ACCESS** None
	MAPS Green Trails *Map 462 (Mount Hood)*, USFS *Mount Hood Wilderness*
TRAFFIC Heavy on summer weekends, moderate otherwise	**FACILITIES** None at trailhead; closest services at Zigzag Store (70171 E. US 26, Rhododendron, OR 97049; 503-622-7681)
TRAIL SURFACE Packed dirt, roots, rocks, ash	
HIKING TIME 3–6 hours	**INFO** Hood River Ranger District, 541-352-6002, **www.fs.usda.gov/mthood**

In Brief

This fairly easy trail to several flower-filled bowls at the tree line on Mount Hood is still more than worth the tedious drive to the trailhead. Since 2011, however, it has a whole new character, as several miles of it burned intensely, giving us all a rare chance to watch a forest regrow. I've given you several options here, but with a map and my hints, you could easily spend two days enjoying this mountain wonderland.

Description

For years, Vista Ridge Trail was inexplicably underused. It's a long drive, and the last section of the road used to be a hassle, but then it was "discovered" in a big way and became massively, and deservedly, popular. Then, in 2011, the Dollar Lake Fire swept over the north side of Mount Hood. In many cases, the effects of forest fires are overstated, but this was, in many places, complete devastation: For some of this hike you'll walk right through the burn, and the experience is utterly fascinating. You'll also see how the fire skipped around and how the forest is recovering—and anyway, the meadows were all spared. So as always, all you have to do is climb slightly for a couple of miles and you're in wildflower heaven. And the hiking options here are plentiful, including abundant chances for an overnighter.

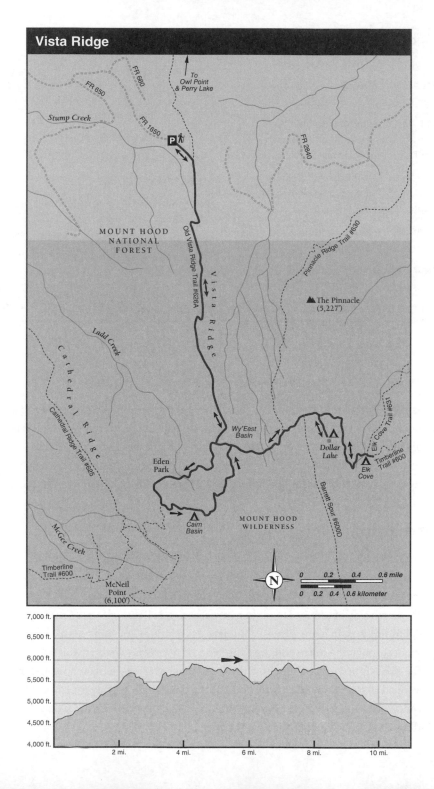

From the trailhead, go 0.2 mile to a sign and wilderness registration at Vista Ridge Trail #626, which is where the burn area starts. To the left here is your first hiking option, which I suggest if you have the whole day or you just don't feel like climbing much.

Owl Point Diversion (4 MILES ROUND-TRIP)

To your left is a section of trail that for years was unmaintained, becoming essentially a "lost" trail.

But in 2007, dedicated volunteers from the Portland Hikers online discussion boards cleared 178 logs from the trail and restored this 2.1-mile section to Owl Point. This event was also a primary factor in the forming of a nonprofit group called Trailkeepers of Oregon. The path is now called Old Vista Ridge Trail #626A, and it offers great views and a rare opportunity for solitude on Mount Hood. The U.S. Forest Service didn't seem too keen on the trail work being done, but it's a nice little hike.

The first 0.8 mile climbs a bit as it traverses the eastern side of Vista Ridge; look in this area for all the sawed-off logs. Look also for remnants of the old phone lines to a fire lookout in the area. A couple of viewpoints are off to the right. A half-mile past this, after you traverse an area of open forest, you'll find huckleberries and beargrass, and descend to a small meadow that can be marshy in early summer and late fall.

After a total of 1.5 miles, you'll reach a signed junction with a rustic side path that leads right 0.1 mile to The Rockpile, a Hood viewpoint with quite the reputation for huckleberries. The first 300 feet of this trip traverse a heather meadow where a faint path heads right to take you the final 300 feet through beargrass to The Rockpile.

Just 0.1 mile farther, Old Vista Ridge Trail intersects Owl Point Trail, a 0.1-mile spur to a viewpoint named for the great horned owls that nest in the area. The path climbs briefly through forest, then emerges to follow the edge of a large talus along a 500-foot cairn-marked route. The expansive view here, which also includes Laurance Lake and the upper Hood River Valley, is probably the best turnaround spot.

Old Vista Ridge Trail continues another 1.2 miles past more viewpoints and on to Perry Lake (more of a pond, really) and the foundation of the old Red Hill guard station and lookout tower. But because this involves rougher trail and another 500 feet of elevation gain getting back, and because Owl Point is the local highlight, you could probably skip this section, unless you're looking for a longer hike.

Vista Ridge Trail to Eden Park, Cairn Basin, and Wy'East Basin (4.8 MILES ONE-WAY)

Back at the wilderness kiosk, turn right and head toward Mount Hood, through the burn. Look for bark peeling off trees, snags turning whiter each summer, and flowers pushing back up through the ash. You also have views all around, which wasn't the case before 2011. When the trail gets just a bit steeper after a couple miles, you're almost there. At 2.5 miles from the kiosk, you'll arrive at Eden Park Trail in an open area, with Hood rising right in front of you. Congratulations: You've now climbed the biggest hill of your day—wasn't much, was it? You can go straight ahead on Eden Park Trail for Wy'East Basin to knock 2 miles off your day, but I suggest turning right for a 2.3-mile loop through Eden Park and Cairn Basin.

You'll briefly plunge downhill and then start heading around to the left, crossing babbling brooks and admiring flowers. After just under a mile of this, you'll cross Ladd Creek, where logs have usually been placed to make a bridge. A quarter-mile on, you'll be in Eden Park, which might be the loveliest mountain meadow you've seen—so far. To preserve the fragile landscape, stay on the trails.

To continue to Cairn Basin, cross Eden Park and follow the trail through the trees as it turns toward Mount Hood. It will climb a small hill, with a view back down to Eden Park, then pass through a notch and arrive 0.2 mile ahead at campsites in Cairn Basin. Here, you can turn right on Timberline Trail #600 to connect with the McNeil Point trip (see Hike 36, page 190), which is just 0.3 mile and a tricky creek crossing away. Or you can go left on Timberline Trail, following a sign for Elk Cove, to complete this longer way to Wy'East Basin. At the far end of the campsites, you'll wade or jump Ladd Creek again—this crossing might be a bit too deep and swift in the early summer—and after that it's basically a flat mile to Wy'East Basin.

Wy'East Basin to Elk Cove (2.4 MILES ROUND-TRIP)

When you arrive in Wy'East Basin, your car is 3 miles to your left (go 0.3 mile to Vista Ridge Trail and turn right) and Elk Cove is to your right. It's easy and beautiful, so go for it. Just 1.2 flat miles away, Elk Cove might be the most spectacular of these destinations; it's certainly the largest, and Mount Hood seems to rise out of its far side all at once. Here, you'll find wildflowers throughout August, huckleberries late in the month, and reddish-orange mountain ash in September. I once spoke to a ranger who had seen elk and black bears in Elk Cove—give them their space, and they won't bother you.

As you head back on Timberline Trail #600, before you get back to Wy'East Basin, keep an eye out for a side trail leading to Dollar Lake. It's unsigned but follows a draw uphill in an area of short trees and a tiny stream that's more of a wet spot in the trail. Look for a rocky area uphill of the trail—if you get back as far as Pinnacle Ridge Trail #630, you've missed it by about 5 minutes. Dollar Lake, so named because it's almost perfectly round, like a silver dollar, probably should be called Half-Dollar Lake; you could wade across it in a minute. The campsites are nice here, and as you'll see, the Dollar Lake Fire didn't burn the area around Dollar Lake!

Barrett Spur Addition (3.6 MILES ROUND-TRIP)

Here's one final option, best for experienced folks who are spending the night in the area. Barrett Spur, named for P. G. Barrett, a 19th-century physician in the Hood River Valley, is the massive ridge you can see on the left side of Mount Hood when looking from Portland. You can get to a little over 7,000 feet on it, using a social trail (labeled Barrett Spur Trail #600D on some maps) that starts from Wy'East Basin. On the way back down, look for a junction that will lead you to Dollar Lake. Rather than take a lot of time describing it here, I'll just refer you to the **Portland Hikers Field Guide,** at **portlandhikersfieldguide.org.**

GPS Information and Directions

N45° 26.531' W121° 43.554'

Take US 26 from Portland, driving 36 miles east of I-205 to Zigzag and turning left on Lolo Pass Road at the Zigzag Store. Drive 10.7 miles and take the second right at Lolo Pass, onto Forest Service Road (FR) 18, which is signed for Lost Lake. After 5.5 miles of gravel, you'll be back on pavement 5 miles beyond that—having driven a total of 10.5 miles on FR 18—make a hairpin right to take the paved FR 16. (A sign at this intersection points to Vista Ridge Trail #626.) Go 5.4 miles and turn right at a large intersection onto FR 1650, which quickly becomes a good gravel road. The trailhead is 3.6 miles ahead, at the end of the road. Note that twice during this stretch, you'll need to stay left and uphill on the bigger of two roads.

45 Wildwood Recreation Site

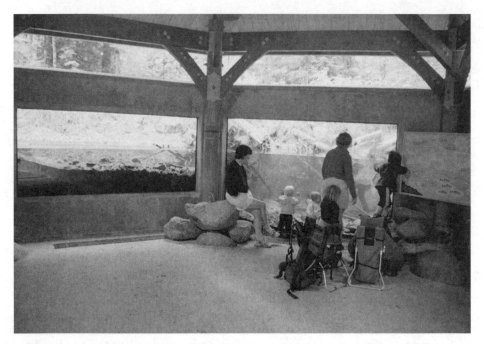

If you've ever wanted to see the world as a fish does, the viewing structure at Wildwood Recreation Site is a good bet.

In Brief

As much an educational experience as a hiking one, this hike offers a glimpse into the Pacific Northwest world of birds, fish, plants, and water. The crown jewel of Wildwood is its underwater-viewing structure, especially when various species of salmon and trout are returning to the area to spawn.

Description

The 33-mile-long Salmon River is the only river in the lower 48 states that is classified as a National Wild and Scenic River from its headwater to its mouth—in this case, from Mount Hood to the Sandy River, 3 miles below Wildwood. As far from the sea as it is, the river still gets several runs each year of anadromous fish—fish that are born in

234

LENGTH Two loops totaling 1.75 miles; 10.6 miles to Huckleberry Mountain

CONFIGURATION Loop or out-and-back

DIFFICULTY Easy for loops, strenuous to Huckleberry Mountain

SCENERY Wetlands, meadows, streams, a big-time summit viewpoint

EXPOSURE Alternately shady and open on loops, sunny on mountain hike

TRAFFIC Moderate–heavy on summer weekends, light otherwise

TRAIL SURFACE Gravel, pavement, boardwalk (loops); packed dirt (hike to mountain)

HIKING TIME 2.5 hours to do both loops, 6 hours for Huckleberry Mountain

DRIVING DISTANCE 43 miles (1 hour) from Pioneer Courthouse Square

SEASON Year-round; see note in Directions about winter parking. The trail up the mountain is generally snow-free June–October.

BEST TIME Late summer and fall

BACKPACKING OPTIONS None in the park. If you're spending the night up in the wilderness, tell park staff which car is yours.

ACCESS $5/vehicle/day

WHEELCHAIR ACCESS Both lower loops

MAPS Free maps in parking-area kiosk

FACILITIES At parking area

INFO Bureau of Land Management, Salem District, 503-622-3696, **blm.gov/or /districts/salem**

freshwater, go to the ocean, and then return to the freshwater of their birth to spawn and die. Although salmon are the most famous of these—and this bend of the Salmon River does get runs of salmon—steelhead do the same thing. Moreover, native trout inhabit this stretch of the river.

To sample this natural wonderland, hike two loop trails: the 1-mile Wetland Boardwalk Trail and the 0.75-mile Cascade Streamwatch Trail. To take Wetland Boardwalk Trail, start to the left of the parking-lot kiosk, where you'll find restrooms and free maps. You'll cross a 190-foot-long wooden bridge over the Salmon River, where in fall and winter you just might see chinook salmon and steelhead spawning below. Once over the bridge, follow the signs onto the boardwalk. You'll visit several lookouts affording views of various parts of the wetland: a cattail marsh, an overgrown beaver dam, an area filled with skunk cabbage, and a wetland stream. At each lookout, a notebook-style informative display describes the area's wildlife. And if you're quiet and go in the morning, there's a good chance you'll even see some wildlife. Be sure to take the gravel Return Trail back to the parking lot, if only to admire the size of some 90-year-old stumps.

Cascade Streamwatch Trail starts at the same kiosk and takes you on a tour of the world of an anadromous fish. In fact, to navigate the trail you just follow the metal fish in the pavement. Along this trail, you'll visit an overlook of the river,

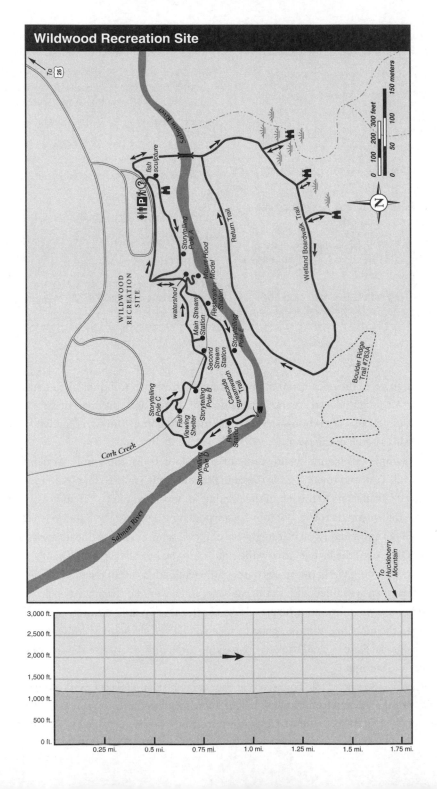

Wildwood Recreation Site

a three-dimensional model of the Mount Hood area, several great picnic areas with grills, and then the fantastic underwater-viewing structure. Here, you can see tiny fish most times of the year and try to identify them using the chart on the wall. From late October to mid-December, you might even catch a glimpse of an adult chinook salmon. You have a better chance of seeing bigger spawning fish a little later on the trail, when it drops to the riverside. Look for winter steelhead in January, spring chinook salmon in March and April, summer steelhead in May, and coho and fall chinook from late September to mid-November. In case you're wondering, the Salmon River is closed to salmon fishing—you can fish for native trout at limited times, but it's all catch-and-release, with artificial lures only.

Now, if it's exercise and a view you're after, take Boulder Ridge Trail #783A up to Huckleberry Mountain—and I do mean up: It climbs 4,100 feet in 5.3 miles to a tremendous viewpoint. Starting at the southwest end of Wetland Boardwalk Trail, you'll climb a series of switchbacks for just less than 2 miles to reach a spot with a nice view of Mount Hood. From here, it's a slightly less severe grade. Another 0.5 mile of climbing puts you at another view from a saddle; from there you'll put in 2 more miles to another saddle, then make a right onto Plaza Trail, heading 1 mile to the summit.

Nearby Activities

Wildwood Recreation Site is a full-service, 600-acre recreation area, with picnic areas for rent (some can be reserved) in addition to ball fields, basketball courts, horseshoe pits, and a play area. For rental information, call 877-444-6777 or visit **recreation.gov.**

GPS Information and Directions

N45° 21.009' W121° 59.523'

Take US 26 from Portland, driving 33 miles east of I-205; turn right at a large sign reading CASCADE STREAMWATCH. It's 0.5 mile past the Mount Hood RV Village. Drive 1 mile past the trailhead sign to the parking area for both trails. The road is gated from the weekend after Thanksgiving until the third Monday in March. During that time, you'll have to park at the gate (no charge) and walk in; restrooms in the park are left open.

46 Zigzag Mountain

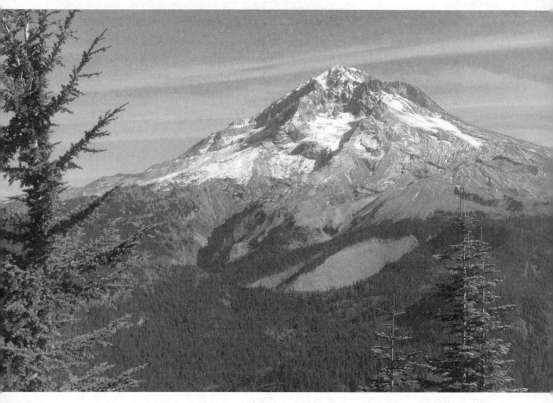

Mount Hood from Zigzag Mountain. With a campsite down at Burnt Lake, this hike would make a great sunset stroll.

In Brief

This is really three hikes in one: a cool, shady amble along a creek; a steady climb to a beautiful lake with a view of Mount Hood; and a strenuous climb to an old lookout site, also with an impressive view of Mount Hood.

Description

Burnt Lake Trail #772 starts in an area where there's no lake and no evidence that anything has ever burned. It's all cool, moist, and shady as you wind your way up through

LENGTH 6.8 miles round-trip to the lake, 9.4 miles round-trip to the mountain	**DRIVING DISTANCE** 54 miles (1 hour, 20 minutes) from Pioneer Courthouse Square
CONFIGURATION Out-and-back	**SEASON** June–October, though there will be some snow higher up in early summer.
DIFFICULTY Easy along the creek, moderate to the lake, strenuous to the mountain	
	BEST TIME August and September
SCENERY Shady creekside forest, a lovely mountain lake, a spectacular summit view	**BACKPACKING OPTIONS** Great sites at the lake
	ACCESS Northwest Forest Pass required (see page 3)
EXPOSURE Some ridgetop walking near the summit	**WHEELCHAIR ACCESS** None
TRAFFIC Heavy on summer weekends, moderate otherwise	**MAPS** Green Trails *Map 461 (Government Camp)*
TRAIL SURFACE Packed dirt, some rocks	**FACILITIES** None at the trailhead— stop in Zigzag on the way.
HIKING TIME 4 hours to the lake, 6 hours to do it all	**INFO** Zigzag Ranger District, 503-622-3191, **www.fs.usda.gov/mthood**

a young forest, with a branch of Lost Creek off to your right. If that name sounds familiar, it's because there are enough things called "Lost" in Oregon (not to mention things called "Salmon," "Elk," and "Huckleberry") to fill a whole hiking book.

Walk 0.25 mile and, just past a big cedar on the right, the forest gets a little more interesting. At just under 0.5 mile, an unmarked trail to the left leads to a cliff-top view toward the main stem of Lost Creek. On the main trail, you'll get your first glimpse of actual water around 1 mile out, and at just under 2 miles you'll hop across a tiny creek.

Continue climbing ever so gently for 0.5 mile, past some old burned-out snags, and look for a trail dipping left to a picnic site by a small waterfall. You've now found the main branch of Lost Creek, and a good place to turn around—2.3 miles out—if you're tired or you have little kids in tow.

Soon you'll make a switchback to the right and climb 1 mile, passing several small creeks, some of them in open areas that offer views back along the valley you've been coming up. You'll see Mount Hood over your right shoulder, but the real views start just after you cross Burnt Lake's outlet creek and arrive at the shores of this local wonder.

You'll immediately realize that lots of folks come up here; even if it's not crowded when you arrive, you'll notice trails leading all over the place. If you're camping, you must stick to designated spots and refrain from making wood fires. If you're just up

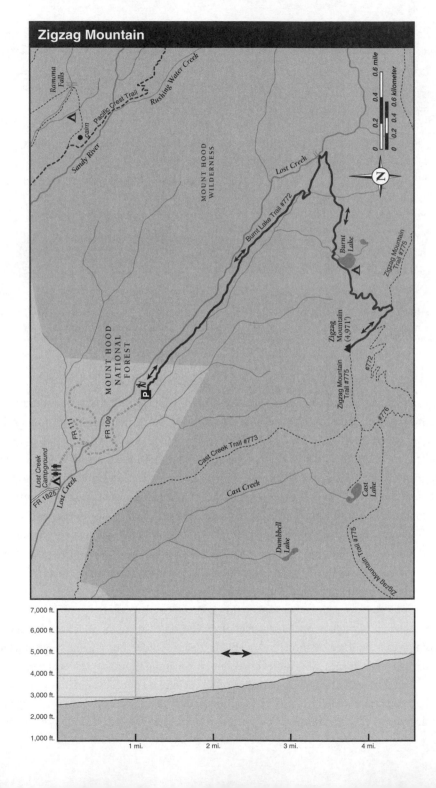

Zigzag Mountain

here for the day, linger a bit, explore the trail around the lake, take a swim, and soak in the rays and the views of Hood. Turn back here, and you have a 6.8-mile day.

To reach the lookout, another 1.3 miles and 800 feet up, continue right on the trail as it leads away from the lake, following a pointer toward Zigzag Mountain Trail #775. Cross a marshy area, then switchback up and out of the lake basin, intersecting Zigzag Mountain Trail after 0.8 mile. Turn right here, and it's quite a steep 0.25 mile climb to a viewpoint of Mount Hood where rhododendrons surround you. After the trail levels, continue straight through another junction and push up the steep final 0.3 mile to the rocky summit.

From the top, your view runs from two-humped Mount Rainier in the north to Mount Jefferson in the south, with Olallie Butte just to the left of it. To the left of Mount Hood, between it and Mount Adams, look for an open stretch alongside a ridge, bisected by a trail—that's Bald Mountain and a section of Timberline Trail, which you can visit on the McNeil Point trip (see Hike 36, page 190). The valley below is that of the Muddy Fork Sandy River, which starts at Sandy Glacier, clearly visible from here, left of the summit. To the right, beyond Zigzag Glacier, you can see dramatic Zigzag Canyon, which you can visit on the Timberline Lodge trip (Hike 41, page 213), and beyond that are two buildings that are part of Timberline Lodge, alongside Palmer Glacier.

So it's a two-creek, one-lake, four-volcano, three-glacier day, and yet you have still more trails up here to explore. The trail you took to the summit, Zigzag Mountain Trail, continues west over the summit toward Cast Lake and a veritable noodle bowl of trails, including the continuation of Burnt Lake Trail #772, which you left behind at the junction just below this summit. So you could make a loop out of all that, or even head for the lookout atop the west end of Zigzag Mountain—if, for some reason, what you've already done isn't enough.

GPS Information and Directions

N45° 22.332' W121° 49.328'

Take US 26 from Portland, driving 36 miles east of I-205 to Zigzag. Turn left (north) onto Lolo Pass Road, which is 0.6 mile past Milepost 41. Go 4.2 miles and turn right on Forest Service Road (FR) 1825, which is 0.1 mile past a sign for Mount Hood National Forest and is marked CAMPGROUNDS AND TRAILHEADS. Stay right at 0.7 mile, cross a bridge, and, 2 miles later, just past Lost Creek Campground, go straight at a junction onto gravel FR 109, continuing 1.3 miles to the trailhead.

THE COAST
AND COAST RANGE

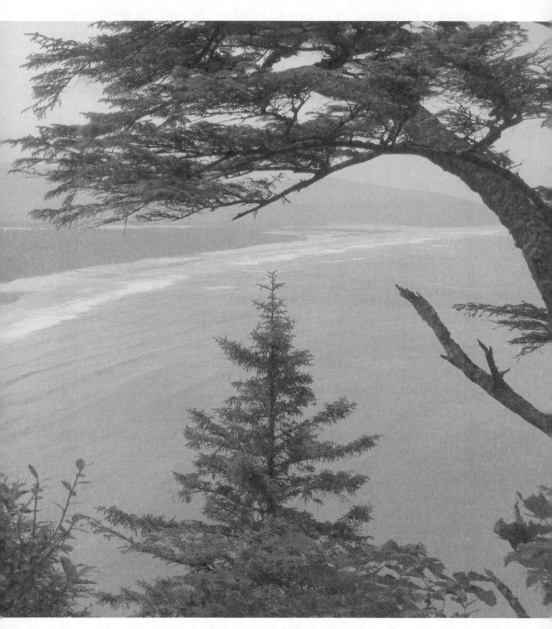

The views just keep getting better as you make your way to the end of Cape Lookout (Hike 47). This one looks south toward South Beach and Sand Lake.

The Coast and Coast Range (Hikes 47–53)

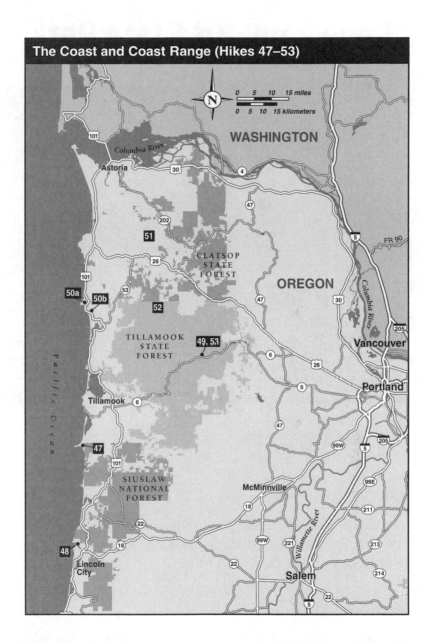

47 Cape Lookout State Park

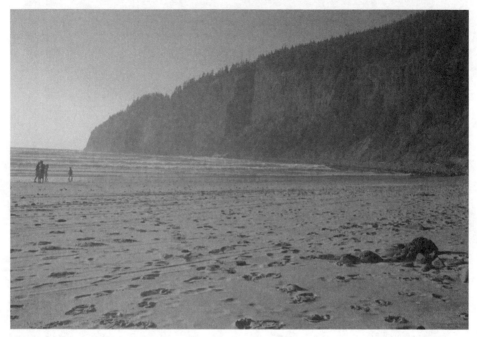

South Beach with Cape Lookout beyond

In Brief

This park offers everything you'd want from the Oregon coast: old-growth forest; secluded beaches; cliff-top views; and wildlife on land, wing, and water. You've got three options from the trailhead, and with a little energy you could do them all.

Description

When you park at this trailhead, you'll have three options to choose from, and it's all downhill from here. Of course, you'll have to come back uphill to get to your car, but even the 800-foot climb from the beach is so well graded, you'll hardly be winded when it's done. (On our elevation profile for this hike, I've included the beach route and the cape route.)

LENGTH 4.8 miles round-trip to end of cape, 3.6 miles round-trip to South Beach, 4.6 miles round-trip to picnic area

CONFIGURATION Three out-and-backs

DIFFICULTY Moderate

SCENERY Old-growth forest, high cliffs, whales in winter and spring

EXPOSURE Shady, open at end

TRAFFIC Heavy on summer weekends, moderate otherwise

TRAIL SURFACE Gravel, dirt, mud

HIKING TIME 3 hours to end of cape, 2.5 hours to South Beach, 3 hours to picnic area

DRIVING DISTANCE 85 miles (1 hour, 40 minutes) from Pioneer Courthouse Square

SEASON Year-round, with mud and storms in winter and spring

BEST TIME July–September for the weather, March and April for the whales

BACKPACKING OPTIONS None

ACCESS No fees or permits at the trailhead, but parking in the day-use area is $3/day.

WHEELCHAIR ACCESS None

MAPS U.S. Geological Survey *Sand Lake*

FACILITIES Portable restroom at trailhead May–September; restrooms, showers, and water at campground

INFO 503-842-4981, **oregonstateparks .org/park_186.php**

SPECIAL COMMENTS This park gets an average of 90 inches of rain annually, compared with Portland's 37.5 inches—you've been warned.

Cape Trail

Start with the best of the three trails. Taking the trail behind the sign at the far end of the lot, continue straight when you get to a junction 100 yards ahead. After a few minutes in younger forest, you'll be hiking through that rarest of treats: a coastal old-growth forest. Some nice Sitka spruces and hemlocks grow here, and the whole thing is as peaceful as can be. Look also for interesting forest features like a split stump, "nurse logs" with new trees growing on them, and "widowmakers" hanging over your head.

At 0.5 mile out, the trail dips down among some giant hemlock trees, and at 0.6 mile you'll come to a plaque honoring the flight crew of a B-17 bomber that crashed into the cape just to the west in 1943. After another 0.5 mile, you'll get a view north; look for the three rocks just off Cape Meares and the town of Oceanside. You can make out an arch in the middle rock—in fact, all three have such arches, and they're called the Three Arch Rocks. When you get to some moderately nerve-wracking dropoffs on the left, along with inspiring views south, you're almost done.

At the tip of the cape, you're looking 270 degrees around and 400 feet straight down at the crashing sea. There's a protective cable at the end of the cape, but in other places

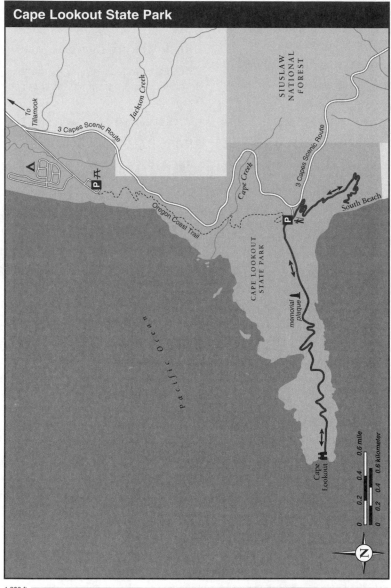

Cape Lookout State Park

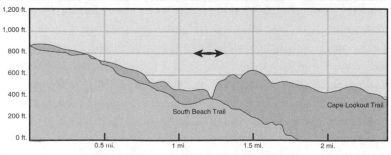

you'll be right at the top of a cliff. On a calm day—which is rare in a place that gets around 90 inches of rain per year—it's not uncommon to see seals or sea lions below.

But the main attraction is the gray whales. Thousands of them make the trip each year from the Bering Sea in Alaska to Baja California in Mexico, a swim of some 6,000 miles. In late December and early January, when they go south, they tend to be farther out. But in March and April, they're on their way back north with newborn calves, so they go slower and stay closer to shore. At these times of year, bring binoculars (and a raincoat), and you might see dozens of whales in a day. For the best viewing, go early in the day, when the sun will be behind you as you look out.

South Beach Trail

At the junction very near the parking lot, heading downhill puts you on the trail to South Beach. Avoid the temptation to take any of the various cutoff trails, as they add to erosion. If the 1.5-mile, 800-foot descent seems a little tedious (like when the beach looks as though it's just right there below you but you're walking more sideways than down), just believe that you'll be thankful for this easier grade on your way back up.

You can also hike down the beach, which extends 4 miles south to Sand Lake, but eventually you'll get into an area where cars are allowed, which sort of detracts from the wilderness feeling.

North Trail

The last option from the trailhead is across the lot, going north on the Oregon Coast Trail. It's 2.3 miles, all downhill, to the picnic area and the nature trail, which are by the campground. You'll pass a couple of viewpoints on the way and probably have the trail largely to yourself.

If you have two cars, put one down at the campground–picnic area. You'll have to pay a $3 day-use fee there, but at the end of the day you can walk downhill just 2.3 miles from the trailhead back to your second car (a total of 11.3 manageable miles for the day). There's also a short nature trail here. If you have only one car, you'll have to come back up at the end of the day, stretching the hike to almost 13 miles, so it might not be worth it.

Nearby Activities

As long as you're in Tillamook, take advantage of its tourist stops, most notably the collection of airplanes at the **Tillamook Air Museum,** south of town (6030 Hangar Rd., Tillamook, OR 97141; 503-842-1130, **tillamookair.com**). Check out dozens of "warbirds," some of which occasionally offer rides.

Two cheese factories are to the north. The **Tillamook Cheese Factory** (4175 US 101 North, Tillamook, OR 97141; 503-815-1300, **tillamook.com**) is the best-known; for slightly more exotic choices, as well as wine tastings and a petting zoo, visit the **Blue Heron French Cheese Company** (2001 Blue Heron Dr., Tillamook, OR 97141; 503-842-8281; **blueheronoregon.com**).

GPS Information and Directions

Cape Trailhead **N45° 20.484' W123° 58.470'**

Day-Use Area **N45° 21.635' W123° 58.168'**

Take US 26 from Portland, driving 20 miles west of I-405, then bear west on OR 6, following a sign for Tillamook. Drive 51 miles to Tillamook and continue straight through the inter-section with US 101. From here on, you'll be following signs for Cape Lookout State Park and the 3 Capes Scenic Route. After crossing US 101, go two blocks and turn left on Stillwell Street. Drive two more blocks and turn right on Third Street. Drive 4.9 miles and turn left. After 5.3 miles, you'll pass the state-park campground and day-use area; this is where you can stash a second car to do the shuttle. The trailhead is 2.7 miles past the campground, on the right. The park's GPS address is 13000 Whiskey Creek Rd. W., Tillamook, OR 97141.

48 Cascade Head

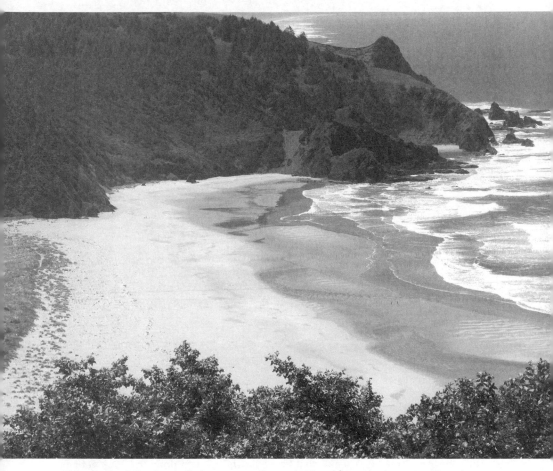

This overlook lies just a little ways up Cascade Head from the lower trailhead. The views are even better up top.

In Brief

Imagine standing high atop a windswept, flower-covered meadow, with the sea and the coast spread out below you and not a tree to block the view. Or imagine peeking into a hidden cove where sea lions bark, a waterfall plunges, and waves crash. Well, you don't have to imagine either scene: You can go to Cascade Head.

LENGTH 5.4 miles round-trip to Harts Cove; 2.5 or 4.5 miles round-trip to Cascade Head Preserve

CONFIGURATION Out-and-back

DIFFICULTY Moderate, with an easy option after July 15

SCENERY Old-growth forest, waterfalls, sea cliffs, wildflowers, wildlife

EXPOSURE In forest at first, then meadows

TRAFFIC Heavy on summer weekends, moderate otherwise

TRAIL SURFACE Packed dirt, some roots

HIKING TIME 3 hours to Harts Cove, 1–2.5 hours for preserve

DRIVING DISTANCE 79 miles (1 hour, 45 minutes) from Pioneer Courthouse Square

SEASON The road to the Harts Cove Trailhead and upper Cascade Head Preserve Trailhead is open July 16–December 31. The lower Cascade Head Preserve Trailhead is open year-round.

BEST TIME July–September

BACKPACKING OPTIONS No camping allowed

ACCESS No fees or permits

WHEELCHAIR ACCESS None

MAPS USGS *Neskowin*

FACILITIES Outhouse at Knight Park, but no facilities at upper trailheads and no drinkable water on the trail

INFO The Nature Conservancy, 503-802-8100, **tinyurl.com/cascadeheadpreserve**; Hebo Ranger District, 503-392-5100, **www.fs.usda.gov/siuslaw**

SPECIAL COMMENTS Dogs are prohibited on both of the trails at Cascade Head Preserve.

Description

Harts Cove Trail

At the start, you might think you've got it made, because it's all downhill and steep— it loses about 500 feet in the first 0.5 mile. Too bad you have to walk back up all that at the end of the hike. The forest here is a young one of mostly Sitka spruce; notice that only the tops of the trees are green—that's because these lower portions don't get any sun, not because they're unhealthy. Notice also the very large stumps; there's one right on the side of the trail that you can get on top of and measure for yourself.

Walk 0.7 mile to cross Cliff Creek and enter a different world. Here you can find out what a Sitka spruce looks like after about 300 years. You'll probably also hear what hundreds of sea lions sound like—they're to the left, and you might get to see some of them later. Now the hiking gets flatter, as you go out to the end of the ridge to a bench with a view of Harts Cove ahead. Wrap back around to the right, through the drainage of Chitwood Creek. A half-mile past the bench, walk under a massive blown-down spruce and then out into the meadows atop the bluff—yet another world.

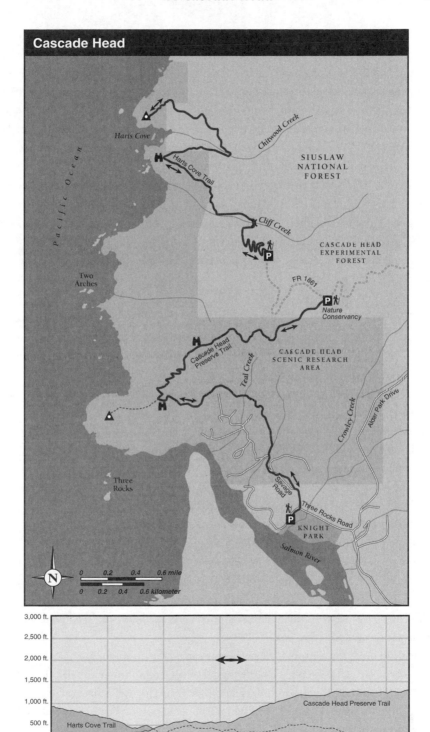

It's important to stay on the trails here; this area is fragile. If you come in July or August, you'll be part of a landscape that looks like it was lifted from the upper reaches of Mount Hood, with goldenrod, lupine, Indian paintbrush, and violets in abundance. Follow the trail that heads for the trees on the left; there's a wonderful spot to sit there, and it has a front-row view into Harts Cove. The waterfall you see is on Chitwood Creek, which you just crossed. As for the louder-than-ever sea lions, they are mostly around the point to the south, but if you have binoculars you might be able to see some of them lounging on rocks or the far beach.

There's no real beach to access here, but you can get close to the water. From the trees, walk west and keep left. Look for a steep trail, almost a slide in spots, that you can descend to the rocky shore. This rock, and all of Cascade Head, in fact, is lava that flowed up through the water. If you make your way to the right 100 yards or so on the rock, you'll have a fabulous view of the headland, Cape Kiwanda to the north, and, farther off, Cape Lookout.

Cascade Head Preserve

If it's after July 15, the upper road is open, and you want an easy, flat, 2.5-mile round-trip hike, start up here. The trail, actually an old roadbed, traverses a young and unexciting forest to the main-attraction meadow.

My advice is to start down below; it's a better, more scenic walk, and effort always makes one more appreciative. From the parking lot at Knight Park, start near the interpretive sign; you'll spot the trailhead directly across Three Rocks Road. The first 0.4-mile stretch crosses private property, switching from boardwalks to trail and occasionally crossing a road, so make sure you stay on the path and don't disturb the landowners—or get run over.

Finally heading into the woods, the trail briefly steepens, over steps and roots, then mellows after 0.1 mile, where a massive spruce guards the path. Enjoy typical coastal scenery—spruces and ferns, skunk cabbage and devil's club, and a small meadow filled with foxglove—as you cross several small streams on boardwalks and continue climbing, now on a more moderate grade. When you reach a trail junction just less than a mile out, keep left, and in a few moments you'll reach a sign telling you you're entering Siuslaw National Forest property. At 1.2 miles, you'll come to a registration station and donation box.

At this point, you'll probably have been hearing the ocean for a while, and at 1.3 miles you'll finally emerge from the tunnel of vegetation to see the Pacific and the mouth of the Salmon River, some 600 feet below you. The trail is flat and wonderful for 0.25 mile—look for elk on the bluffs and bald eagles in the sky. At a switchback to the right, the path starts to climb more steeply.

In summer, you'll climb through waist-high flowers, with birds chirping, swallows swooping, butterflies fluttering, and bumblebees buzzing. From any of the switchbacks, wander out, carefully, toward the cliff edge to peer north; you might spot sea lions below. When you see a sign reading D A N G E R : H A Z A R D O U S   C L I F F S, you've gone 2 miles and gained 1,000 feet. Only 0.25 mile and a couple hundred feet to the top! The spot where the upper trail emerges from the woods is 0.3 mile past the summit.

As you take it all in from the top of the hill, consider this: Back in the 1960s, this meadow was slated to become a housing development, but conservation-minded folks banded together, bought it, and donated it to The Nature Conservancy. Now also designated as a United Nations Biosphere Reserve, it's protected as the home of the Oregon silverspot butterfly, whose caterpillar eats only a rare violet that lives in these meadows. That's why Forest Service Road (FR) 1861 and the upper part of the trail are closed January 1–July 15. The silverspots emerge in late August and hang out here for about a month.

Nearby Activities

Back on OR 18, a mile before you reached US 101, you passed through the town of Otis. You might not have noticed it—it has only about a dozen buildings—but it's the home of an Oregon coast tradition, the **Otis Cafe** (1259 Salmon River Hwy., Otis, OR 97368), where you'll find 28 seats, a line outside, and the biggest portions this side of a logging camp. Famous for its sourdough pancakes, German potatoes, and whole-wheat molasses toast, the café also makes wonderful pies. More info: 541-994-2813, **otiscafe.com**.

GPS Information and Directions

Cascade Head Preserve (Lower Trailhead) **N45° 2.506' W123° 59.556'**
Cascade Head Preserve (Upper Trailhead) **N45° 3.641' W123° 59.305'**
Harts Cove Trailhead **N45° 3.893' W123° 59.723'**

Take I-5 from downtown Portland, driving 6 miles south to Exit 294/Tigard-Newberg. Bear right on OR 99 West and follow it 22 miles. Just before the town of McMinnville, turn left on OR 18 (following signs for the coast) and follow it 53 miles to its intersection with US 101. Turn right (north) on US 101. For the lower, year-round trailhead to Cascade Head Preserve, go 1 mile north and turn left on Three Rocks Road. Follow this 2 miles, turn left, and park at Knight Park. To reach the trailhead, follow a trail along the road behind the info sign.

For the two upper trailheads, drive 3.8 miles north of OR 18 on US 101 and turn left onto unsigned FR 1861, just before the top of a hill on US 101. Stay left at 2.4 miles, still on FR 1861. The upper Cascade Head Preserve Trailhead is 0.8 mile past this turn, on the left. The Harts Cove Trailhead is at the end of the road, 1 mile ahead.

49 Kings Mountain and Elk Mountain

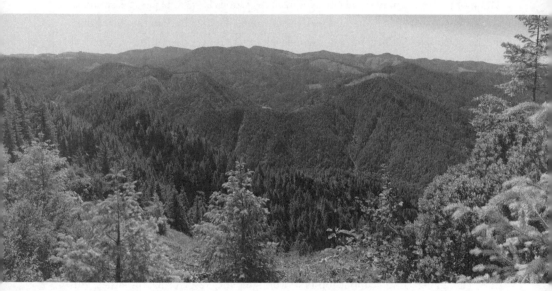

This panorama from Elk Mountain shows little evidence of how hard it is to reach this spot!

In Brief

I've laid out four options for you: a steep hike up Kings Mountain, a *really* steep scramble up Elk Mountain, a killer loop that includes both, and a more casual (though lengthy) trip along Elk Creek. With a campground at one trailhead, why not spend the night and do a couple of hikes?

Description

All of these hikes are in Tillamook State Forest. At first glance, this locale might not sound terribly impressive compared with a national park or wilderness area, but the forest has a fascinating story behind it.

On a hot August day in 1933, a fire started at a logging operation in Gales Creek Canyon. The temperatures had been in the 90s for weeks, and humidity was at an

LENGTH Options from 5.2 to 13.4 miles	**SEASON** Year-round, but there will often be snow on top in winter. Recent rains make some slopes very slippery.
CONFIGURATION Loop, out-and-back	
DIFFICULTY Moderate–strenuous	
SCENERY Second-growth forest, regrowth after fires, wildflower meadows, a couple of panoramas on top	**BEST TIME** May and June, for the wildflowers
	BACKPACKING OPTIONS None
EXPOSURE Shady on the way up, open on top; some dangerous sections up above, especially if it's wet	**ACCESS** No fees or permits
	WHEELCHAIR ACCESS None
	MAPS USGS *Jordan Creek*
TRAFFIC Moderate on summer weekends, light otherwise	**FACILITIES** Restrooms and water at Elk Creek Campground; vault toilet at Kings Mountain Trailhead
TRAIL SURFACE Packed dirt, with some rock; sheer rock and steep scrambles on Elk Mountain	
	INFO Tillamook State Forest, 503-357-2191, **oregon.gov/odf/tillamookstateforest**
HIKING TIME 3.5 hours to Kings Mountain, 8 hours for either loop	**SPECIAL COMMENTS** Because of the mountain terrain, you should avoid these hikes if it's been raining or there's snow on the ground.
DRIVING DISTANCE 47 miles (55 minutes) from Pioneer Courthouse Square	

all-time low. The forest, therefore, was a bomb waiting to go off. The Gales Creek fire started as a fairly standard conflagration, but then a hot, dry wind came in from the east, and the 40,000-acre fire turned, in less than 24 hours, into a 240,000-acre fire. This "explosion" threw up a mushroom cloud 40 miles wide that rained 2 feet of debris on a 30-mile stretch of the Oregon coast.

A major fire burned every six years until 1951, by which time 355,000 acres and 13 billion board feet of timber—enough for more than a million large homes—had been completely destroyed. Logging came to a halt, wildlife was decimated, rivers were choked with sediment and debris, and, most importantly for the forest, seed cones were annihilated, meaning that the forest wouldn't grow back on its own.

But a recovery effort was launched with a bond measure in 1949. Eventually, more than 72 million seedlings were hand-planted, and in 1973 what had been known as the Tillamook Burn was renamed Tillamook State Forest. Now the question facing the state is whether or not to start logging it again.

These hikes offer you a chance to explore one or two of the highest points in the forest and have a look at how the place has recovered. Keep an eye out for charred logs, for example, and remember that 50 years ago most of this area was bare.

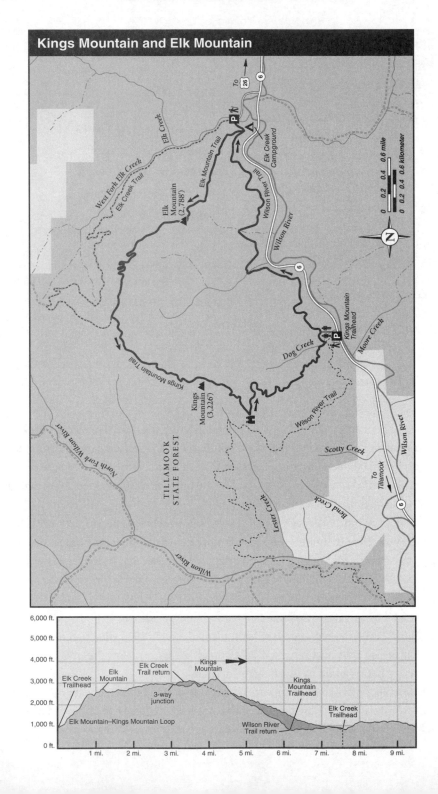

Kings Mountain and Elk Mountain

Kings Mountain Trail (5.2 MILES ROUND-TRIP; STRENUOUS)

This hike gives you the most reward for your effort. It's a tough, 2.6-mile climb, but compared with Elk Mountain it does have the advantage of taking you along a legitimate trail the whole time.

From the Kings Mountain Trailhead on OR 6, set out through a forest of alder and fern—replanted after the big burns—with a small, unnamed creek off to your right. At 0.1 mile, you'll see, but not take, Wilson River Trail on your right; if you're interested in that one, its entire 21-mile length is described in detail starting on page 276. It's also the return portion of a killer loop described later.

Around 1 mile, things get nasty-steep; the next mile gains about 1,300 feet, as opposed to the 800 feet you've gained in the first mile. When your trail makes a sharp turn to the right, look for a small trail to the left, leading to a peak called "Kings Jr." Go a few feet out there for your first real view to the north. Lester Creek, below you, flows into the Wilson River to your left; Kings Mountain rises directly behind you, higher than the rocky peak you can see from here. There are also some large, charred stumps on this ridge. The live trees were all planted after the big fires, and some of the seeds were dispersed by helicopter.

The last 0.6 mile of this hike gains about 900 feet, so just take your time and believe it's worth the effort. If you're here in May or June, you'll have no doubt about that when you walk past a picnic table (many thanks to Troop 299 from Tigard!) and out into the meadows, which in early summer are filled with beargrass, lupine, Indian paintbrush, and seemingly a billion other tiny flowers. The summit is now just 0.3 mile straight ahead, marked by a sign. The view stretches from the ocean to the Cascades; be sure to sign the trail register, one of the few in Oregon.

If you want to do both peaks, I strongly suggest starting with Elk Mountain, profiled next, and coming back this way.

Elk Mountain Trail (3 MILES ONE-WAY; STRENUOUS)

For one stretch, this is the steepest, roughest trail in this book. It climbs 1,900 feet in 1.5 miles, making it considerably steeper than Dog Mountain, for example. If you ascend this trail, don't come back down it—return on Kings Mountain Trail or the easier Elk Creek Trail.

From the trailhead at Elk Creek, head up Wilson River Trail 0.2 mile, then take off up Elk Mountain Trail. There's an immediate big step; get used to it. I don't know what to tell you about the next 1.5 miles, except that the view is worth it. You'll get some views along the way, and some spring-summer flowers, but mainly there's a whole lot of up.

You'll pass a sign on a tree indicating 2,500 feet elevation, which is nice except that then the trail starts back down. The real summit, at 2,788 feet, has a great register placed by the Mazamas, who also maintain the trails in this area. If you face the Wilson River on the summit, Kings Mountain is the peak off to your right.

If you really want to descend the way you just came, have at it. My advice is to continue on the trail, which dives steeply off the summit and becomes a little rocky and brushy in places; then it goes up and down and all around for a mile until it enters an old roadbed.

Eventually you pop out onto a sunny ridge with views to the south and a three-way trail junction with the Kings Mountain and Elk Creek Trails. Here you have a choice to make. Oh, and you've actually gained 200 feet since topping out on Elk Mountain!

Elk Mountain–Kings Mountain Loop
(11.2 MILES, 7.5 MILES WITH SHUTTLE; VERY STRENUOUS)

This traverse means business. If you have a second car at the Kings Mountain Trailhead, the loop is only 7.5 miles. Without that shuttle, you'll have to hike 3.7 more miles to return on Wilson River Trail. Either way, it's a challenge.

As if going up Elk Mountain and then scrambling over to Kings Mountain Trail wasn't enough work, you're now faced with a 1.3-mile ridgetop traverse that even in dry weather could stir up a fear of heights. The spookiest section is along the top of cliffs on the north side of the ridge, where snow lingers later than in other places.

The good news is, there's only one trail and it sticks to the ridge, so you won't get lost. Also, in recent years somebody added a rope on at least one section, to help with traction. When you get to Kings Mountain at 4.9 miles, enjoy that view, then head down the steep trail described above. If you have a car at that trailhead, good for you; if not, turn left on Wilson River Trail to follow it 3.7 miles back to your starting point.

Elk Creek Trail (4 MILES ONE-WAY; MODERATE)

This is the least challenging of the four options, of interest mostly as a safer, saner return trip from Elk Mountain. To do that, it's a pretty uneventful 4 miles and very easy to follow from the three-way junction described above. If you're looking for a chill hike to do with the kids, go up this one from the Elk Creek Trailhead.

Ascending, you'll walk along the main creek, which has a steelhead run (river otters have reportedly been sighted here). Several side trails offer access to the water. At 0.5 mile, you'll come to the confluence of the main Elk Creek and its West Fork; head up the West Fork 1 mile before starting your climb out of the canyon. After 2.5 miles of gradual uphill walking, you'll arrive at the junction with Elk Mountain Trail.

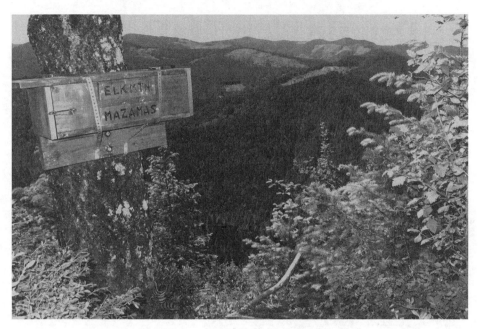

The Portland-based Mazamas maintain a summit register at Elk Mountain. Be sure to read it for some entertainment.

Doing the summit loop up and down this way is 13.4 tedious miles, so go ahead and tackle the steep part going up if you want to do Elk Mountain.

Whichever of these hikes you choose, I say you deserve the next day or two off!

GPS Information and Directions

Elk Creek Trailhead N45° 36.618' W123° 27.999'

Kings Mountain Trailhead N45° 35.814' W123° 30.378'

Take US 26 from Portland, driving 20 miles west of I-405; then bear west on OR 6, following a sign for Tillamook. To start at Elk Mountain, go 23 miles to Elk Creek Campground, on the right just past Milepost 28. The road will be gated in winter, but it's only 0.3 mile to the trailhead, which is on the right just beyond the campground. For Kings Mountain, continue 3 more miles on OR 6 to the trailhead, on the right just before Milepost 25.

50 Oswald West State Park

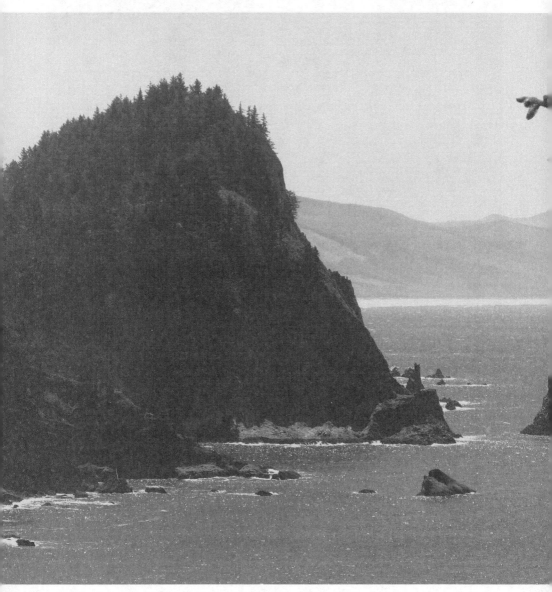

There are a whole lot of rocky headlands, and maybe some sea lions, in view from the Cape Falcon Trail.

LENGTH 6 miles round-trip to Cape Falcon, 2.5–9 miles round-trip to Neahkahnie Mountain	**HIKING TIME** 3 hours to Cape Falcon, up to 5 hours for the mountain
CONFIGURATION Out-and-back	**DRIVING DISTANCE** 89 miles (1 hour, 40 minutes) from Pioneer Courthouse Square
DIFFICULTY Easy to Cape Falcon, strenuous to Neahkahnie Mountain	**SEASON** Year-round, but wet in winter
SCENERY Old-growth forest, waterfalls, several cliff-top vistas of the sea	**BEST TIME** Whenever it's not raining
	BACKPACKING OPTIONS None
EXPOSURE Shady, except for cliff tops at the cape and a rocky scramble at the mountain summit	**ACCESS** No fees or permits
	WHEELCHAIR ACCESS None
	MAPS USGS *Arch Cape*
TRAFFIC Heavy all summer, especially weekends; moderate otherwise	**FACILITIES** Restrooms and drinking water near second parking area off US 101 (see page 265)
TRAIL SURFACE Packed dirt, with some gravel; brief rock-scrambling on Neahkahnie	**INFO** 503-368-3575, **oregonstateparks .org/park_195.php**

In Brief

This ultra-popular state park includes two of the best hikes on the northern Oregon coast: a nearly flat stroll through old-growth forest to a cliff-top ocean view, and a vigorous hike to a peak with a grand panorama.

Description

Cape Falcon

About five steps from the parking lot, you'll find yourself in a rare old-growth coastal forest, walking a wide, mostly flat path with Short Sand Creek down on your left. You'll cruise 0.5 mile to a junction, where Short Sand Beach will be to your left and downhill about 0.3 mile; Cape Falcon will be to your right. Straight ahead is a nice view of Smugglers Cove.

Turn right, cross a small creek, and start winding along the contours of the land. Around 0.8 mile, where the trail makes a sharp left turn, a downed tree on the right has left a large, disfigured stump. Some more-imaginative hiking friends of mine dubbed this stump "The Throne of the Forest King." Assume the throne to survey your kingdom, which includes a nice little grove of Sitka spruce and hemlock.

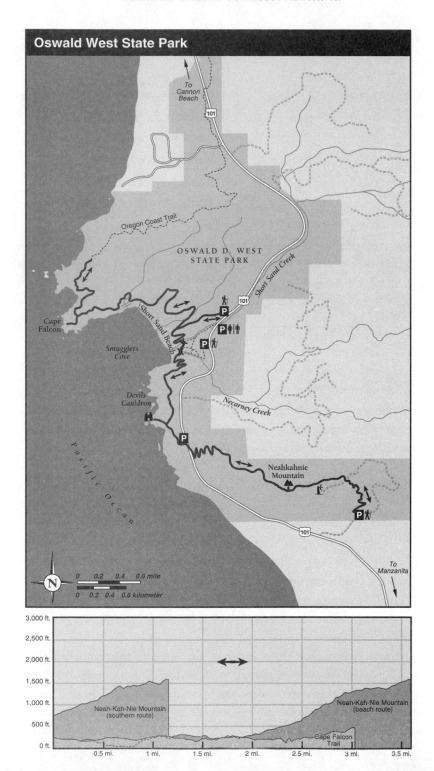

Oswald West State Park

A half-mile past that goofiness, ignore a trail that plunges down to the left. It accesses the beach but is too steep to fool with—especially at the end. On the main trail, just after a footbridge over a creek, a brushy path to the left leads 100 feet to a view of a tiny hidden waterfall. If you take this trail left another 100 yards or so, often having to nearly crawl through the brush, you'll find yourself at the top of an even larger falls that goes right down to the ocean. Just be careful of your footing, or you'll wind up in a heap on the rocks some 50 feet below.

A short distance later, back on the main trail, you'll start out toward the end of Cape Falcon itself. You'll get nice views back into Smugglers Cove and up to Neahkahnie Mountain; then you'll descend through the trees once more to a junction at the edge of a brushy, largely treeless area. For the end of the cape, turn left and walk about 0.2 mile through the gauntlet of brush. Out at the end, you'll find yourself atop an unrailed 200-foot cliff, with the sea below and Falcon Rock out in front of you. You'll find some good picnicking spots under the trees. In late May and early June, the grassy bluffs here are awash in Indian paintbrush and irises. Look for seals and sea lions below. Make sure to get up to the very top of the hill to see the views north.

When you head back to the main trail, walk left for a bit to add more scenery to your day. This is the Oregon Coast Trail, which stretches (in one form or another) from California to the Columbia River. In this next mile or so, you'll get three more views of the sea. When the trail starts climbing inland, you might as well turn back, unless the old-growth magic has you in its grip. There are no more ocean views for a while, but there are plenty of big trees, and not many people.

Neahkahnie Mountain

Perhaps all these trailheads have you confused. Well, don't be. It's really very simple. Neahkahnie Mountain has a killer view from 1,600 feet above the ocean, and you have two good options for getting there: The simplest is a 2.5-mile round-trip from the southernmost trailhead, gaining 850 feet; the longer option starts at the beach and offers more to see as it gains 1,600 feet in 3.3 miles. With two cars, you could do both and put in only 4.5 one-way miles.

First, the shortest option, starting at the southernmost trailhead: Switchback up through open areas filled with tasty red thimbleberries in late summer, and, after 0.7 mile, you'll reach a junction with a road that leads left to some radio towers. Cross the road and follow the trail. You'll climb gradually another 0.3 mile, pass to the north of (and below) the radio towers, and then, in 0.2 mile, come to the summit trail. Right where you pop out into the open, after you cross to the west side of the ridgeline, you'll see a little trail heading up and to your right: That's it. It's a little rocky scramble, nothing intense.

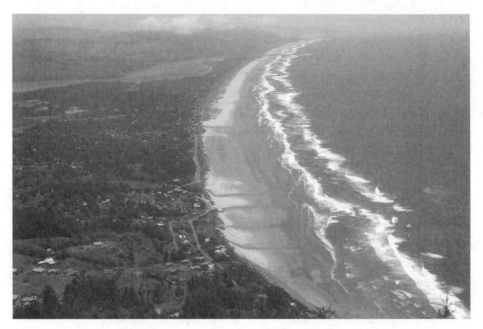

From the rocky top of Neahkahnie Mountain, it feels like you can throw a rock to the town of Manzanita.

For the beach option, which is the best and most scenic route, start at the west-side parking lot for Oswald West State Park. Walk 0.1 mile down the trail, among some awesome Sitka spruces, toward Short Sand Beach to reach a junction offering a choice between beach and campground; choose beach. Walk 0.1 mile, turn left at another junction, and this time cross a wonderfully bouncy suspension bridge over Necarney Creek. Take a few minutes to explore the lovely beach, which has some pretty decent tidepools around to the left.

Now, back on the trail to Neahkahnie Mountain, you'll climb a ridge covered with fantastic trees. About 0.2 mile up the trail, you'll actually go through a Sitka spruce. After this the trail flattens, and when the walk-through tree is 0.3 mile behind you, look for a large Western red cedar just by the trail on the left; just beyond that are two ridiculously large Sitka spruces, with foot-thick branches that have turned upward to become trees in their own right. If you think they can't get any bigger, just wait: The largest spruce of the hike, which has several trunks, is 0.2 mile ahead.

When you pop out into the open, in a meadow more than 200 feet above the sea, you'll have come 1.3 miles since leaving your car. Just ahead you'll see two trails splitting off to the right—ignore the first one you come to; the second one leads to a cliff-top viewpoint among the trees, looking down at Devils Cauldron. And don't wander around in these meadows. I know a guy who fell into a 15-foot hole here and had to be pulled out with a rope.

When you reach US 101, cross it carefully and start into the woods at a trail sign. Climb 0.6 mile in the open before reentering the trees. At this point, you're about 1,000 feet above sea level. You'll climb gradually after this, but if the trail seems to drop a little, don't worry—you're just walking around to the far side of the mountain, where the view is. When you come around a corner and hear the ocean again, you have a mile to walk and 300 feet to gain. Eventually, you'll be back in the open and see a small, rocky trail heading up to the left; that's the summit.

From the top of Neahkahnie, you can see all the way south to Cape Meares; look for Three Arch Rocks offshore there. If it's a really clear day, you might make out Cape Lookout, south of Cape Meares. The beach town seemingly at your feet is Manzanita, and the body of water beyond it is Nehalem Bay. During the invasion-scare days of World War II, the Coast Guard had a lookout up here, while soldiers patrolled the beaches on horseback and blimps from Tillamook cruised offshore.

If you have a car at the southern trailhead, time your arrival on the summit for just before sundown. It's quite a show from up here, and even at dusk you'll have no problem getting back to your car, especially if you came the short way.

Nearby Activities

I have a soft spot for the family-operated **Ecola Seafoods Restaurant & Market** in Cannon Beach, 11 miles north of the trailhead on US 101. (*Ecola,* by the way, is the Chinookan word for "whale.") I feel quite strongly that they serve the best clam chowder around, and they always have lots of fresh seafood. You can find them at 208 N. Spruce St., right across from the visitor center; contact them at 503-436-9130 or **ecolaseafoods.com.**

GPS Information and Directions

Southern Trailhead **N45° 44.448' W123° 56.0752'**
Campground Trailhead **N45° 45.787' W123° 57.580'**
West Parking Area **N45° 45.595' W123° 57.562'**

Take US 26 from Portland, traveling 74 miles west of I-405; turn south on US 101. The trailhead is 14 miles ahead, on the right. There are actually four parking areas in succession here: The first (unmarked) one on the right is for Cape Falcon, distinguished by a small median strip along the highway. The second one, 0.1 mile ahead on the left, is where the restrooms are. For the shortest trip to Neahkahnie Mountain, drive 2 miles past the restrooms and turn left onto a gravel road by a brown hiker sign. The trailhead is 0.4 mile up, on the left.

51 Saddle Mountain

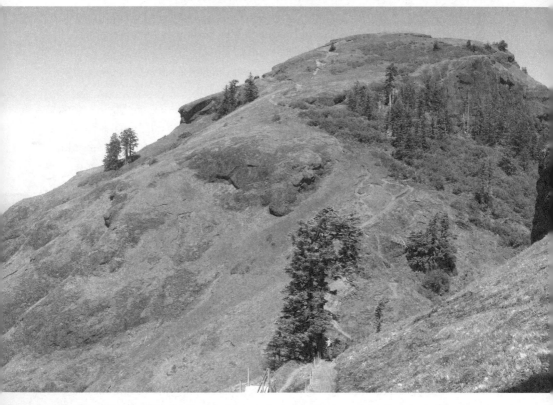

The last bit of trail to the Saddle Mountain summit is less daunting, but often more flowery, than this picture implies.

In Brief

The highest point in northwest Oregon, Saddle Mountain is also one of the most popular hiking trails in the state. Traversing flower-filled meadows unparalleled in this part of the state, it affords a view from the top that stretches from the ocean to the mouth of the Columbia River to the Cascades.

Description

Saddle Mountain just doesn't seem to belong in its surroundings. It's the highest point in this part of the state, but the hills around it aren't even close. It doesn't even

LENGTH 5.2 miles

CONFIGURATION Out-and-back

DIFFICULTY Strenuous

SCENERY Deep forest, wildflowers, panoramic view

EXPOSURE In the forest, then out in the open on top; occasionally steep on some loose rocks and metal fencing—slippery if there's been rain or snow

TRAFFIC Very heavy on summer weekends, heavy on other summer days, moderate otherwise

TRAIL SURFACE Packed dirt with rocks, then just rocks

HIKING TIME 3.5 hours

DRIVING DISTANCE 74 miles (1 hour, 30 minutes) from Pioneer Courthouse Square

SEASON Year-round but does get snow in winter

BEST TIME June and July, for the flowers

BACKPACKING OPTIONS None on trail; campground at trailhead open March–October

ACCESS No fees or permits

WHEELCHAIR ACCESS None

MAPS USGS *Saddle Mountain*

FACILITIES Restrooms at trailhead; closed November–February

INFO Saddle Mountain State Natural Area, 503-368-5943, **tinyurl.com /saddlemountain**

resemble them, with its two-headed, rocky summit of "pillow lava," which looks like that because it erupted under water, millions of years ago when this area was the sea floor. When you get on top of Saddle Mountain, you might think you're on Mount Hood, with the faraway views and abundant wildflowers. Of course, as crowded as it gets on summer weekends, you might think you're in a city park right after quitting time on a weekday. Whatever—it's a great hike, so start early in the morning and get there before everybody else.

When you get out of your car, you might be a little intimidated as you look up at the mountain. You might even see some speck-sized people up there. The good news is, you'll be up there soon enough; the bad news is, that's not the summit.

Things start out mellow, in a young forest filled with big old stumps—relics of logging in the 1920s and fires in the 1930s. After you've hiked 0.2 mile, you'll see a side trail to the right, which leads 0.1 mile to a great view of all of Saddle Mountain—the only one in the park, oddly enough. At 0.7 mile, you'll pass through an area where storms took down a bunch of trees. Then you'll start climbing, gaining about 1,100 feet in the next 1.4 miles, and occasionally walking on a combination of rocks and metal grating put in for traction. You'll also start to catch glimpses of the rocky world you're headed for, and you'll pass a picnic table in an unlikely spot. Somebody even

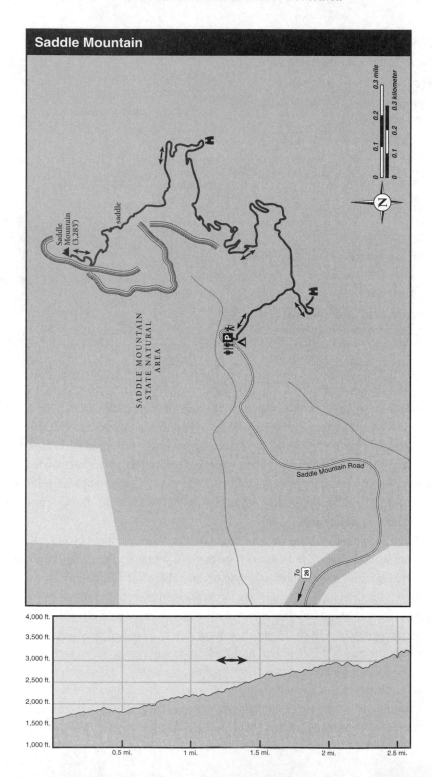

put in mileage markers on this trail! When it passes a table (where once was a shelter) and flattens, you'll be at 2,900 feet, just 300 feet below the summit.

Now you're out in the serious flower meadows. Several rare species grow here, such as Saddle Mountain saxifrage and Saddle Mountain bittercress—species that survived the last ice age on these slopes. Stay on the trail and on the footbridges, and remember that it's illegal to pick the flowers. You'll descend briefly and cross the saddle—this is the point you can see from the car, which is now visible, if very small, on your left—and then climb the last, steep scramble to the summit, in places with handrails to hold onto.

On a clear day, you can see from the volcanoes of the Cascades to the Pacific, and to the mouth of the Columbia just beyond Astoria to the north. See if you can spot the Astoria Tower. On a (rare) really clear day, you can make out the mountains of the Olympic Peninsula beyond that. I also once spotted Saddle Mountain from Chinidere Mountain in the Columbia River Gorge (see Hike 5, page 36). Needless to say, I've never seen Chinidere from Saddle Mountain.

Nearby Activities

You no doubt noticed **Camp 18** (42362 Highway 26, Elsie, OR 97138) a few miles before the turnoff from US 26—and how could you not? It might look like a logging museum, and it is, but it's also a restaurant with famously filling portions and log decorations. As one newspaper story put it, "You can throw on one serious feedbag." It's not a bad way to prepare for (or recover from) an assault on Saddle Mountain. Find out more at 503-755-1818 or **camp18restaurant.com.**

GPS Information and Directions

N45° 57.767' W123° 41.391'

Take US 26 from Portland, traveling 66 miles west of I-405, and turn right at a sign for Saddle Mountain State Park. The trailhead is 7 miles ahead, at the end of Saddle Mountain Road.

52 Salmonberry River

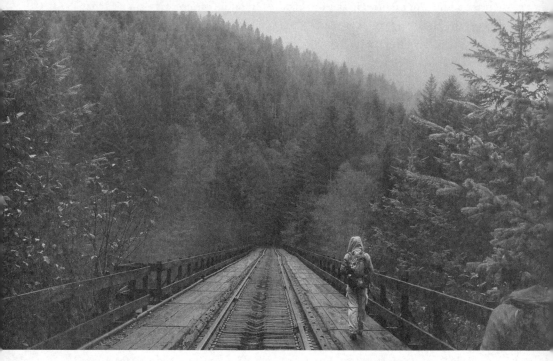

Walking on bridges like the Big Baldwin is part of what makes this hike such a unique adventure.

In Brief

Ever wanted to wander off down the railroad tracks? This is your chance. This rail line was destroyed by floods in 2007, and access is allowed all the way through its remote 16-mile canyon. While it's possible to do the whole thing with a car shuttle—our map shows a point-to-point route from the upper end to the lower—what I've described here are two walks starting on each end, each offering an easy tour through history and a chance to watch nature reclaim an area in slow motion.

Description

For years, the Port of Tillamook Bay allowed people to walk on these tracks, even when it had trains going through, and in fact I included this hike in two earlier editions

LENGTH 12 miles for the lower section, 10 miles for the upper; more if you want it	**SEASON** Year-round, but some snow in winter
CONFIGURATION Out-and-back or point-to-point with shuttle	**BEST TIME** Spring or late fall, when the foliage is down
DIFFICULTY Easy terrain, moderate difficulty due to length and odd surfaces	**BACKPACKING OPTIONS** Several sites
SCENERY Remote forested canyon, mountain streams, high bridges, tunnels, and abandoned railroad tracks	**ACCESS** No fees or permits
	WHEELCHAIR ACCESS None
EXPOSURE In and out of the sun, with some weird footing and high bridges (with handrails)	**MAPS** USGS *Cook Peak* and *Rogers Creek*
	FACILITIES Campgrounds on the way to each trailhead
TRAFFIC Light	**INFO** Oregon Department of Forestry, Tillamook District; 503-842-2545, **tinyurl .com/odftillamook**
TRAIL SURFACE Dirt, rocks, railroad tracks, some creek fords	
HIKING TIME 5 hours for the lower section, 4 for the upper section	**SPECIAL COMMENTS** Bring a flashlight for this one, as you'll be going through some tunnels. If you're afraid of heights, this might not be your best choice. And sometimes the upper section in particular is closed for logging activity.
DRIVING DISTANCE From Pioneer Courthouse Square, Cochran is 48 miles (1 hour, 5 minutes) and Salmonberry is 77 miles (1 hour, 35 minutes).	

of this book. But a catastrophic flood in December 2007 meant no more trains—and now the state is considering a long-term plan to convert the whole line, from Lake Oswego to the Coast, into a trail.

That's probably decades away, so for now let's go see what's left of this hobo adventure. This hike has a decaying-industry feel about it, with train cars left behind, tracks twisted around or suspended in the air, trestles still standing—oh, and a beautiful Coast Range forest and a clear-running river. And with a grade of something like 100 feet per mile, you can't imagine a hike that is any closer to being truly flat.

Just understand: This isn't a trail. You're actually walking on the tracks most of the time, and the ties can get slick. In other places they're simply gone or buried, so you have to use makeshift trails and/or thrash through brush. There's at least one creek crossing where you may get your feet wet. Of course, there's another word for all of this: *adventure!* Come in the spring for lush greenery and roaring water, or in October for fall colors and migrating salmon. Either way, you're likely to have the place to yourself, at least until word of this gem starts to spread.

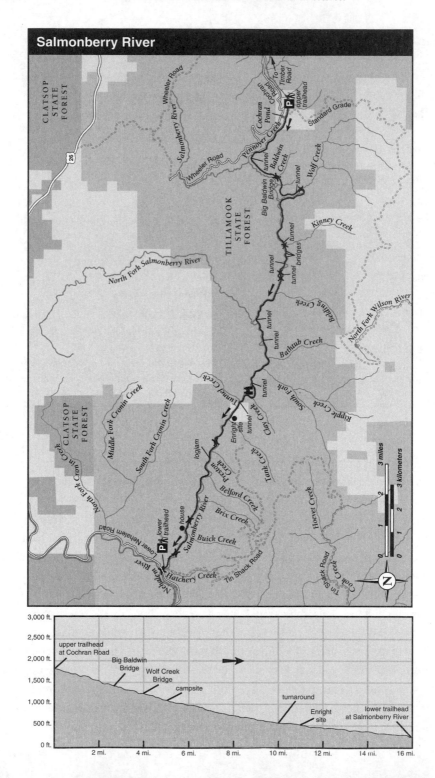

The Lower End (12 MILES)

For the lower loop, start at the confluence of the Salmonberry and Nehalem Rivers, and before you go, check out the road bridge over the Salmonberry. For a little perspective, the 2007 flood took that thing out! Essentially what happened is that tributaries, scarred by roads and logging and the railroad itself, unleashed massive slides into the Salmonberry. In some cases they plugged tunnels and dammed up the river, and when that gave way . . . well, this bridge was a victim, and you'll see more evidence later on.

The lower hike is better for views of and access to the Salmonberry. It used to be quite the salmon and steelhead river before all the floods. There are also some fancy houses across the way, and near the trailhead there is some private property to avoid. Just stick to the tracks, or a little trail next to them.

The first few miles are pretty straightforward, the first highlight being a 1925 bridge about 0.6 mile out. In this stretch you'll also see several washouts where the rails remain but the ground under them vanished. In other areas, enormous piles of wood and rock now cover the tracks.

The challenges in here are twofold: footing and brush. The footing makes it hard to pick your head up and look around while you're walking. Smooth sailing is pretty rare, but none of it is hard. Sometimes you have to walk on the ties when there's nothing between or below them, but it's no worry unless you're afraid of heights.

There are also tunnels, but they're pretty cool. You'll want to bring a flashlight, just in case. These were *much* more interesting when a train might be coming through!

About 1.3 miles out, you can actually catch a glimpse of a house across the river, with cables (presumably) to run supplies over. Who lives in here I don't know, but it would be a mighty remote existence! No map I've seen shows road access to that side of the river.

You'll cross a few more bridges; then, at 3.6 miles, you'll have to take a trail around an impressive logjam on the tracks. Look around for a second and think about this: Those logs came down the river! At 5 miles, you can spot a big water tower, and then—rail cars. And houses! Crazy, huh?

This is Enright, an old logging and railroad town, which actually had a post office from 1932 to 1943. Two private homes remain and are clearly still in use, so don't go poking around them. The cars, as well as some machinery you'll see along the way, just happened to be in there when the flood hit.

You could turn around at Enright and have a 10-mile day, but give it another mile to Clay Creek (named for a 1960s Forest Service employee), where you'll make a slightly tricky crossing, but nothing serious. Just after passing through a tunnel, look

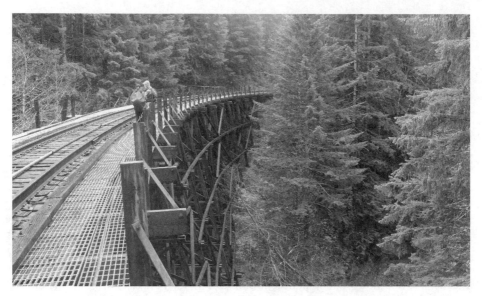

The trestle at Wolf Creek provides a direct path into the tree canopy.

down in the creek for sections of track all twisted up and scattered around. Some flood, huh? Just beyond Clay Creek is a place with a lovely river view, and where one rail actually got stacked on top of another—imagine the force it took to do that. It also makes a nice seat for lunch with a view of the river.

The worst of the rail damage and creek crossings lies ahead, so unless you're doing a one-way superadventure with a car shuttle, call it good here and head back down the rails to Salmonberry.

The Upper End (10 MILES)

The upper loop is closer to Portland and more spectacular in some ways: Basically, you trade seeing the main Salmonberry for going over some awesome trestles.

For the first 0.7 mile you'll actually have a trail next to the tracks, and right away you pass Cochran Pond, a man-made structure presumably related to old logging operations in the area. About a mile down, you'll encounter the first of many small tunnels; these are no big deal, but a light will help with footing. Just beyond one of them is an old kiosk that used to offer information to fishermen walking the tracks. The creek off to the right here is actually Pennoyer Creek, not the Salmonberry.

At 2.3 miles, you'll pass a series of mini-bridges and some cool rock formations; then, at 2.6 miles, you come to the highest trestle on the line, the Big Baldwin Bridge. It's 167 feet high and 520 feet long, and it was finished in 1911. And what a thing it is to walk over! There are grates and handrails, but those with a fear of heights might decide to call it a day here. Below you flows Baldwin Creek, another Salmonberry tributary. I assume the water tanks here were for fighting fires on the trestle. In fact, a hose goes from one of these tanks to another trestle, some 1.6 miles down the line.

At 3.7 miles, you'll start winding around the drainage of Wolf Creek, where one of the biggest slides occurred in 2007. If you look across the way, you'll see a section of tracks that you'll be walking on in a mile or so. The debris down in Wolf Creek should give you some idea of what happens here in a big storm. You'll cross Wolf Creek on another, all-wood trestle. It's pretty amazing that this one withstood the floods.

Continuing another 1.3 miles will give you a nice view back through the trees to the Wolf Creek Bridge, then at 5 miles bring you down to very near the Salmonberry. Here you'll find a nice little campsite with a bench, a fire pit, and easy river access. You could go another 0.5 mile to a tricky crossing of Kinney Creek, but this is a nice turnaround spot for today.

By the way, I'm told there are two more trestles in the 1.2 miles west from Cochran, but I haven't seen them.

Two more random notes of interest: The mileage markers along the tracks indicate distance on the line from San Francisco. And the Nehalem River actually starts just on the other side of Cochran; flows through the town of Timber, on the east side of the Coast Range; and then travels some 100 miles in a great northern loop through four counties to get to Salmonberry, at the bottom of this canyon, only 16 miles from where it started. Then it flows into the ocean.

GPS Information and Directions

Upper Trailhead **N45° 42.272' W123° 24.667'**
Lower Trailhead **N45° 44.994' W123° 39.137'**

For the upper trailhead at Cochran, from Portland on US 26, drive 37 miles west of I-405 to Timber Junction and turn left onto Timber Road—at this point, it's best to zero your odometer. Drive 3 miles to the town of Timber and turn right onto Cochran Road. The pavement will end in 0.5 mile. Stay right at a junction at 3.7 miles, pass Reeher's Camp at 5.5 miles, stay left just after that, and then go right at a junction at 7.1 miles. At 10.2 miles, go left onto Giveout Grade Road, then at 10.3 miles take the left-hand road at a three-way intersection. Park 0.1 mile ahead, just before the road crosses the tracks, and outside the gate.

For the lower trailhead, at the confluence of the Salmonberry and Nehalem Rivers, stay on US 26 for 18 more miles and turn left onto Lower Nehalem Road, following a sign for Lower Nehalem River. Follow this for 13 miles, some of it unpaved but just fine, and park on the left, just before the road crosses the Nehalem River.

53 Wilson River

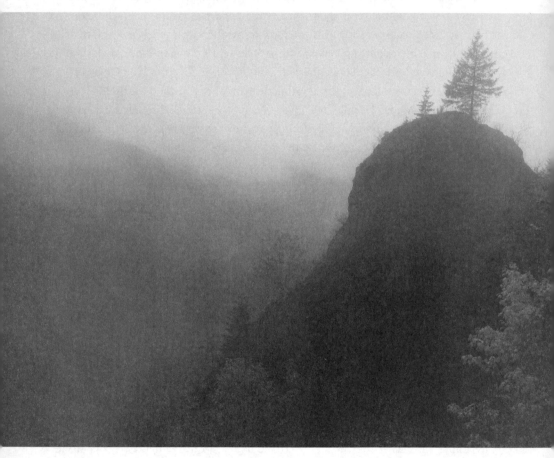

Rock formation between the Kings Mountain and Jones Creek Trailheads. I think it's required by law that you have to take a picture here!

In Brief

This relatively new trail explores the canyon of the Wilson River, where salmon and steelhead come to spawn. For many years, it was known to those who don't fish as "that river along Highway 6 on your way to Tillamook," but with a trail and a forest center now in place, plus a healthy forest making a comeback after catastrophic fires, the Wilson is a destination all its own.

LENGTH 20.6 miles one-way, with sections 3.5–7.4 miles in length	**SEASON** Year-round, but might get snow in winter, especially the Kings–Jones section
CONFIGURATION Out-and-back or point-to-point with shuttle	**BEST TIME** March and April for flowers, October for fall colors
DIFFICULTY Easy–strenuous—it's up to you.	**BACKPACKING OPTIONS** None
SCENERY Second-growth forest, a river, occasional views from up high	**ACCESS** No fees or permits
EXPOSURE In the forest the whole way	**WHEELCHAIR ACCESS** Only around Tillamook Forest Center (see Nearby Activities)
TRAFFIC Moderate on summer weekends, light otherwise	
TRAIL SURFACE Packed dirt, some rocks	**MAPS** Free brochures available from Tillamook State Forest
HIKING TIME 12 hours for the whole thing; varies for each section	**FACILITIES** At Elk Creek and Jones Creek Campgrounds, both closed in winter
DRIVING DISTANCE About 50 miles (1 hour) from Pioneer Courthouse Square, depending on which trailhead you choose	**INFO** Tillamook State Forest, 503-357-2191, **oregon.gov/odf/tillamookstateforest**

Description

This is a great year-round hike that's close to Portland and offers something for everybody: steep hills, flat sections, solitude, picnic areas, forests, views, you name it. There's a pretty good chance that the Kings–Jones or Footbridge–Keenig section will have snow in winter, but otherwise it should be open. Come in spring for flowers and maximum water flow, or in October for amazing fall colors.

If you want to do this whole nearly-21-mile thing at once, stash a car at Keenig Creek, start your hike at Elk Creek, and know that you'll have my respect and admiration, for whatever it's worth. Otherwise, pick a section and have at it. I do advise a car shuttle, though—it's easy to work out, and it means you don't have to backtrack.

ELK CREEK TO KINGS MOUNTAIN is a 3.7-mile stretch most often done as part of the formidable Elk Mountain–Kings Mountain loop (see Hike 49, page 254). But it's a nice forest stroll on its own, with the highlight being a series of meadows just 0.5 mile from the Kings Mountain Trailhead.

From the Elk Creek Trailhead, you'll ascend a steep 0.2 mile to reach the even steeper Elk Mountain Trail. Continue on Wilson River Trail, and the grade will let up a bit before the path becomes a long, mostly flat traverse. At 2 miles, just after a switchback that seems like a dramatic change, descend to a bridge over Dog Creek.

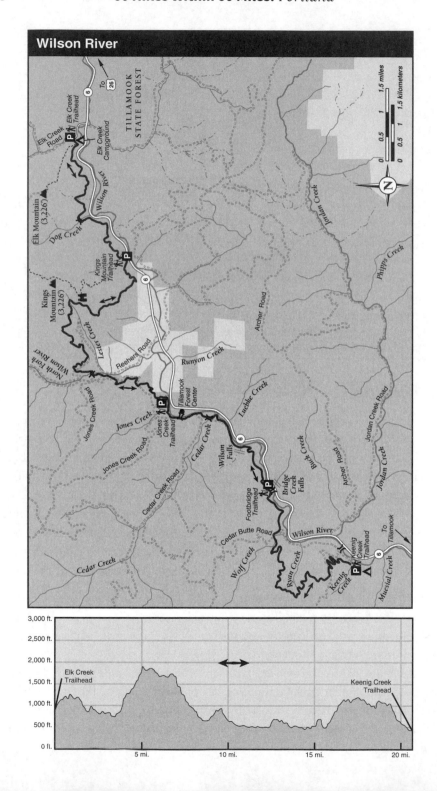

Wilson River

The next mile is more of the same, until you descend to the meadows at 3.2 miles. Try to get here in the morning or late afternoon, and if you're quiet you might see some elk. Another 0.5 mile brings you to Kings Mountain Trail, where you can turn left and descend 0.1 mile to that trailhead. Or keep going.

KINGS MOUNTAIN TO JONES CREEK, at 7.4 miles, is the toughest, highest, and most scenic section of Wilson River Trail. It also, somewhat ironically, never visits the Wilson River. The reason is that a bloc of private land along the river necessitates a big climb up the slopes of Kings Mountain, but you get some nice views from up there.

Leaving Kings Mountain Trail, which is 0.1 mile up from Kings Mountain trail-head, you'll first cross a jeep track with a sign reading KINGS MT. JR., then start to climb. You'll put in 1,200 feet in 1.5 miles on a steady grade. Just before the hilltop is a nice lunch spot, a trailside log where some old roadbeds intersect.

Past there, you'll start generally downhill, making lots of tiny creek crossings. You're going around a side canyon, that of Lester Creek. Around 3 miles, you'll come to a big rock formation with a tree growing atop it. My friends and I joked that, despite all the forest scenery so far, this was The Only Interesting Thing on the Hike. (Perhaps that's true only if you're doing this in the rain and didn't expect that 1,200 foot climb!) You'll find two good viewpoints here, and a chance to head out (carefully) to the rock itself.

A half-mile later, hike down steeply and, at 4 miles total, traverse a tiny meadow where several more old roads intersect. These roads are steep, aren't they? Imagine driving a truck loaded with logs down one of those things.

Keep moseying along, drop through a particularly lush area with a sea of sword ferns, and, at 5.5 miles, cross the North Fork Wilson River on a large, scenic bridge. At the far end are a picnic table and a side trail leading down to the river. You'll see a sign here reading TILLAMOOK COUNTY WATER TRAIL—this is a combined effort of local citizens with the Tillamook Estuaries Partnership to develop maps and guides for the whopping 1,800 miles of navigable water in the county. Check out **tbnep .org** to see how they're doing.

You may also, in this area, hear off-road vehicles. Fear not: They can't come on your trail. Follow the path downstream and, after 100 yards, pass Lester Creek Falls across the Wilson, finely adorned with a bright-orange NO TRESPASSING sign. Over the next 1.9 miles, you'll cross two roads and a small ridge, then pop out at Jones Creek Trailhead. Keep an eye out in this section for some amazing anthills and "legacy" trees that survived the forest fires last century.

JONES CREEK TO FOOTBRIDGE, at 3.5 miles, is the most popular section, owing to its ease of access, lack of big hills, and proximity to the river. The Jones Creek area has a campground nearby and a series of picnic sites along the first stretch of the trail.

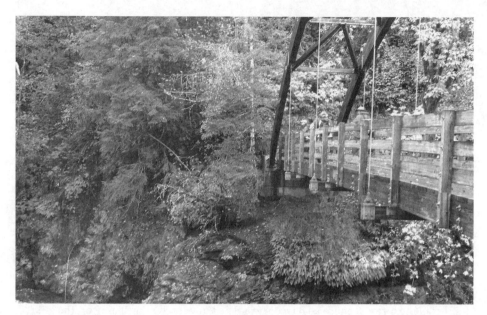

This lovely hikers' bridge crosses the North Fork Wilson River.

After 0.3 mile—some of which will certainly go into the river one day—you'll reach a big bridge leading over to Tillamook Forest Center, which has exhibits about the forest and its history (see Nearby Activities). The trail stays on the north side of the river, occasionally on roads, and after a mile swings away from the river a bit to cross Cedar Creek on a one-log bridge over a deep pool that looks like a good place for a dip.

Just past the bridge, keep left to avoid power lines, and at 1.3 miles look for a social trail leading down to a rocky area along the river. A quarter-mile ahead is a better trail to a sandier beach. Soon after, you'll have a bit of a hill to get up. You'll climb for about 1 mile to pass the 100-foot Wilson Falls, which may seem overrated if it hasn't rained lately.

The last 1.5 miles of this section traces a fern-filled bowl, then makes a long, gradual descent to the trail over to Footbridge. Even if you intend to keep going, it's worth a trip down to the river here. There's a huge logjam; a nice swimming hole, with a rock outcropping and a swing rigged from a log; and the footbridge itself, which crosses the Wilson at a deep, placid pool in a small gorge.

To get to the trailhead from here, turn left at the far end of the bridge and walk 100 (protected) yards along the shoulder of the highway.

FOOTBRIDGE TO KEENIG CREEK is a lonesome 6.1-mile stretch with another big hill, but lots of cool scenery. If you're starting at Footbridge, walk up the road from the parking lot, cross the bridge, and follow the trail across the creek bed and into the woods. Turn left on Wilson River Trail and you're on your way.

In the first mile, you'll cross a log bridge and then head up to a rock bluff with views of the Wilson. At 1 mile, you join Wolf Creek Road for about 500 feet; head to the right, up the road to the north, to find the trail. At the creek just below, you'll find a nice log bench for a break—which you'll need.

After Wolf Creek, things get steep for a mile and then the grade relents a bit. A few creeks and waterfalls break up the monotony before you cross a ridge at 2 miles to start a 3-mile traverse in and out of side canyons.

When you hit Cedar Butte Road, it's only 1.5 downhill miles through switchbacks and a recent clearcut. Nothing much to see, in other words, but by this time you're probably just ready to be done—especially if you're one of those 21-miles-in-a-day folks!

Nearby Activities

Tillamook Forest Center is open in spring and fall, Wednesday–Sunday, 10 a.m.–4 p.m.; summer hours are 10 a.m.–5 p.m. daily; closed in winter. Admission and programs are free. One thing to remember, though: If you park here and go hiking, your car will be stuck if you don't return before the gates are locked at closing time. See **tillamookforestcenter.org** for more info.

GPS Information and Directions

Elk Mountain Trailhead N45° 36.619' W123° 27.998'
Keenig Creek Trailhead N45° 32.605' W123° 36.733'

Take US 26 from Portland, driving 20 miles west of I-405, then bear west on OR 6, following a sign for Tillamook. The trailheads are all along the right side of the highway. For Elk Mountain, go 23 miles to Elk Creek Campground, just past Milepost 28; the trailhead is 100 yards past the campground. Kings Mountain Trailhead is 3 miles farther along, just before Milepost 25. Jones Creek Trailhead is in a day-use area between Mileposts 22 and 23; head for the campground, then turn left just after a bridge. Footbridge Trailhead is a parking area on the right at Milepost 20. For Keenig Creek Trailhead, go 2 miles past Footbridge, turn right on Cedar Butte Road, cross the bridge, and go left onto Muesial Creek Road. The trailhead is 0.2 mile ahead, on the right.

PORTLAND AND THE WILLAMETTE VALLEY

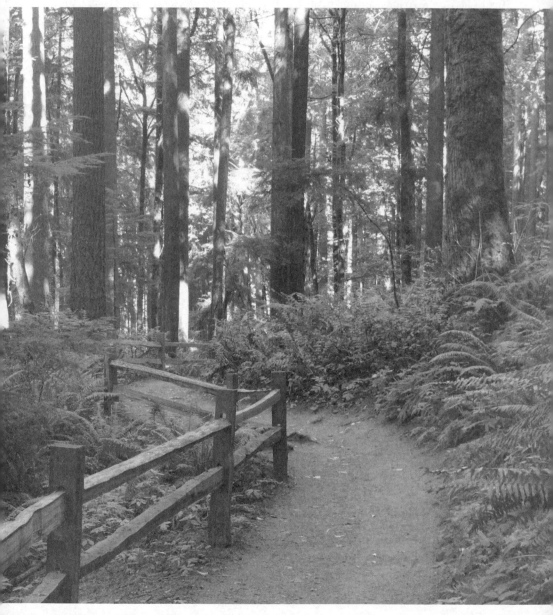

A wild spot in the middle of the city, the Upper Macleay Trail (see Hike 54) winds its forested way toward Pittock Mansion.

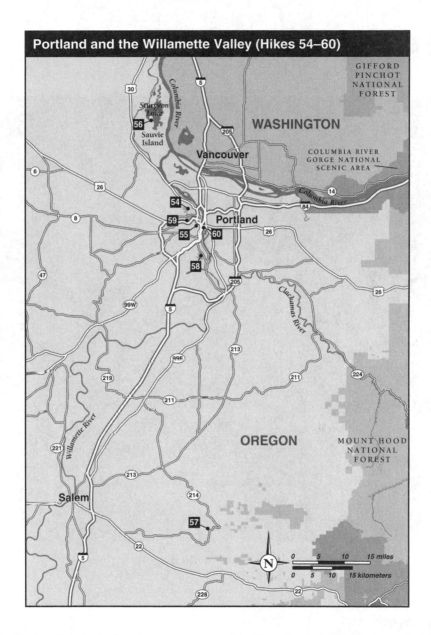

Portland and the Willamette Valley (Hikes 54–60)

GIFFORD PINCHOT NATIONAL FOREST

WASHINGTON

Vancouver

COLUMBIA RIVER GORGE NATIONAL SCENIC AREA

Columbia River

Sturgeon Lake

Sauvie Island

Portland

OREGON

Clackamas River

MOUNT HOOD NATIONAL FOREST

Willamette River

Salem

0 5 10 15 miles

0 5 10 15 kilometers

N

54 Macleay Trail

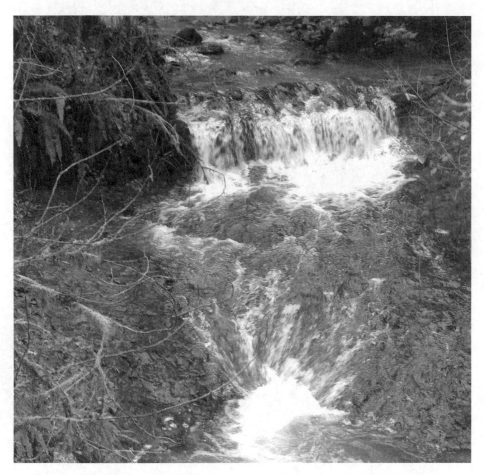

Falls on Balch Creek, which is home to wild cutthroat trout

In Brief

If you just take the easier trip to the Audubon Society, you'll get some quiet time along a creek in the woods, where you'll see two monumental trees, and enjoy close-up views of (caged) wildlife. If you put in a little more effort, you'll get that and some history with a great view—and another monumental tree. Heck, you can even connect this with another hike in the book. And it's all right in the middle of town!

LENGTH 2.2 miles round-trip to Upper Macleay Park and Audubon Society, 4.5 miles round-trip to Pittock Mansion	**DRIVING DISTANCE** 3 miles (10 minutes) from Pioneer Courthouse Square
CONFIGURATION Out-and-back	**SEASON** Daily, 5 a.m.–10 p.m., year-round
DIFFICULTY Easy to Upper Macleay Park and Audubon Society, moderate to Pittock Mansion	**BEST TIME** Any clear day, for the view
	BACKPACKING OPTIONS None
SCENERY Quiet woods, predatory birds (in cages), three must-see trees	**ACCESS** No fees or permits
EXPOSURE Shady all the way; 1 road crossing	**WHEELCHAIR ACCESS** Lower 0.25 mile is paved; mansion area is entirely accessible.
TRAFFIC Moderate on the trail weekdays; heavy on weekends and at mansion	**MAPS** Forest Park maps at Audubon Society
TRAIL SURFACE Packed dirt, with some gravel	**FACILITIES** Water and restrooms at trailhead, Audubon Society, and mansion
HIKING TIME 1 hour to Audubon Society, 2.5 hours for the whole thing	**INFO** Portland Parks and Recreation, 503-823-7529, **tinyurl.com/macleaypark**

Description

First, if the headquarters of the No Ivy League (at the trailhead) is open, it's worth a look inside. The project has cleared, as of 2013, more than 100 acres of ivy and saved some 30,000 trees in Forest Park from invasive English ivy, which creates "deserts" where no native plants can survive. In this building the crews house some of their trophies—ivy roots bigger than you can imagine such things being. Gawk, get some water, and head up the trail.

What you're walking up here is Balch Creek, named for the man who once owned this land—and also the first man in Portland to be tried and hanged for murder. Small as it is, the creek was the original water supply for the city of Portland. And if that doesn't amaze you, consider that in 1987 the Oregon Department of Fish and Game discovered a native population of cutthroat trout living in this tiny stream. Balch Creek is one of only two year-round streams in all of Forest Park. Check some of the deeper pools, and you just may see some of the (quite small) fish. Please keep your dog on a leash and out of the water.

This land, by the way, was sold by the Balch family and eventually wound up being donated to the city by a prominent Scottish merchant in town named Donald Macleay—apparently because he was tired of paying taxes on it. One of the conditions

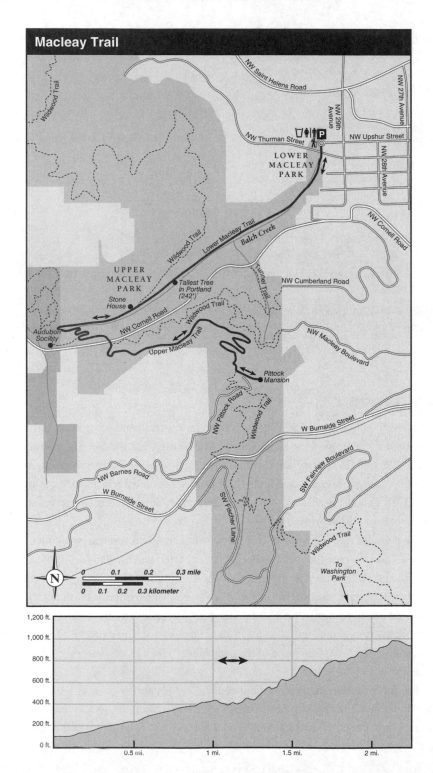

Macleay Trail

of Macleay's gift was that the paths be wide enough for hospital patients to be wheeled through in the summertime.

The path is still wide and now adorned with rails, bridges, benches, and stumps for sitting to admire the creek. At 0.8 mile, look for a Douglas-fir on your left that is marked with a plaque identifying it as a Portland Heritage Tree, one of some 300 such trees around town to be forever protected from the saw. This one happens to be the tallest tree in the city of Portland—last measured at 242 feet in 1997—and is thought to be the tallest in any major U.S. city.

At 0.9 mile, you'll join the 30-mile Wildwood Trail at the Stone House, built by the Works Progress Administration during the 1930s; it was a restroom until the early 1960s, when a storm destroyed its pipes by uprooting numerous trees. In fact, legend has it that the building is also the scene of nocturnal battles between the ghosts of Danford Balch and his victim, Mortimer Stump, a neighbor who had eloped with Balch's teenage daughter. (If there's a better Old Portland name than "Mortimer Stump," I want to know what it is.)

Stay straight (upstream), now joining Wildwood Trail, and in the next 0.5 mile you'll cross the creek and climb to Upper Macleay Park. Whether you're headed for Pittock Mansion or not, make a right here and walk 100 yards to the Portland Audubon Society. They rehabilitate injured owls and hawks here, and you can view the caged birds for no charge; they also have an extensive collection of mounted animals and an excellent gift shop plus bookstore. Three loop trails explore sanctuaries from here; free maps of those and all of Forest Park are available at the gift shop. Particularly worth visiting is a shelter overlooking a pond, just below the headquarters. You can impress your friends by telling them that the massive sequoia beside the parking lot is actually less than 100 years old. They grow quickly at first.

To do a hike of just 2.2 miles, head back to the car. To add another 2.3 miles (and just over 400 feet in elevation), stay on Wildwood Trail by walking along Macleay Park's parking lot, crossing busy NW Cornell Road at a crosswalk, and reentering the forest. After 100 yards, turn right on Upper Macleay Trail. This trail climbs about 0.2 mile, then flattens. At 0.5 mile, you'll find a wooden bench with a cool pattern on it. Just past that, rejoin Wildwood Trail, turning right and uphill for the final 0.6 mile to the Pittock Mansion parking lot.

The home (see Nearby Activities) is to your left. Wander out to the front yard to enjoy the roses and a view of city and mountains, and admire yet another spectacular tree: a European white birch that offers pleasant shade to two benches with great views.

If you took the bus, you don't have to walk back down the trail. You can, instead, walk down the road from the mansion to West Burnside Street, about 0.3 mile away, cross it (carefully!), and take the #20 (Burnside/Stark) bus downtown.

You can also continue 1 mile on Wildwood Trail, descending 300 feet to connect with the Washington Park and Hoyt Arboretum hike (see Hike 59, page 309). To do that, follow the paved path around the house, head down the driveway about 50 yards, and look for Wildwood Trail heading down and to the left. It dives down to West Burnside, across which you're in Washington Park. A flat 0.5 mile gets you to a junction that's part of the Hoyt Arboretum hike. You can also just follow signs for 0.55 mile to the visitor center, and from there another 0.4 mile to the Washington Park MAX Station.

Nearby Activities

Pittock Mansion, built in 1914 by the owner-publisher of *The Oregonian* and founder of the Portland Rose Festival, is open for tours daily (3229 NW Pittock Dr., Portland, OR 97210). For more information, call 503-823-3623 or visit **pittockmansion.org.**

GPS Information and Directions

N45° 32.151' W122° 42.751'

From downtown Portland, drive 1 mile west on West Burnside Street and turn right onto NW 23rd Avenue. Proceed 0.8 mile and turn left onto NW Thurman Street. Go six blocks to NW 28th Avenue and turn right. Go one block, turn left onto NW Upshur Street, and follow it three blocks to the trailhead, at the end of the road.

This trailhead can also be reached by TriMet: From downtown, take Bus #15 (Belmont/ NW 23rd), but make sure it's headed for NW Thurman Street and not Montgomery Park. Get off at Thurman and NW 29th Avenue, walk one more block, and descend a flight of steps beside the bridge.

55 Marquam Trail to Council Crest

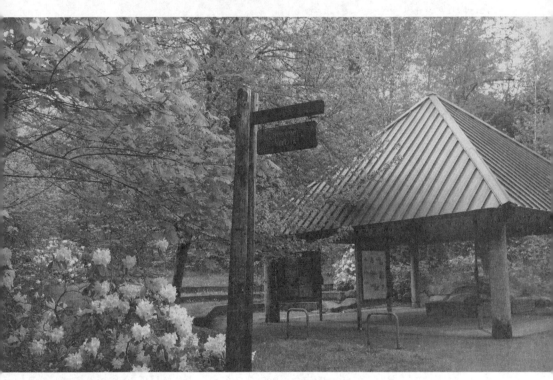

The Marquam Shelter marks the beginning of the trail.

In Brief

This pleasant trail through a wooded gulch just minutes from downtown leads to the highest point in Portland: a park where you can take in a view of four volcanoes. What a city we live in!

Description

Council Crest got its name in 1898 when a group of visiting ministers met there after a 2-hour wagon drive. They assumed the Native Americans must have held many

LENGTH 3.7 miles

CONFIGURATION Out-and-back with side loop

DIFFICULTY Easy on Nature Loop Trail, moderate to Council Crest

SCENERY Woods, impressive homes, and a sweeping vista on top

EXPOSURE Shady all the way up, open on top, a couple of street crossings

TRAFFIC Heavy on weekends and work-day evenings, moderate otherwise

TRAIL SURFACE Packed dirt, gravel

HIKING TIME 2 hours

DRIVING DISTANCE 1 mile (5 minutes) from Pioneer Courthouse Square

SEASON Daily, 5 a.m.–midnight, year-round

BEST TIME Any clear day

BACKPACKING OPTIONS None

ACCESS No fees or permits

WHEELCHAIR ACCESS None

MAPS Available at trailhead

FACILITIES Water at trailhead and at Council Crest

INFO Portland Parks and Recreation, 503-823-7529, **tinyurl.com/marquam naturepark;** Friends of Marquam Nature Park, **fmnp.org**

a council there. It turns out they probably didn't, but the name stuck. In the early and mid–20th century, you could ride a trolley to the top and visit an amusement park. Today you can get here by car or bus, but the best way is to walk up Marquam Trail through the woods.

At the trailhead shelter, two signs lead you to Marquam Trail, a 7-mile stretch of the 40-Mile Loop that passes through Marquam Nature Park, running from Willamette Park to Washington Park. The Nature Loop is a 1.2-mile interpretive traverse that meets Marquam Trail and returns to the shelter. If you got a brochure and feel like adding the Nature Loop, take the path on the left that says 0.7 MILE instead of the one on the right that says 0.4 MILE. The Nature Loop, to the left, leads you 0.3 mile up the creek to a junction—here, turn right; numbered signs along the way point out various local flora and fauna as you head 0.4 mile back to the right to reach Marquam Trail.

Whichever way you went to start with, you'll get to this same junction. From here, if you don't feel like going up the hill, go down the Shelter Trail and walk 0.4 mile back to your car (this is the right-hand trail you skipped at the trailhead). But for the best view in town, continue up and follow the trail 0.5 mile up Marquam Gulch, then make a left turn, following the signs to Council Crest. At this point the trail climbs a bit. Just before you cross the next road (SW Sherwood Drive), there's an extremely cool treehouse on your left. Oh, to be a kid in a neighborhood like this! Another 0.4 mile on, you'll cross SW Fairmount Boulevard and then continue uphill.

Marquam Trail to Council Crest

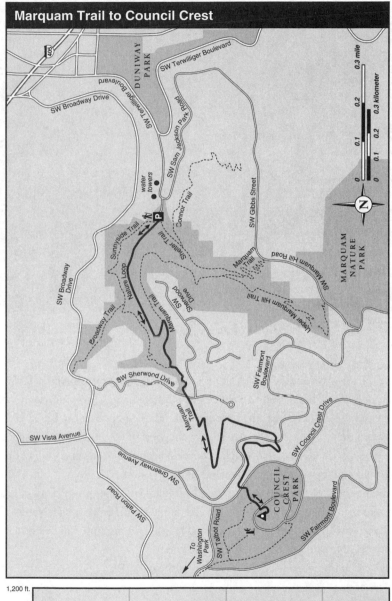

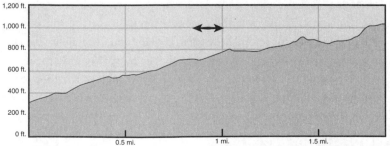

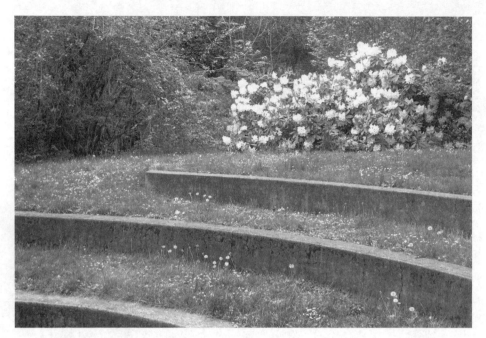

Amphitheater in Marquam Nature Park

After crossing yet another road (Greenway Avenue), in an area planted decades ago with May-blooming rhododendrons, you'll walk uphill to reach the wide, open area atop Council Crest, where couples come to snuggle and kids come to throw a Frisbee. Rest a moment on the two benches there to admire the view of Mount Hood—and check out the dates inscribed here. The benches were dedicated to Frank and Nadia Munk, a couple who both made it to age 98, dying within a year of each other. Nadia Munk, in whose dining room plans were made to save Marquam Gulch 40-plus years ago, was one of the park's cofounders. That group, which became Friends of Marquam Nature Park, stopped plans for apartments in the ravine and lobbied for multiple trailheads to make the area accessible as a retreat from the urban world.

Now, climb to the stone circle at the top of the park. Plaques there point out the four volcanoes and give the native name for each. To the east you can see into the Columbia River Gorge. The view to the west goes out to Beaverton and, on a clear day, the Coast Range. Finally, for an odd little treat, find the small metal disc in the middle of this stone enclosure, stand on it facing Portland, and say, "Portland rocks."

You can connect this trail to the Washington Park trip (see Hike 59, page 309), if you're up for something a little longer. As you start back down the trail, take a left just after you enter the trees, turning to the north. This trail will traverse the hill briefly before descending to the right, eventually reaching the intersection of SW Talbot Road and Fairmount Boulevard. Walk down Talbot about 0.3 mile to the intersection with SW Patton Road. Turn right onto the sidewalk on the far side of Patton; 200 feet ahead, you'll see a trail descending to the left. Follow it 1 mile through the forest until you reach an access road along US 26. Walk left 50 yards, cross the bridge over the expressway, then look on the left for a trail going up the hill, into the trees again. This will lead you through a meadow, behind the World Forestry Center, and eventually, in 0.2 mile or so, to an intersection with Wildwood Trail. (This is also the end of Marquam Trail.) Turn right on Wildwood Trail, and in 0.1 mile you'll be at the parking lot; across that is the MAX station, where you can catch a train back to town if you don't want to keep hiking. You could also keep going on Wildwood . . . for another 30 miles or so!

To return from Council Crest, head 1.3 miles back down the trail, following signs for Marquam Shelter, and when you get to a junction pointing left 0.4 mile to Marquam Park, take it. That's the shorter route back to the car that you skipped earlier in favor of Nature Loop Trail.

Nearby Activities

If it's a Saturday from mid-March to late December, don't miss the **Portland Farmer's Market** at Portland State University, just a few blocks north of Marquam Nature Park. It runs 8:30 a.m.–2 p.m. March–October, 10 a.m. 2 p.m. November and December, in the South Park Blocks. Call 503-241-0032 or check **portlandfarmersmarket.org** for the latest.

GPS Information and Directions

N45° 30.170' W122° 41.513'

From downtown Portland, drive south on Broadway Avenue. After it crosses I-405, take the second right onto SW 6th Avenue, following the blue H signs leading to the hospital. (Don't take the right signed COUNCIL CREST.) Continue straight through three lights in the next 0.5 mile, passing two large concrete water towers on your right. When the road cuts back to the left, turn right on SW Marquam Street to enter a parking lot. You can also take TriMet Bus #8 to the third light, SW Terwilliger Boulevard and Sam Jackson Park Road, and walk 200 yards to the trailhead.

56 Sauvie Island

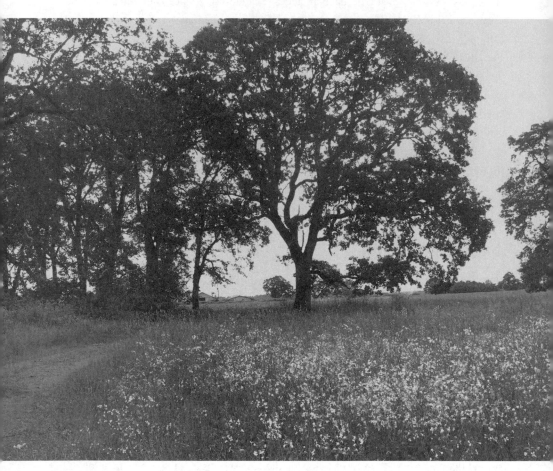

A walk at Oak Island delivers country lanes, flowers, birds, and, well, oaks.

In Brief

Two casual strolls on the edge of the city offer a glimpse into the local world of wild-life—and back into the past. Both of them are easy to reach and easy to do, and there's plenty of other stuff to experience on the island while you're out here.

LENGTH 3 miles for Oak Island, 7 miles for Warrior Rock

CONFIGURATION Oak Island, loop; Warrior Rock, out-and-back

DIFFICULTY Easy

SCENERY Lakeshore, woods, meadows, beaches, and birds

EXPOSURE Oak Island, mostly open; Warrior Rock, mostly wooded

TRAFFIC Moderate on summer weekends, light otherwise

TRAIL SURFACE Packed dirt, grass, and some beach

HIKING TIME 1 hour for Oak Island, 3 hours for Warrior Rock

DRIVING DISTANCE Oak Island is 19 miles (30 minutes) from Pioneer Courthouse Square, Warrior Rock 22 miles (45 minutes).

SEASON Oak Island, April 15–September 30; Warrior Rock, year-round

BEST TIME Mid-April–May for Oak Island, fall for Warrior Rock

BACKPACKING OPTIONS None

ACCESS Parking on the island is $7 per day or $22 for the season. Buy passes at Cracker Barrel Grocery (15005 NW Sauvie Island Rd., Portland, OR 97231; 503-621-3960).

WHEELCHAIR ACCESS None

MAPS USGS *St. Helens;* free map on-site and at **tinyurl.com/oakislandtrailmap**

FACILITIES Outhouse at each trailhead; nearest water at Cracker Barrel Grocery

INFO Sauvie Island Wildlife Area, 503-621-3488, **tinyurl.com /sauvieislandwildlifearea**

Description

Oak Island

Oak Island is actually a peninsula in a lake on an island in a river.

Some hikes are in the wilderness, some are walks through history, some are educational, some offer a distant view. This one is out in the country, or so it feels. You'll even pass crops. The whole scene might remind you of visiting your grandparents in the country. But even the crops are part of a plan by the Oregon Department of Fish and Wildlife to manage waterfowl in this area—and waterfowl are what Oak Island is all about.

Sauvie Island (named for Laurent Sauvé, a French Canadian employee of the Hudson's Bay Company) has, for thousands of years, been a rest stop for migratory birds. At the peak of the fall migration, some 150,000 ducks and geese alight here, along with several thousand sandhill cranes. In all, about 250 species of birds spend time on the island each year, including bald eagles by the score in the winter. So if you were to go to Oak Island in the middle of a summer day, you might wonder what the big deal is. But if you come in the spring or fall, or early on a summer day when the

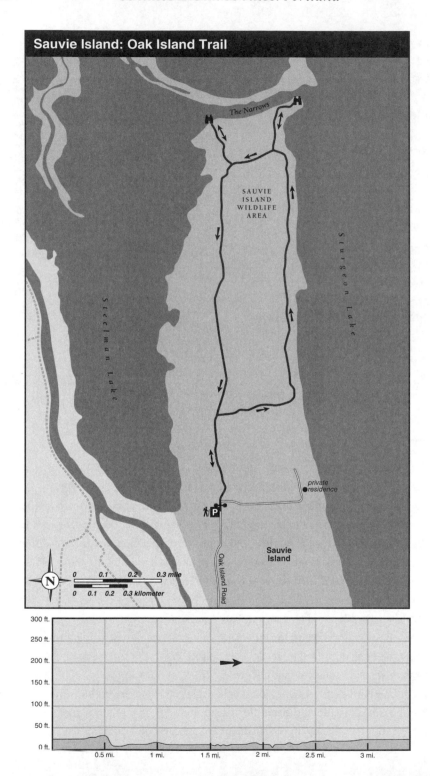

animals haven't hidden from the heat yet, you just might see a whole different world. And, in fact, even though the bulk of the migratory birds are gone when the trail is open, numerous songbirds hang out here, in addition to ducks, geese, and even bald eagles that spend the whole summer.

From the trailhead, head around the gate and walk a few minutes on the mowed roadway–trail to a junction. Be sure to grab a guide from the box; it explains several signs around the trail. Head in either direction, or strike off into the grassy meadows or woods. If you stay on the trail, going right will take you to a view of Sturgeon Lake, which at some times of year might be a long way off because it's so shallow. Turn left here, hike 0.9 mile, and, when the signed trail turns left, follow another trail to the right, continuing 200 yards to The Narrows, a—you guessed it—narrow body of water that connects Sturgeon Lake to the east with Steelman Lake to the west.

Continuing on the loop trail, you'll head back to the left and walk along a plowed area; Oregon Fish and Wildlife actually farms some 1,000 acres of its land on Sauvie Island as part of a cycle that brings alfalfa, corn, millet, and other foods to migratory birds in the winter and cattle in the summer.

Warrior Rock

In the fall of 1805, Lewis and Clark's Corps of Discovery floated down the Columbia River and managed to miss the Willamette River entirely. It wasn't that they were fools; it's just that the Willamette's entry was blocked from view by the forested wetland now called Sauvie Island. While much of it has long since been diked and some is now farmed, about half of it is managed by the Oregon Department of Fish and Wildlife.

Lewis and Clark, while exploring the island that was the summer and fall home of the Multnomah Indians, camped on the beach that's just beyond the parking area. If for some reason you would like to skip the beach entirely, walk over a low point in the fence at the southern end of the parking lot, then walk through the pasture, parallel to the river, to the trees. You'll find the road here.

To start on the beach, follow the trail out onto it and stroll along, considering what it must have looked like in 1805 but also how quiet it is today. Look for animal tracks leading from the woods to the water; raccoons and deer are common here. But those critters move around mostly at night, and if the hunters and fishermen aren't out, you may have the place to yourself.

If it's late summer or early fall, when the river is low, you can make it almost the whole 3 miles to the lighthouse on Warrior Rock by walking the beach. Otherwise, go as far as you can, or wish to, and then look for a place to head up into the woods. Up on the bluff, you'll encounter a trail that once served as a service road to the

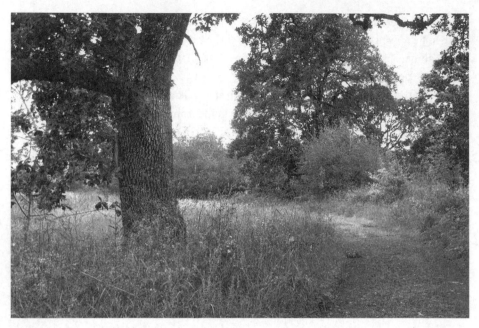

To hike Oak Island is to take an old-fashioned walk in the countryside.

lighthouse. Follow it through a world of blackberry, oak, alder, and maple. After about 2.5 miles, at a point where the trail is right at the top of the bluff, look to the right for an old shipwreck on the beach. Just a few minutes later, you'll come to a large meadow; keep right for 0.2 mile to the lighthouse.

Warrior Rock got its name when members of a 1792 English expedition up the Columbia (the party that named the river for their ship, and Mount Hood for the head of the English navy) found themselves surrounded on this rock by dozens of native warriors. They cleverly made peace and lived to tell the tale. The lighthouse is maintained by the U.S. Coast Guard. And speaking of ships, there's a decent chance you'll see an oceangoing vessel making its way roughly 70 river miles from Portland to the Pacific Ocean at Astoria.

A hundred yards up the sandy beach to the left, somebody cut a perfect little bench into a large piece of driftwood; with any luck, the river will not have reclaimed it before you get here. A few minutes beyond that, at the northwestern tip of Sauvie Island, you'll come to old pilings that no one seems able to explain. Leading theories are that it was a fish-processing plant, a boat works, or a loading dock for shipping milk from island dairies. Whatever it was, it offers a viewpoint of the town of St. Helens, which was founded in 1845—and in case you're wondering why the town and the nearby mountain are called St. Helens, well, the same English sailors who named Mount Hood and the Columbia River named the volcano for the English ambassador to Spain at the time, a certain Baron St. Helens. His real name was Alleyne Fitzherbert—thank goodness they chose his noble title.

Nothing like some useless trivia to contemplate while you're walking back to the car. Speaking of which, if you stay on the trail the whole way, you'll come to the cow pasture above the beach where you started. Just walk across it—careful where you step—to the fenced parking area and step over the low portion of the fence to your right, next to the hunters' check-in stand.

And, for the record, Lewis and Clark saw the Willamette on the way home, in the spring of 1806. Clark stood on a bluff near where the University of Portland is today; from there, he saw and named Mount Jefferson.

Nearby Activities

Many of the farms on Sauvie Island are "you pick 'em" operations, with treats such as berries, flowers, pumpkins, and corn mazes. You can't miss it. Stop and get a little something for dinner on your way home, if you don't get lost.

GPS Information and Directions

N45° 42.846' W122° 49.247'

Take US 30 from Portland, driving 10 miles west of I-405. Turn right to cross Sauvie Island Bridge. Cracker Barrel Grocery (where you'll buy your parking pass) is on your left, on NW Sauvie Island Road, 0.1 mile beyond the bridge. Go 2 more miles on NW Sauvie Island Road and turn right on NW Reeder Road.

Oak Island: Drive 1.3 miles on NW Reeder Road, then turn left on NW Oak Island Road— although, since Reeder heads right here, it's more like continuing straight. After 1.9 miles you'll leave the pavement, and 0.8 mile farther you'll cross a dike. At the bottom of the dike, go left; the trailhead is 0.4 mile ahead, at the end of the road.

Warrior Rock: After 10 miles on NW Reeder Road, you'll leave the pavement and reach a series of parking areas for Welton Beach, just over the dike to your right. Past that is parking for Collins Beach—which happens to be clothing-optional but is blocked from the road by forest. At 2.3 miles after you leave the pavement, the road ends at the parking area for Warrior Rock.

57 Silver Falls State Park

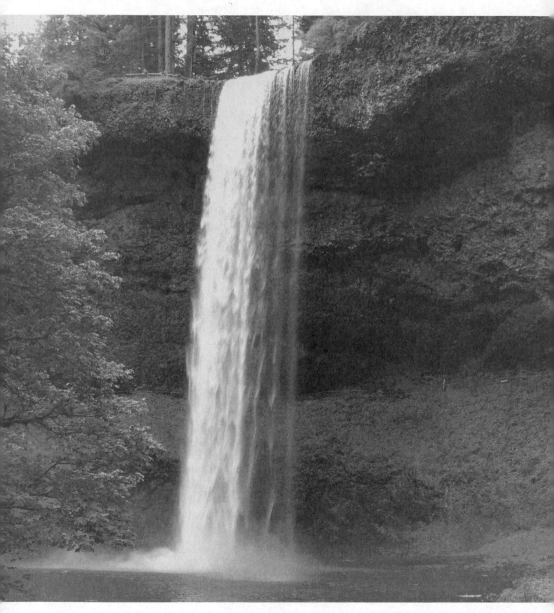

It takes little effort at all to visit, and walk behind, magnificent South Falls. This view is just minutes from the historic lodge.

LENGTH Anything up to 7 miles	**BACKPACKING OPTIONS** None
CONFIGURATION Loop	**ACCESS** $3/vehicle/day. If the toll booth isn't open, self-pay at the dropbox at the trailhead.
DIFFICULTY Easy–moderate	
SCENERY Every type of waterfall, in a forested canyon	**WHEELCHAIR ACCESS** Much of the recommended loop is not accessible, but some falls are, as are many other trails.
EXPOSURE Shady all the way	
TRAFFIC Heavy spring, summer, and fall; light–moderate otherwise	**MAPS** USGS *Drake Crossing;* free maps in South Falls Lodge and at trailheads
TRAIL SURFACE Pavement, gravel, dirt	**FACILITIES** Water, restrooms, snack bar, and gift shop at South Falls Trailhead
HIKING TIME Up to 4 hours	
DRIVING DISTANCE 61 miles (1 hour, 30 minutes) from Pioneer Courthouse Square	**INFO** Silver Falls State Park, 503-873-8681, **oregonstateparks.org/park_211.php**
SEASON Year-round, but wet in winter and spring, with occasional snow or ice	**SPECIAL COMMENTS** Dogs, even on a leash, are not allowed on Canyon Trail, described here. They are welcome (if leashed) on other trails in the park.
BEST TIME March and April for big water, September and October for fall colors	

In Brief

If it's waterfalls you're after—especially the chance to get behind them—this is the hike of your dreams. It's an easy loop that's known as Trail of Ten Falls. You can also hike several shorter loops, all of which take in views of one or more waterfalls.

Description

This is the crown jewel of the Oregon State Parks system; it's also one of the most visited parks in the state. Unless it's a rainy weekday in the winter, you probably won't be close to alone here, but it hardly matters. It's one of the finest walks around, especially if you're into waterfalls.

By the way, Silver Creek was named not for its color but for a pioneer named James Smith who settled here in the 1840s. He was known as "Silver" because it was said that he brought a bushel of silver dollars with him from back East.

Be sure to visit South Falls Lodge, 0.1 mile from the parking lot. It was built of native stone and wood by the Civilian Conservation Corps (CCC) in 1941. Warm yourself by two massive fireplaces, enjoy photos of the park and some of the tools used

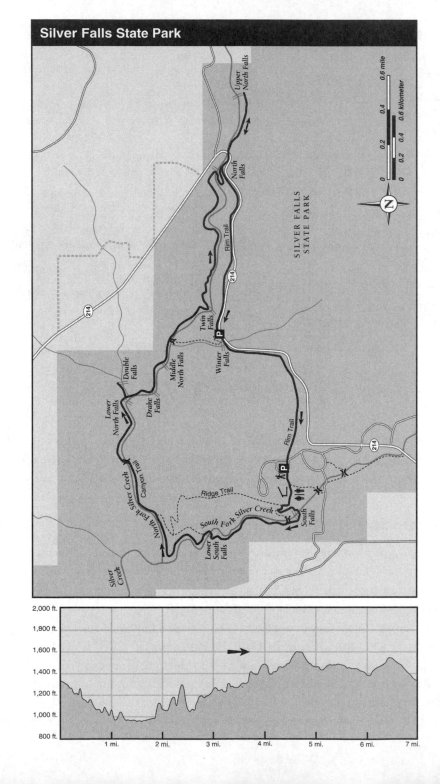

Silver Falls State Park

by the CCC, and take advantage of that most modern of conveniences: a snack bar with an espresso stand.

With your hot drink in hand, walk toward 177-foot South Falls, take in the view from the top, and contemplate the fact that in the 1920s a man named D. E. Geiser used to send old automobiles over the falls as a Fourth of July stunt. It's said that fishermen were pulling car parts out of the pool for decades. Now take the trail behind the sign. (*Note:* This is as far as your dogs can go, even if they're on a leash.) The trail will switchback down 0.2 mile, then go behind South Falls. The cavelike setting was created over the millennia by water seeping through the rocks above, freezing and expanding, and then cracking away the rocks that now lie at your feet. Even in the middle of summer, you'll get a little spray here; in winter or early spring, you may get soaked.

When the trail comes to a bridge 100 yards ahead, you can cross it to finish a 0.6-mile loop—the first of several opportunities to cut the loop short. But continue 0.7 mile to see the 93-foot Lower South Falls. Here, the trail descends a number of steps, often wet even in summer, and passes behind this falls, which is a combination of curtain and cascade falls.

After another 0.2 mile, you'll come to your second chance to cut the loop short. Turn right and it's 1 mile along Ridge Trail back to the lodge; continue straight and it's 0.7 mile to the 30-foot Lower North Falls. At this point you've left the South Fork of Silver Creek for the North Fork; the two combine downstream from here to form Silver Creek—this is why you're suddenly walking upstream rather than down. (I like to pose this "mystery" to fellow hikers, to see who's paying attention.) Keep an eye out for deer and beaver, both of which live in the park. Human treecutters left their mark, too; on some of the big cedar stumps, you can still make out springboard slots, where loggers stood to cut the trees by hand.

Just past Lower North Falls, make sure to go left for a 0.1-mile side trip to see Double Falls, at 178 feet. Its shallow splash pool, which you can get in if you like, almost always hosts a rainbow when the sun is out. Back on the main trail, you'll pass the 27-foot Drake Falls (named for a photographer whose images were instrumental to the creation of the park) and 103-foot Middle North Falls (which you can go behind to visit a small cave) in the next 0.4 mile. When you get to a bridge—the halfway point for the full loop—you can turn right for one last chance to cut the loop short. To do that, take this trail 0.3 mile to Winter Falls, then continue past it; turn right on Rim Trail and walk 1.2 miles back to the lodge to end your day at 4.2 miles.

If you ignore the bridge and continue straight, you'll walk 0.3 mile to reach the 31-foot Twin Falls, which at low-water times of year is just one falls, but which does have the hike's best picnic spot, right at the creek's edge. Another 0.9 mile along (look for the rocks in the creek with ferns growing on top), you'll reach North Falls, which you'll see before you get there and which is probably the most spectacular falls in the park. Once again, the trail takes you behind the falls. Back there, look for the columns in the rock overhead, left when lava cooled around trees and then the trees rotted—15 million years ago!

After examining that, climb some steps, then head up along a railing with another view back down to North Falls. When you get to Rim Trail, on the right, go ahead and put in the 0.4-mile loop to Upper North Falls, a less-visited 65-foot drop in an area with ample opportunity to rock-hop and explore.

On Rim Trail's 2.3-mile trip back to the lodge, you'll pass by the top of Winter Falls—more of a damp spot in the late summer and fall, but worth descending to—and through some pleasant forest, where I have encountered deer on three occasions. Look also for some jaw-dropping massive old trees in here. When you get to the picnic area, continue straight on a nice new trail, and you'll be back at the lodge in no time. I recommend another coffee drink.

Nearby Activities

Just upstream from the South Falls parking area, there's an official swimming area in Silver Creek. The kids will love it, and if it's a hot day, grown-ups might like to take a dip as well. The park also has campsites and cabins you can rent for the night; horses can be rented between May and September.

GPS Information and Directions

N44° 52.769' W122° 39.268'

Take I-5 from Portland, driving 17 miles south of I-205 to Exit 271/Woodburn. Turn left and drive 14 miles on OR 214 to Silverton. Note that you'll be turning right at 2.7 miles, then left at 3.9 miles—both intersections have signs, so watch for them. In Silverton, follow signs for Silver Falls State Park, continuing 15 miles on OR 214. After entering the park, drive 2.3 miles on OR 214 and park on the right, at the South Falls parking area.

58 Tryon Creek
State Natural Area

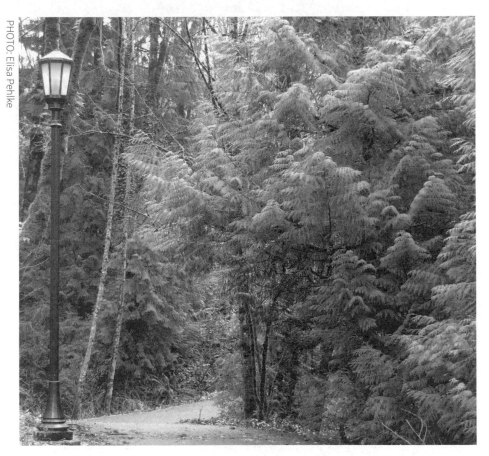

PHOTO: Elisa Pehlke

You'll find peaceful paths aplenty at Tryon Creek State Natural Area.

In Brief

Tryon Creek—Oregon's only state park in a major city—is the kind of place you want
to visit over and over, just to see what's going on. Are the steelhead in? Are the trees
wearing their fall colors yet? Are the trilliums in bloom? Any beavers around?

LENGTH 3 miles; 8 total miles of hiking trails in the park	**BEST TIME** April, for the trillium bloom
	BACKPACKING OPTIONS None
CONFIGURATION Loop	**ACCESS** No fees or permits
DIFFICULTY Easy	**WHEELCHAIR ACCESS** The 0.4-mile Trillium Trail offers two barrier-free loops.
SCENERY A woodsy ravine with a creek, lots of springtime wildflowers	
	MAPS Free maps at Nature Center
EXPOSURE Shady	**FACILITIES** Water and restrooms at Nature Center
TRAFFIC Heavy on weekends, moderate otherwise	**INFO** Tryon Creek State Natural Area, 503-636-9886, **oregonstateparks.org/park_144.php**
TRAIL SURFACE Packed dirt, gravel	
HIKING TIME 1 hour for this loop	**SPECIAL COMMENTS** The nonprofit **Friends of Tryon Creek** puts on numerous events in the park, from day camps to nighttime hikes to classes and lectures. To find out what's going on, call 503-636-4398 or visit **tryonfriends.org.**
DRIVING DISTANCE 6 miles (15 minutes) from Pioneer Courthouse Square	
SEASON Year-round, 7 a.m.–dusk daily; Nature Center open 9 a.m.–4 p.m. daily	

Description

An iron company logged this whole area in the 1880s to provide fuel for its smelter, so what you see today is what's known as second-growth forest. But it's certainly not a second-class forest; if nothing else, some of those old tree trunks are amazing! This 670-acre park, in a ravine between Portland and Lake Oswego, hosts 50 species of birds, plus deer, beaver, fox, coyote, barred owl, and a winter steelhead-trout run, in addition to resident steelhead and cutthroat trout.

Numerous hiking options start at the Nature Center, so pick up a free map and make your own way, or call the park for a schedule of ranger-led activities. For our suggested loop, when you come out of the Nature Center, turn left, walk past Jackson Shelter, and start on Maple Ridge Trail. As the name implies, this area is home to many vine maples, which put on quite a red-and-orange show in late October and early November.

Hike 0.2 mile, then take a right on Middle Creek Trail. Descend 0.2 mile to cross Tryon Creek at High Bridge. It's worth it to turn right here and explore up the 0.4-mile North Creek Trail, if only to see the astonishing fields of impatiens (also known as jewelweed) and a few places to access the creek, one of them a deep pool at a bend. Return to Middle Creek Trail and follow it 0.2 mile to an intersection with Cedar Trail. Follow this trail to the right as it crosses a horse trail (careful where you step!) and

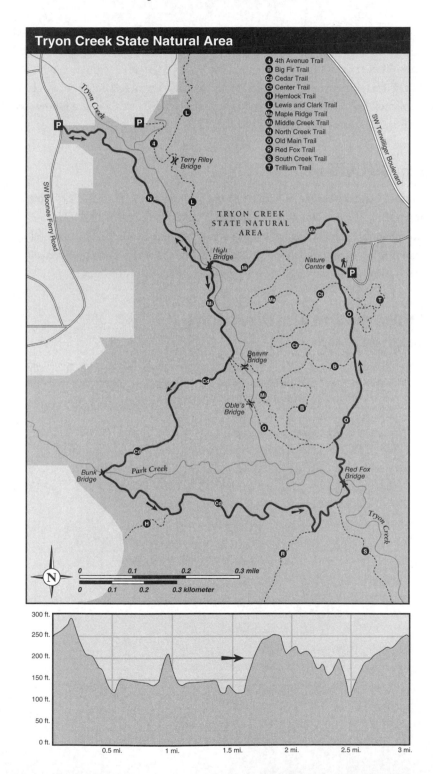

Tryon Creek State Natural Area

- **4** 4th Avenue Trail
- **B** Big Fir Trail
- **Cd** Cedar Trail
- **Cl** Center Trail
- **H** Hemlock Trail
- **L** Lewis and Clark Trail
- **Ma** Maple Ridge Trail
- **Mi** Middle Creek Trail
- **N** North Creek Trail
- **O** Old Main Trail
- **R** Red Fox Trail
- **S** South Creek Trail
- **T** Trillium Trail

TRYON CREEK
STATE NATURAL
AREA

Tryon Creek

SW Terwilliger Boulevard

SW Boones Ferry Road

Terry Riley
Bridge

High
Bridge

Nature
Center

Beaver
Bridge

Oble's
Bridge

Bunk
Bridge

Park Creek

Red Fox
Bridge

Tryon Creek

N

0   0.1   0.2   0.3 mile
0   0.1   0.2   0.3 kilometer

300 ft.
250 ft.
200 ft.
150 ft.
100 ft.
50 ft.
0 ft.

0.5 mi.   1 mi.   1.5 mi.   2 mi.   2.5 mi.   3 mi.

then climbs a short ways into a more open forest. Keep an eye out for a downed cedar trunk on the right that has obviously been explored by many an adventuresome child.

Cedar Trail crosses Bunk Bridge, then continues 0.8 mile to a junction with Red Fox Trail. Turn left here and cross Red Fox Bridge; if it's winter, keep an eye out for spawning steelhead. Climb briefly to Old Main Trail, then turn right and follow it back to the Nature Center.

Nearby Activities

The Original Pancake House, founded in 1953, isn't far away (8601 SW 24th Ave., Portland, OR 97219; 503-246-9007, **originalpancakehouse.com**). This third-generation family business has spawned more than 120 franchises in 28 states (along with one location each in Japan and South Korea). Go there, get an apple pancake or a Dutch baby, and discover the joy of breakfast. It's cash-only, though.

GPS Information and Directions

N45° 26.495' W122° 40.542'

Take I-5 south from Portland, driving 3 miles to Exit 297/Terwilliger-Bertha. Turn right at the end of the ramp, then take the first right on SW Terwilliger Boulevard. Stay on Terwilliger 2.5 miles; the main entrance to the park is on the right.

59 Washington Park and Hoyt Arboretum

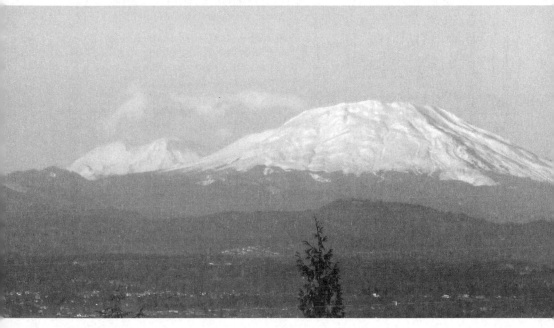

A viewpoint just off Wildwood Trail affords a prime view of Mounts Rainier and St. Helens.

In Brief

A family could spend a weekend in Washington Park and never run out of things to do. The park has a zoo, a children's museum, the World Forestry Center, the Vietnam Veterans of Oregon Memorial, a world-class Japanese garden, Hoyt Arboretum, and miles of hiking trails. TriMet runs a shuttle bus that connects it all. The loop described here is only a suggestion.

Description

This loop hike can be your base for exploring and an introduction to all that Washington Park has to offer. From a hiker's perspective, the heart of the park is

LENGTH 4 miles

CONFIGURATION Loop

DIFFICULTY Easy

SCENERY 1,400 species and varieties of plants, more than 5,000 labeled trees and shrubs

EXPOSURE Shady, with the occasional open spot for city views

TRAFFIC Heavy on weekends, moderate during the workday or bad weather

TRAIL SURFACE Pavement, packed dirt, gravel

HIKING TIME 2 hours for the recommended loop

DRIVING DISTANCE 2 miles (5 minutes) from Pioneer Courthouse Square

SEASON Year-round

BEST TIME Spring for the blooms, fall for colors

BACKPACKING OPTIONS None

ACCESS No fees to hike, but parking is $1.60/hour up to $4/day October–March and $6.40/day April–September.

WHEELCHAIR ACCESS Several barrier-free trails run through the area; ask at the Hoyt Arboretum Visitor Center.

MAPS Trail guide at visitor center

FACILITIES Water and restrooms at visitor center

INFO Hoyt Arboretum, 503-865-8733, **hoytarboretum.org**

Hoyt Arboretum (literally meaning "tree museum"), founded in 1928 on land that was completely clearcut in the early 20th century. Stop in the visitor center (which is on this loop) for a helpful map.

Beginning your walk at the Vietnam Veterans of Oregon Memorial, follow the trail under and then across the bridge and through a circular series of memorials describing events at home and in Southeast Asia from 1959 to 1972. Follow the trail out of the memorial, and then turn left onto Wildwood Trail. (To your right is the beginning of this "wonder trail," which wanders some 30 miles through Washington and Forest Parks.

Stay on Wildwood Trail 0.4 mile as it circles to the right, crosses a road, and climbs a small hill to a viewpoint between two water towers. Look for Mount St. Helens and Mount Rainier, and then turn left on Holly Trail and walk 100 yards to the visitor center, where you'll find water, restrooms, really nice people, and a mountain of information. Return to the viewpoint and turn left to continue on Wildwood Trail. In about 200 feet you'll come to Magnolia Trail on the left; take it 0.3 mile to the Winter Garden if you'd like to cut about 1.6 miles off your hike and stay in the arboretum. For a pleasant, woodsy stroll and access to other Washington Park attractions, stay on Wildwood Trail.

The wide, flat Wildwood Trail loops out 1.5 miles, with access along the way to the Hawthorne, Walnut, and Maple Trails. At the 1.2-mile mark, you will have a view down to the right of the waterfall area of the Japanese garden; just after that, a trail on

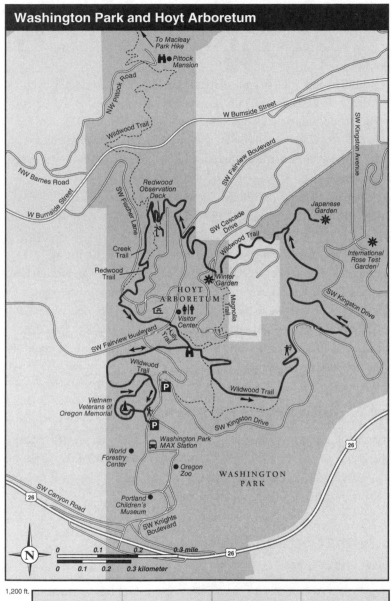

Washington Park and Hoyt Arboretum

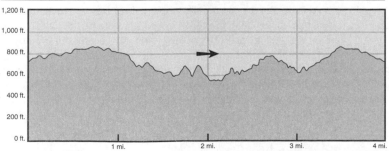

the right leads to the garden, the largest in the world outside Japan and a must-see. Just down a hill beyond that is the International Rose Test Garden, with 8,000 rose-bushes in more than 550 varieties. Did I mention you could spend quite a while in Washington Park?

Back on Wildwood Trail, 0.3 mile past the Japanese Garden Trail, you enter Winter Garden, where Magnolia Trail reenters. Just 0.6 mile later on Wildwood Trail, after passing a wonderful viewing platform, take a left on Redwood Trail to explore the sequoia collection. Shortly beyond that, you'll enter the redwood collection, which includes a specimen of the dawn redwood, which, until a few decades ago, was thought to be extinct.

Note: If you were to stay on Wildwood Trail here, you could add a 2.4-mile out-and-back trip to Pittock Mansion, which stands atop Macleay Trail (see Hike 54, page 284).

Back on Redwood Trail, when you come to a trail on the right marked TO CREEK TRAIL, take that, then go left on Creek Trail. It dead-ends at a road; pick up Redwood Trail at the far side and you'll pass through the larch collection on your way to the picnic shelter. Cross the road, and you're back at the visitor center. Turn right, take Holly Trail back to Wildwood Trail, turn right on it, and follow it 0.5 mile back to your car.

Or just get a map at the visitor center and explore on your own. As you'll see on the map, this loop is just a beginning.

Nearby Activities

The **Portland Children's Museum** (4015 SW Canyon Rd., Portland, OR 97221) features hands-on exhibits in a "center for creativity, designed for kids age 6 months through 12 years old." Kids can climb, swim, toss balls, act in a play, and even produce a movie. More info: 503-223-6500, **portlandcm.org.**

GPS Information and Directions

N45° 30.689' W122° 43.044'

The best way to get to this trailhead is to take MAX Light Rail. It takes you to the deepest transit station in North America—at 260 feet, the second-deepest in the world—which features artwork and displays on the geological history of the region. An elevator puts you right next to the World Forestry Center; turn right when you're facing the center, and the trailhead is across the road and about 100 yards uphill. To drive here from downtown Portland, head west on US 26 and take Exit 72/Zoo after 1.3 miles. At the end of the ramp, turn right on SW Canyon Road. Then stay to the left, circling the parking lot, and turn left at the MAX station. Our trailhead is at the Vietnam Veterans of Oregon Memorial, 0.1 mile ahead on your left.

60 Willamette River Greenway

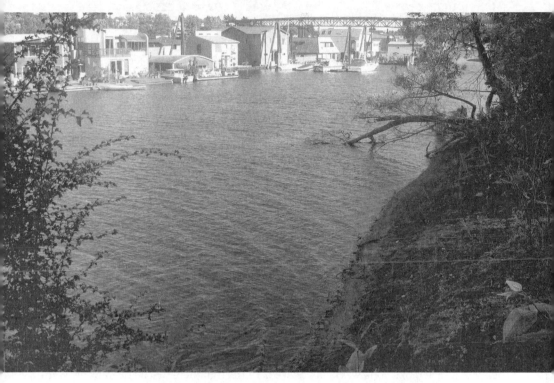

One of numerous points of interest along the greenway, Butterfly Park offers a semisecret view of the Willamette River.

In Brief

Tour central Portland and the Willamette River on a series of paved walkways. You can piece this one together on different days, mixing in tourist activities, or do it all in a pleasant day of wandering. Whatever you do, it's a fine introduction to some of Portland's cooler elements, combining city access with peaceful natural spaces.

Description

I've broken this hike into several different sections, each with access points from the Portland Streetcar, MAX Light Rail, or TriMet Bus.

LENGTH Options of up to 12.2 miles

CONFIGURATION One-way, out-and-back, or a big loop

DIFFICULTY Easy terrain, moderate difficulty depending on how far you go

SCENERY City, river, forests, an amusement park—you name it.

EXPOSURE In and out of the sun

TRAFFIC Moderate–heavy

TRAIL SURFACE Paved

HIKING TIME 6 hours to do it all

DRIVING DISTANCE None—see Description for transit access.

SEASON Year-round

BEST TIME Anytime you want

BACKPACKING OPTIONS None

ACCESS Parking fees or TriMet pass ($2.50 ages 18–64, $1 seniors 65+)

WHEELCHAIR ACCESS All of it!

MAPS Available from the Travel Portland Visitor Information Center, in Pioneer Courthouse Square (701 SW 6th Ave., Portland, OR 97204)

FACILITIES Several places along the way

INFO Travel Portland, 503-275-8355, **travelportland.com**

SPECIAL COMMENTS A few sections of this walk will be affected by bridge construction until perhaps 2016, but detours are in place.

Portland Aerial Tram to Steel Bridge (2.4 MILES)

South Access Portland Streetcar, SW Moody/Gibbs Stop (#12760)
North Access MAX Light Rail, Old Town/Chinatown Station (#8339)

From the base of the Portland Aerial Tram, start out walking north on SW Moody Avenue. You'll pass under the tram and then intersect a new MAX line, which was being built when this book was being revised. To the right here will be the new bridge, which was also being built at this writing. Someday you'll be able to cut across the river here to get to the Oregon Museum of Science and Industry (OMSI). Otherwise, keep trucking up Moody, passing under the Ross Island Bridge and soon coming to River Parkway, 0.8 mile north of the tram. Turn right on River Parkway and look for where the path resumes, at a viewpoint under the I-5 Marquam Bridge.

The next section of trail passes along condos and apartments, as well as side trails going down to the water, and you'll reach South Waterfront Garden in 0.3 mile; here, you can walk to the right, down a dock to Newport Bay Restaurant, which is open spring–fall. Even if it isn't open, it affords nice access to the river. The path continues through the RiverPlace neighborhood, passing shops and tables and benches, before coming onto the large (and often goose-filled) lawn that marks the beginning of Tom McCall Waterfront Park. Just beyond this expanse of green is the Hawthorne Bridge, where you can find restrooms as well as stairs that access the bridge. Walk across the river to pick up another section of this walk on the other side.

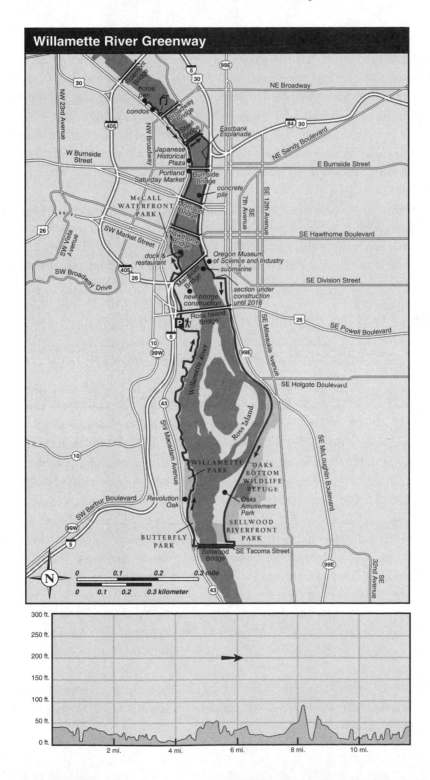

Willamette River Greenway

The path now enters a much-loved stretch of land that says something about Portland's character: McCall Park was once a highway, but that was torn out to create a grassy, riverside expanse that's home to picnickers, disc tossers, and a series of festivals. You may also notice huge steel bollards; these secure ships during the annual Rose Festival, when McCall is filled with an amusement park. Along this stretch, you'll pass the Morrison Bridge, the *Portland Spirit* tour boat, the Salmon Street Fountain, the Oregon Maritime Museum, and the Battleship *Oregon* Memorial, eventually arriving at the Burnside Bridge and the site of the Portland Saturday Market, which actually happens both weekend days from March through Christmas.

Just on the other side of the Burnside is the Japanese Historical Plaza, whose cherry trees provide a burst of hope and color to rain-soaked locals each March, and at the other end of that—1 mile north of the Hawthorne—you reach the Steel Bridge and the end of this section. The Old Town/Chinatown MAX Station is one block west, on NW Davis Street.

North of the Steel Bridge (1.4 MILES ROUND-TRIP)

South Access MAX Light Rail, Old Town/Chinatown Station (#8339)
North Access Portland Streetcar, NW 10th/Northrup Stop (#13604)

This little extension of the Willamette Greenway Trail is either an out-and-back for those doing the full loop, or another exit that will leave you in the Pearl District. Either way, it's a nice and relatively quiet little trip, and highly recommended.

From the Steel Bridge, just walk north across the railroad tracks, then look for a WILLAMETTE GREENWAY TRAIL sign leading to the right, toward a river beach. You'll immediately notice that this area seems quieter, since most of the joggers and cyclists have gone over the Steel Bridge. Follow the path north, between condos and the river, and take note of the reminders that there's a *port* in *Portland:* the grain elevators across the way, and the seagoing vessels being serviced along the other side of the Willamette. Also look across the way for the arenas in the Rose Quarter.

The path soon turns to boardwalk and you pass under the Broadway Bridge, then reach a great viewing platform at the corner of the 1909 Albers Mill Building, once home to the largest flour-milling operation on the West Coast. Past that, you'll come to much-more-modern condos and their fancy glass and water features; then the trail ends at the corner of NW 9th Avenue and Naito Parkway, where a pen houses police horses.

To reach Portland Streetcar Stop #13604, near Tanner Springs Park in the Pearl, just walk across Naito Parkway and the railroad tracks on NW Ninth Avenue, walk one block, and turn right onto NW Northrup Street.

Steel Bridge to OMSI (1.5 MILES)

North Access MAX Light Rail, Old Town/Chinatown Station (#8339)
South Access Portland Streetcar, SE Water/OMSI Stop (#13615)

As you walk across the Steel Bridge, consider this: It's the only double-deck bridge with independent lifts in the world. In other words, they can lift just the lower part, where the trains go, and let traffic and light rail keep going on the upper part. You can cross on either the upper or lower section.

At the east end of the 890-foot walkway, turn right and you'll be on the Eastbank Esplanade. Enjoy some of the 280 trees and 43,695 shrubs (most native) planted along the trail; local beavers sure did when they first went in, so now many of them are covered by fencing (the plants, not the beavers). Also, enjoy the 13 "urban markers" along the way; they mark where streets are, and each marker has a unique light fixture.

In just a few minutes, you'll come to the fanciest feature of the Esplanade: the floating walkway. At 1,200 feet, it's the longest in the world. It's held in place by 65 pylons, each one sunk 30 feet into the bottom of the river. Each section of the walkway weighs 800,000 pounds, yet you can still feel it bobbing up and down when the wind tosses up the river.

If you want to head back to the west side, you can do so on the Burnside Bridge via a staircase on the south side.

Just north of the Morrison Bridge, you'll see what looks like a strange rock formation; in fact, this is leftover concrete, dumped when the Morrison Bridge was being built. What kind of fine do you think that would generate these days?

If you're wondering about the little bumps on the seats of benches, those are to keep skateboarders from practicing tricks on them.

Just past the Hawthorne Bridge, which has a nice lookout point on the north side and access to cross back over the river, you'll come to OMSI. The path goes right across the front of OMSI (past the submarine); if you like, you can step inside for a snack, a drink, or some education. (I especially recommend the Omnimax Theater.)

OMSI to Sellwood Bridge (3.9 MILES)

North Access Portland Streetcar, SE Water/OMSI Stop (#13615)
South Access TriMet Bus, SE 13th/Tacoma Stop (#6709)

This is the other section being affected by bridge construction. The path has a detour until 2016 because of work on the east end of the bridge from here to South Waterfront. Whenever you're reading this, follow the path south from OMSI and, in 0.6 mile, enter the Springwater Corridor Trail, one of the very few to have a walkthrough entrance sign. It also has mile markers.

Around the first mile marker, after passing under Ross Island Bridge, you'll come to a series of grassy areas on the right with benches and an art installation by Linda Wysong. Around here you'll notice it gets considerably quieter—except for where you pass by the Ross Island Sand and Gravel Company.

A third of a mile later, look for a trail leading right, into the woods, and take it for a respite from the concrete and bikers. You'll wander 0.6 mile through cottonwood forest with several views of the river, then rejoin the main path at an entrance for Oaks Bottom Wildlife Refuge. Here, you can stick with the main, paved path to the right or cross under the tracks to continue your woodsy wanderings in the refuge. To do that, just make a couple of right turns in the refuge, walking along a large pond and then cutting back over to this path.

Either way, you'll arrive at Oaks Amusement Park and, just past that, hit SE Spokane Street. The Springwater Corridor Trail keeps going about 18 miles to the town of Boring, and you can explore that way if you like. We'll go left on Spokane for two blocks, right on SE Sixth Avenue, and right on SE Tacoma Street to head over Sellwood Bridge. Or left for a world of coffee shops, cafés, and antiques dealers in Sellwood.

Sellwood Bridge to OSHU Tram (2.9 MILES)

South Access TriMet Bus, SE 13th/Tacoma Stop (#6709)
North Access Portland Streetcar, SW Moody/Gibbs Stop (#12760)

Yes, you can walk across Sellwood Bridge, even during construction that's replacing it. And yes, it's among the scarier walks in this book. But it has a terrific view toward downtown Portland, and it offers access to a lovely stretch of trail on the west side.

At the west end of the bridge, follow the path down and around and back onto the Willamette River Greenway. This section was also diverted for construction when the book was written, so you might have to walk along SW Macadam Avenue for a bit. If not, you'll get to visit Butterfly Park (who knew?) and eventually enter Willamette Park. Be sure to stop to admire the Revolution Oak, a massive Oregon white oak recognized for being alive during the Revolutionary Way. It's one of some 300 Portland Heritage Trees, and you'll find it at the southern end of the park by some playground equipment.

Now we're back to an open riverside path, winding through Willamette Park, passing the Willamette Sailing Club, and then reentering the world of condos. At the very first condo, which you walk around, check out that wisteria! The 1.2 miles north of Willamette Park are wide-open, with constant views of the river, and you'll pass a series of benches, boat docks, and beaches.

At 1.2 miles north of the park, you'll have to get around some private property by cutting through an office park, but the signs are easy to follow. You'll arrive at

SW Bancroft Street, back in the up-and-coming South Waterfront neighborhood. If you're hungry, head north on SW Lowell Street to several food carts. Otherwise, go a block east and walk three blocks up SW Bond Avenue to SW Gaines Street, then walk two blocks east to get back to the river.

Pass a series of benches along a walkway, and a riverside area that was being constructed as this book went to press. After coming to a viewpoint of the Ross Island Bridge, turn west along SW Curry Street, passing a dahlia garden and pumpkin patch, then cut through Elizabeth Caruthers Park to reach the Oregon Health & Science University Center for Health & Healing, at the base of the Portland Aerial Tram. Inside you'll find a coffee bar and restrooms.

GPS Information and Directions

N45° 29.917' W122° 40.311'

Please see the public-transit access points for each section in the Description.

Appendix A: Hiking Stores

Columbia Sportswear
columbia.com

Main Store
911 SW Broadway
Portland, OR 97201
503-226-6800

Outlet
1323 SE Tacoma St.
Portland, OR 97202
503-238-0118

The Mountain Shop
mountainshop.net

1510 NE 37th Ave.
Portland, OR 97232
503-288-6768

Next Adventure
nextadventure.net
(Sells some used items)

426 SE Grand Ave.
Portland, OR 97214
503-233-0706

Oregon Mountain Community
omcgear.com

2975 NE Sandy Blvd.
Portland, OR 97232
503-227-1038

Patagonia
patagonia.com

907 NW Irving St.
Portland, OR 97209
503-525-2552

REI
rei.com

Clackamas Town Center
12160 SE 82nd Ave.
Portland, OR 97086
503-659-1156

Hillsboro
2235 NW Allie Ave.
(NW 194th Avenue at Cornell Road)
Hillsboro, OR 97124
503-617-6072

Portland
1405 NW Johnson St.
Portland, OR 97209
503-221-1938

Tualatin
7410 SW Bridgeport Rd.
Portland, OR 97209
503-624-8600

Appendix B:
Places to Buy Maps

Green Trails Maps
greentrailsmaps.com

Oregon Mountain Community
omcgear.com

2975 NE Sandy Blvd.
Portland, OR 97232
503-227-1038

REI
rei.com

Clackamas Town Center
12160 SE 82nd Ave.
Portland, OR 97086
503-659-1156

Hillsboro
2235 NW Allie Ave.
(NW 194th Avenue at Cornell Road)
Hillsboro, OR 97124
503-617-6072

Portland
1405 NW Johnson St.
Portland, OR 97209
503-221-1938

Tualatin
7410 SW Bridgeport Rd.
Portland, OR 97209
503-624-8600

Appendix C: Hiking Clubs

Bergfreunde Ski Club
503-245-8543, bergfreunde.org

Columbia River Volkssport Club
walking4fun.org
Facebook: tinyurl.com/columbiavolkssport
Hikes scheduled at www.meetup.com/walking-oregon-and-sw-washington

Forest Park Conservancy
210 NW 17th Ave., Ste. 201, Portland, OR 97209; 503-223-5449,
forestparkconservancy.org
Facebook: facebook.com/forestparkconservancy; *Twitter:* twitter.com/pdxforestpark

Friends of the Columbia Gorge
522 SW 5th Ave., Ste. 720, Portland, OR 97204; 503-241-3762, gorgefriends.org
Facebook: facebook.com/gorgefriends; *Twitter:* twitter.com/gorgefriends

Mazamas
527 SE 43rd Ave., Portland, OR 97215; 503-227-2345, mazamas.org
Facebook: tinyurl.com/mazamaspdx; *Twitter:* twitter.com/mazamas

Portland Parks & Recreation
503-823-PLAY (7529), portlandparks.org
Facebook: facebook.com/portlandparks; *Twitter:* twitter.com/pdxparksandrec

Sierra Club, Oregon Chapter
1821 SE Ankeny St., Portland, OR 97214; 503-238-0442, oregon.sierraclub.org
Facebook: facebook.com/orsierraclub; *Twitter:* twitter.com/orsierraclub
Hikes scheduled at www.meetup.com/the-portland-vancouver-sierra-club-outings

Trails Club of Oregon
503-233-2740, trailsclub.org
Facebook: tinyurl.com/ortrailsclub
Hikes scheduled at www.meetup.com/trails-club-of-oregon

Appendix D: Online Resources

My *website,* **paulgerald.com,** features my blog, regular hike reviews, and information on trail conditions, public appearances, and guided hiking trips. You can also find me at **facebook.com/hikerpaul** and **twitter.com/60hikesportland.**

Here are more excellent online resources:

- **GREEN TRAILS MAPS** (**greentrailsmaps.com**) sells some terrific recreation maps.
- **MEETUP.COM** hosts a dozen or so local groups related to hiking and outdoor adventures (see opposite page for a few examples).
- **NORTHWEST HIKER** (**nwhiker.com**) is an excellent guide to area hikes, with photos.
- Find searchable listings of all **OREGON STATE PARKS** at **oregonstateparks.org** (*Facebook:* **tinyurl.com/orstateparks,** *Twitter:* **twitter.com/orstateparks**).
- On the **NWHIKERS.NET** discussion boards, thousands of members post trip reports and trail conditions from all over the Pacific Northwest.
- **PORTLAND HIKERS** (**portlandhikers.org**) is an invaluable resource for finding up-to-date conditions, trail descriptions, and people to go hiking with in the Portland area. (Say hello to OneSpeed there—he wrote this book.)
- **TRAILKEEPERS OF OREGON** (**trailkeepersoforegon.org, facebook.com/trailkeepers oregon**) is a nonprofit dedicated to protecting and enhancing the Oregon hiking experience through advocacy, stewardship, outreach, and education. If you've ever wanted to do some work on an Oregon trail to keep it in shape—and that would be a fine thing to do—get in touch with these folks.
- The massive **SUMMITPOST.ORG** message boards discuss mountain ranges all over the world, from the Absarokas in Wyoming to the Zlatibor Massif in Serbia. Seriously.
- The **U.S. FOREST SERVICE** operates the following websites for national forests within the scope of this book: **Columbia River Gorge National Scenic Area, www .fs.usda.gov/crgnsa; Gifford Pinchot National Forest, www.fs.usda.gov/giffordpinchot; Mount Hood National Forest, www.fs.usda.gov/mthood; Siuslaw National Forest, www .fs.usda.gov/siuslaw;** and **Willamette National Forest, www.fs.usda.gov/willamette.**
- Find information on **WASHINGTON STATE PARKS** at **parks.wa.gov, facebook.com /washingtonstateparks,** and **twitter.com/wastatepks.**
- Finally, the **WASHINGTON TRAILS ASSOCIATION** (**wta.org, facebook.com/washington trails, twitter.com/wta_hikers**) promotes hiking, leads trips, and coordinates trail maintenance.

Index

DEAR CUSTOMERS AND FRIENDS,

SUPPORTING YOUR INTEREST IN OUTDOOR ADVENTURE, travel, and an active lifestyle is central to our operations, from the authors we choose to the locations we detail to the way we design our books. Menasha Ridge Press was incorporated in 1982 by a group of veteran outdoorsmen and professional outfitters. For many years now, we've specialized in creating books that benefit the outdoors enthusiast.

Almost immediately, Menasha Ridge Press earned a reputation for revolutionizing outdoors- and travel-guidebook publishing. For such activities as canoeing, kayaking, hiking, backpacking, and mountain biking, we established new standards of quality that transformed the whole genre, resulting in outdoor-recreation guides of great sophistication and solid content. Menasha Ridge continues to be outdoor publishing's greatest innovator.

The folks at Menasha Ridge Press are as at home on a whitewater river or mountain trail as they are editing a manuscript. The books we build for you are the best they can be, because we're responding to your needs. Plus, we use and depend on them ourselves.

We look forward to seeing you on the river or the trail. If you'd like to contact us directly, join in at trekalong.com or visit us at menasharidge .com. We thank you for your interest in our books and the natural world around us all.

SAFE TRAVELS,

BOB SEHLINGER
PUBLISHER